AGING, IMMUNITY, AND INFECTION

Douglas C. Powers, MD, is a staff physician at the St. Louis VA Geriatric Research, Education and Clinical Center, and an Assistant Professor of Medicine at Saint Louis University, where he holds appointments in the Divisions of Geriatric Medicine and of Immunology and Infectious Diseases. His research interests include immune senescence and vaccination of the elderly.

John E. Morley, MB, BCh, is Dammert Professor of Gerontology at Saint Louis University, and Director of the Geriatric Research, Education and Clinical Center at the St. Louis VA Medical Center. He has written more than 500 scientific articles and edited 6 books. He was among the top 100 most cited scientists in the world during 1981 to 1988. He has received the Mead and Johnson Award of the American Institute of Nutrition for his work in appetite regulation. His current research interests include the role of neuropeptides in the regulation of memory function, nutrition in the elderly, and hormonal changes with aging. He is associate editor of the *Journal of the American Geriatrics Society,* and the editor of the aging section of the *Yearbook of Endocrinology.*

Rodney M. Coe, PhD, is Professor and Chairman, Department of Community and Family Medicine, with appointments in the Division of Geriatric Medicine, Department of Internal Medicine, and the School of Public Health, Saint Louis University, and the Geriatric Research, Education and Clinical Center, St. Louis VA Medical Center. He is the author of several books and articles on various aspects of gerontology and geriatrics. His current research investigates factors affecting health status and use of health services by the elderly, and patterns of communication and outcomes of encounters between health care providers and elderly patients.

AGING, IMMUNITY, AND INFECTION

Douglas C. Powers, MD
John E. Morley, MB, BCh
Rodney M. Coe, PhD
Editors

Springer Publishing Company
New York

Copyright © 1994 by Springer Publishing Company, Inc.

Springer Publishing Company, Inc.
536 Broadway
New York, NY 10012–3955

94 95 96 97 98 / 5 4 3 2 1

Library of Congress Cataloging-in-Publication Data

Aging, immunity and infection / Douglas C. Powers, John E. Morley, Rodney M. Coe, editors.
    p. cm.
    Includes bibliographical references and index.
    ISBN 0–8261–8180–5
    1. Communicable diseases in old age—Immunological aspects—Congresses. 2. Aging—Immunological aspects—Congresses. 3. Immune system—Aging—Congresses. I. Powers, Douglas C. II. Morley, John E. III. Coe, Rodney M.
    [DNLM: 1. Aging—immunology—congresses. 2. Infection—congresses. 3. Communicable Diseases—immunology—congresses. 4. Communicable Diseases—in old age—congresses. WT 104 A 26758 1994]
    RC112.A36 1994
    618.97′079—dc20
    DNLM/DLC
    for Library of Congress   93–42177
                                   CIP

Printed in the United States of America

Contents

Contributors   *ix*

Preface   *xiii*

Acknowledgments   *xvii*

1. Infectious Diseases, Immunity, and Aging: Perspectives
   and Prospects   1
   T. T. Yoshikawa

Part I   Aging and Host Defenses: From Bedside to Bench

2. Tuberculosis in Elderly Persons   15
   W. W. Stead

3. Senescence of Cellular Immunity to Tuberculosis
   Infection in the Mouse: Some Radical Departures
   From Previous Thinking   27
   I. M. Orme

4. Immunity to Influenza in the Elderly   41
   D. C. Powers

5. Influenza in Aged Mice   56
   B. S. Bender

6. Immune Deficiency of Aging   66
   W. H. Adler, L. Song, J. E. Nagel, R. K. Chopra,
   R. A. Windchurch, K. S. Waggie, and J. E. Nagel

7. Alterations in T-Cell Heterogeneity and Responsiveness
    in Aging Mice   82
        R. A. Miller, S. Li, H. R. Patel, J. Shi, and
        J. M. Witkowski

**Part II   Psychoneuroendocrine Modulation of Immunity:
            Implications for the Elderly**

8. Reversibility of Age-Related Thymic Involution by
    Hormonal and Nutritional Interventions   97
        N. Fabris

9. Age-Related Alterations in Noradrenergic Sympathetic
    Innervation of the Immune System   114
        D. L. Bellinger, K. S. Madden, S. Y. Felten, and
        D. L. Felten

10. Endogenous Opioids, Immune Function, and Aging   133
        J. E. Morley

11. Aging, Stress, and Immune Function: Neural Regulation
    of Natural Killer Cell Activity   140
        M. Irwin

12. Immunologic and Psychological Correlates in Older
    Females   152
        D. Benton and G. F. Solomon

13. The Pineal Aging Clock: An Approach to Age-Delaying
    Strategies   166
        W. Pierpaoli

**Part III   Infectious Syndromes in the Elderly: Cause,
             Course, and Treatment**

14. Urinary Tract Infection in the Elderly   179
        S. L. Berk

15. Pneumonia in the Elderly   191
        D. J. Kennedy

16. Methicillin-Resistant *Staphylococcus aureus* (MRSA):
    Epidemiology and Control in the Long-Term Care
    Setting   199
    S. F. Bradley

17. *Clostridium difficile* Infection in the Elderly   216
    R. G. Bennett

Part IV   Preventive and Therapeutic Strategies

18. Aging, Nutrition, and Immunity   233
    J. S. Goodwin and E. L. Burns

19. Options for Control of Influenza in Long-Term Care
    Facilities   248
    S. Gravenstein, B. A. Miller, and P. J. Drinka

20. Strategies for Improving Vaccine Delivery to Targeted
    Groups   265
    C. M. Wade, J. Karuza, E. Calkins, and J. Feather

21. Withholding Antibiotics as a Form of Care: An Ethical
    Perspective   283
    D. K. Miller

Index   299

Contributors

William H. Adler, MD
Gerontology Research Center
National Institutes on Aging
Baltimore, MD

Denise L. Bellinger, PhD
School of Medicine
University of Rochester
Rochester, NY

Bradley S. Bender, MD
GRECC, Gainesville VA Medical
  Center and Department of
  Medicine
University of Florida College of
  Medicine
Gainesville, FL

Richard G. Bennett, MD
Division of Geriatric Medicine and
  Gerontology
The Johns Hopkins University School
  of Medicine
Baltimore, MD

Donna Benton, PhD
GRECC, Sepulveda VA Medical
  Center and Department of
  Psychiatry and Biobehavioral
  Sciences
UCLA School of Medicine
Los Angeles, CA

Steven L. Berk, MD
Department of Internal Medicine
East Tennessee State University
Johnson City, TN

Suzanne F. Bradley, MD
GRECC, Ann Arbor VA Medical
  Center and Department of Internal
  Medicine
University of Michigan Medical
  School
Ann Arbor, MI

Edith L. Burns, MD
Department of Medicine
University of Wisconsin Medical
  School
Milwaukee, WI

Evan Calkins, MD
Western New York Geriatric
  Education Center
State University of New York
Buffalo, NY

Rajesh K. Chopra, PhD
Department of Environmental Health
  Sciences
The Johns Hopkins School of Hygiene
  and Public Health
Baltimore, MD

Paul J. Drinka, MD
Department of Medicine
University of Wisconsin and GRECC,
    Middleton VA Medical Center
Madison, WI

Nicola Fabris, MD, PhD
Italian National Research Centers on
    Aging and Faculty of Immunology
University of Pavia
Ancona, Italy

John Feather, PhD
Western New York Geriatric
    Education Center
State University of New York
Buffalo, NY

David L. Felten, MD, PhD
School of Medicine
University of Rochester
Rochester, NY

Suzanne Y. Felten, PhD
School of Medicine
University of Rochester
Rochester, NY

James S. Goodwin, MD
Division of Geriatrics and Center on
    Aging
University of Texas Medical Branch
Galveston, TX

Stefan Gravenstein, MD
Department of Medicine
University of Wisconsin and GRECC,
    Middleton VA Medical Center
Madison, WI

Michael Irwin, MD
Department of Psychiatry
University of San Diego and San
    Diego VA Medical Center
San Diego, CA

Jurgis Karuza, PhD
Western New York Geriatric
    Education Center
State University of New York
Buffalo, NY

Donald J. Kennedy, MD
Department of Internal Medicine
Saint Louis University School of
    Medicine
St. Louis, MO

Shaokang Li, PhD
Institute of Gerontology
University of Michigan
Ann Arbor, MI

Kelley S. Madden, PhD
School of Medicine
University of Rochester
Rochester, NY

Barbara A. Miller, RN
Department of Medicine
University of Wisconsin and GRECC,
    Middleton VA Medical Center
Madison, WI

Douglas K. Miller, MD
Division of Geriatric Medicine
Saint Louis University School of
    Medicine
St. Louis, MO

Richard A. Miller, MD, PhD
Department of Pathology
Institute of Gerontology and VA
    Medical Center
University of Michigan
Ann Arbor, MI

James E. Nagel, MD
Gerontology Research Center
National Institutes on Aging
Baltimore, MD

Ian M. Orme, PhD
Department of Microbiology
Colorado State University
Fort Collins, CO

Hiren R. Patel, PhD
Department of Microbiology
University of Michigan
Ann Arbor, MI

Walter Pierpaoli, MD, PhD
Institute for Biomedical Research
Quartino, Switzerland

Jia Shi, MD, PhD
Department of Pathology
Institute of Gerontology
University of Michigan
Ann Arbor, MI

George F. Solomon, MD
GRECC, Sepulveda VA Medical
Center and Department of
Psychiatry and Biobehavioral
Sciences
UCLA School of Medicine
Los Angeles, CA

Lijun Song, MD
Gerontology Research Center
National Institutes on Aging
Baltimore, MD

William W. Stead, MD
Arkansas Department of Health and
Department of Medicine
University of Arkansas for Medical
Sciences
Little Rock, AR

Cassandra M. Wade, MS
Western New York Geriatric
Education Center
State University of New York
Buffalo, NY

Kimberley S. Waggie, PhD, DVM
Division of Comparative Medicine
The Johns Hopkins University
Baltimore, MD

Richard A. Winchurch, PhD
Department of Surgery
The Johns Hopkins University School
of Medicine
Baltimore, MD

Jacek M. Witkowski, MD, PhD
Department of Pathology
University of Michigan
Ann Arbor, MI

Thomas T. Yoshikawa, MD
Office of Geriatrics and Extended
Care
U.S. Department of Veterans Affairs
Washington, DC

Preface

The association between increasing age and prevalence of chronic diseases is well known and discussed in professional and lay publications. This emphasis often obscures the fact that infectious diseases also frequently afflict older people, often with more serious, even fatal results. In part, the susceptibility of the elderly to serious complications following infection is due to a well-documented but little understood age-related decline in the immune function. This book examines the mechanisms of immune dysregulation in the aging host, and issues pertaining to the cause, course, and treatment of selected infectious diseases in older adults.

In chapter 1, T. Yoshikawa puts the development of theories and practices regarding immunity in a historical context and then applies them to the specific situation of older people. Presentations in Part I reflect the interplay between clinical care and bench research by examples of application of knowledge about immune function to treatment of infectious diseases. W. Stead draws attention to the impact of tuberculosis on older adults who are at higher risk of reactivation disease by virtue of waning immunity to this pathogen. Of particular concern is that many older people develop the disease undetected (especially in nursing homes) until they put health workers and family at risk. Using a murine model of tuberculosis, I. Orme has examined the cellular immune basis for the increased susceptibility to infection in old mice. He presents data suggesting that functional immune cells in aged animals have defective expression of surface homing receptors and are thereby prevented from focusing quickly at sites of mycobacterial implantation. Thus, the earlier hypothesis of the decline in T-cell function with age gives way to an alternative hypothesis of defective mobilization of resources, which offers the potential for alternative therapeutic interventions.

D. Powers examines the effect of aging on humoral and cellular immunity to influenza virus. These studies may help to explain why elderly adults experience most of the serious morbidity and mortality during influenza epidemics, despite having lower infection rates than in younger people. Influenza immunization provides protection that attenuates the severity of infection more effectively than preventing its occurrence. B. Bender reports on laboratory investigations with mice showing that influenza cytotoxic T lymphocyte (CTL) activity, which is important for recovery from viral infections, is reduced with age. These observations corroborate those of Powers and may help explain the excess morbidity and mortality in older people. W. Adler and colleagues emphasize the complexity of immune senescence. They illustrate how not all immune parameters exhibit a decline with age; some are known to increase, particularly in association with inflammatory responses. R. Miller and associates conclude the section with a brief review of their studies of phenotypic and functional heterogeneity within naive and memory pools of cells in old and young mice in which the fraction T lymphocytes expressing high levels of P-glycoprotein increase with age. Separating T cells based on differences in P-glycoprotein expression has yielded new information on age-dependent differences in the cell-activation process.

Chapters 8–13 in Part II examine some dimensions of the relatively new field of psychoneuroimmunology. N. Fabris reviews research on neuroendocrinologic pathways, and evidence for the hypothesis is that these connections do not experience intrinsic and irreversible declines with age, again suggesting the possibility for some degree of recovery through interventions. Specifically, the focus is on hormonal and nutritional interventions to restore certain functions of the thymus that impinge on the neuroendocrine system. D. Felten reports that the loss with age of noradrenergic innervation of spleen and lymph nodes contributes to altered immunologic reactivity seen in old animals. J. Morley reports that aging in mice is associated with declines in β-endorphin effects on the immune system. In humans, increases in natural killer (NK) cells are mediated by β-endorphins, suggesting that endogenous opioids and age interact to produce age-related changes in the immune system. M. Irwin hypothesizes that age-related and age-dependent factors have a negative effect on the immune system. Studies of the effects of age on corticotropin-releasing hormone (CRH) in rats showed that the abnormal regulation of the autonomic nervous system may contribute to suppression of the natural cytotoxicity in older compared with younger rats. D. Benton and G. Solomon also studied NK cells as a function of the immune system, this time in response to stressful life events in older humans. During a 5-year study both psychological function and immune function have remained stable, with good psychological status accompanied by good immune status. W. Pierpaoli concludes this section with a provocative hypothesis, suggesting that decline in pineal functioning is responsible for many immune deficits associated with aging. This is based on findings that melatonin can prolong life in rodents and that the tripeptide thyrotropin-releasing factor may play a role in modulating this process.

Part III reviews the cause, course, and treatment for infectious diseases commonly found among older people. Chapters by S. Beck and D. Kennedy summarize clinical strategies for infections of the urinary and respiratory tracts, respectively. As noted by both authors, therapeutic choices have to recognize alterations in host defense mechanisms, associated systemic disease, and age-related physiologic changes that influence drug side-effects. S. Bradley comments on the particular problems of controlling methicillin-resistant *Staphylococcus aureus* (MRSA) in the long-term care setting. Infection control policies in acute care settings are difficult to implement in nursing homes, and antibiotics for decolonization have not been effective in this population. R. Bennett reviews the epidemiology and proposed treatment of *Clostridium difficile* in older populations, particularly in nursing homes. An important aspect of this treatable infection is its deleterious effect on nutritional status of older persons.

Finally, the chapters in Part IV examine some preventive and therapeutic strategies concerning infections. J. Goodwin and E. Burns examine the possible contribution of nutritional deficiencies to the decline in T-cell function and the role of "nutrients as drugs" (doses greatly exceeding recommended daily allowance levels) in reversing or slowing decline in immune functions. S. Gravenstein and colleagues consider ways to limit the spread of influenza in nursing homes. They emphasize that institutions can protect residents in part by screening visitors and encouraging ill employees to stay home. Influenza epidemics within a long-term care facility can be limited by institutional policies that promote widespread vaccination plus judicious use of drugs (amantadine). C. Wade and colleagues focus on physician behaviors as a means to increase the proportion of community-dwelling older persons who are appropriately vaccinated against influenza. Their study reported significant increases in compliance with influenza-vaccination guidelines in the experimental group that used postcard reminders and printed literature in physicians' offices. Quite a different meaning of therapeutic strategy is discussed by D. Miller, who addresses ethical issues of withholding or withdrawing antibiotics from critically ill patients. A key judgment involves whether prolongation of life through use of antibiotics will improve the quality of life.

Acknowledgments

The preparation of this book was aided by several sources of assistance. The symposium at which these chapters were presented was supported by a grant from the Department of Veterans Affairs Office of Geriatrics and Extended Care. Administrative support was provided from the Geriatric Research, Education and Clinical Center, and the Continuing Education Center, St. Louis VA Medical Center, Saint Louis University Schools of Medicine and Nursing, St. Louis College of Pharmacy, the SSM Rehabilitation Institute, and the Missouri Gateway Geriatric Education Center, St. Louis, Missouri. We are especially indebted to Derry Bowling and Carolyn Cole for their exemplary handling of the many details associated with the symposium. We also received helpful professional advice from the editorial staff of Springer Publishing Company. Finally, we thank the contributors to this book.

Infectious Diseases, Immunity, and Aging

Perspectives and Prospects

Thomas T. Yoshikawa

PERSPECTIVES

Infectious diseases have been with humankind since the beginning of civilization. Until the mid-20th century, infections were the major causes of death throughout the world. Well-known diseases such as plague, typhus, cholera, typhoid fever, diphtheria, smallpox, and tuberculosis (TB) caused major epidemics and pandemics, and accounted for the deaths of countless of millions of humans. Similarly, leprosy, syphilis, rheumatic fever, scarlet fever, measles, pertussis, and poliomyelitis caused not only death but severe disabilities, deformities, limitation of function, and social rejection (Lyons & Petrucelli, 1978). Up until the early 1900s, infectious diseases generally comprised one half of the top 10 causes of deaths in the United States. TB was the leading cause of death at the turn of the 20th century (Yoshikawa, 1992). Not surprisingly, life expectancy in the United States in 1900 was relatively short. The average life expectancies for a white male and female born in 1900 were approximately 47 and 50 years, respectively.

However, today, infection is only one of the top 10 causes of deaths among Americans (pneumonia and influenza together being the fourth

1

leading cause of death). Moreover, life expectancy has drastically increased during the past three quarters of a century. Presently, the life expectancies at birth for non-Hispanic white males and females are 73 and 80 years, respectively. In contrast to 4% of the population being 65 years and older in 1900, older Americans (65 years and older) currently comprise approximately 12.6% of the total population (U.S. Senate Special Committee on Aging, 1991). By the year 2030, the percentage of older Americans is expected to increase to nearly 22%. Moreover, aging persons have also increased their life expectancies—although not as dramatically as younger persons—over the last 75 years. A white male age 65 can expect to live, on the average, another 14 years, and a white female at 65 has a life expectancy of another 19 years.

What are the reasons for such changes in longevity? Certainly, the early discoveries of the germ theory, asepsis, antisepsis, vaccination, antimicrobials, and public health measures paved the way for the modern practice of infectious diseases and reduced the role of infections as the major life-shortening process (Yoshikawa, 1983). The outcome of these discoveries led to the reduction of infant and child mortality as well as death in younger adults—hence, the improvement in life expectancy. However, increased longevity has brought other causes of morbidity and mortality such as cardiovascular disease, cancer, diabetes mellitus, osteoporosis, chronic joint diseases, and stroke. Many of the age-associated illnesses, in concert with the aging process itself, have placed the older adult at higher risk for acquiring infections as well as suffering death and complications. Table 1.1 lists infections that increase in frequency with age (Yoshikawa, 1981). Table 1.2 summarizes the relatively greater rate of death in older persons compared with young adults for various infections (Yoshikawa & Norman, 1987).

TABLE 1.1   Infections that Increase in Frequency with Age

• Pneumonia	• Tuberculosis
• Urinary tract infection	• Herpes zoster
• Skin and soft tissue infection	• Cholecystitis
• Sepsis	• Diverticulitis
• Infective endocarditis	• Liver abscess

TABLE 1.2 Relationship of Infectious Mortality and Aging

Infection	Elderly Patient Mortality Compared to Young Adults*
Pneumonia	3
Kidney infection	5-10
Sepsis	3
Appendicitis	15-20
Cholecystitis	2-8
Tuberculosis	10
Infective endocarditis	2-3
Bacterial meningitis	3

*Relative rate, e.g., 3 means 3 times higher.

Immunity

The term *immunity* originated from the Latin words *immunitas* and *immunes*, which were originally used in a legal context to mean exception from service or duty. Later in Middle Ages, immunity applied to the Church (i.e., "exemption" of the church and its properties and personnel from civil control) (Silverstein, 1989).

The first use of the term immunity in a biologic context was by the Roman Marcus Annaeus Lucanus (A.D. 39–65) in his epic poem "Pharsalia" in which "immunes" is described as the famous resistance to snakebite of the Psylli tribe of North Africa (Silverstein, 1989). The term was employed only intermittently thereafter, and it did not obtain great usage until the 19th century following Edward Jenner's discovery of smallpox vaccination. However, throughout recorded history, two of the most fearful causes of death were pestilence (infection) and poison (which incidentally was universally known by its Latin name *virus*). These experiences with pestilence and poison, the observation that man can recover from diseases and illness, and survival from certain diseases that "exempted" a person from further involvement on second exposure led to the development of concepts of disease and immunity.

The concept of acquired immunity in early times was explained by the Hippocratic school theory of diseases (i.e., an imbalance of the four humors: blood, phlegm, yellow bile, and black bile). A former Islamic physician named Aku Bekr Mohammad ibn Zakariya al-Razi (A.D. 880–932) gave the first modern clinical description of smallpox and observed that survival from smallpox infection conferred lasting immunity. He explained that smallpox is due to fermentation of the blood because of its "excess moisture" (Silverstein, 1989). Smallpox pustules that break and release fluid were a mechanism by the body to expel "excess moisture" from blood. A second infection would be impossible because "excess moisture" of the blood to support the disease would have been expelled with the first attack (hence lasting immunity). This was the first such theory of *acquired immunity.*

As small pox swept into Western Europe at the end of the 17th century, parts of Eastern Europe had been practicing *variolation*. This is an early form of immunization against smallpox in which mild infection is established by inserting crusts derived from pustules of active but mild cases of smallpox into the skin of uninfected persons. This induced lasting immunity. Variolation was an important step in preventing smallpox, a disease that killed 50 million people in Europe during a span of 100 years in the 18th century (Silverstein, 1989). It was later in 1796 that Jenner inoculated the cowpox virus into a young boy named James Phipps, and 6 weeks later inoculated him with the smallpox virus more than 20 times. The boy did not contract the disease, and thus vaccination was first established.

Louis Pasteur, in the 1870s, demonstrated acquired immunity to fowl cholera by using attenuated organisms for vaccine prophylaxis. This finding served as the foundation for the new science of immunology as well as the modern theory for acquired immunity. However, Pasteur explained immunity on the basis of a depletion theory (similar to al-Razi's theory for smallpox immunity). He thought infection caused depletion of the body's nutrients, which then prevented reinfection (because organisms required nutrients to survive). It was not until the late 1880s when Elie Metchnikoff's cellular theory of immunity and Emil Von Behring's discovery of antibodies to diphtheria and tetanus were published that acquired immunity finally was correctly explained (Brock, 1975).

Infection, Immunity, and Aging

Elie Metchnikoff, as mentioned earlier, is credited with developing the theory of cellular immunity. However, he also developed the first theory of aging because of infection and immunity (Bibel, 1988). (He is also credited with coining "gerontology.") Metchnikoff theorized that the intestinal flora influenced the outcome of an infection caused by another pathogen, as well as being responsible for chronic toxin production, which hastened atrophy and aging of the body. He reasoned that low levels of toxins released by microbial flora chronically escaped detoxification by the kidneys and liver. Toxins damaged tissue, which would activate phagocytes to attack the body's tissue (autoimmunity). Metchnikoff's theory of old age was the following (Bibel, 1988):

> Old age is an infectious chronic disease which is manifested by a degeneration or an enfeebling of the noble elements, and by excessive activity of the macrophages. These modifications cause a disturbance of the equilibrium of the cells composing our body and set up a struggle within our organism which ends in a precocious aging and in premature death, contrary to nature.

Later, Metchnikoff believed that changing the intestinal microflora would inhibit growth of organisms producing toxins and thus prevent premature aging. He suggested changing the intestinal microflora by feeding lactobacilli through foods such as yogurt and sour milk. This concept reached the public and the demand for fermented milk products, especially yogurt, reached extraordinary levels in Europe for many years. Eventually, the lactobacillus theory was disproven, and by the 1940s other theories of aging became more prominent.

State of the Art

Much has evolved during the past 25 years in our understanding of the interrelationship, interaction, pathogenesis, and consequences of aging, immunity, and infection. The many scientific publications, journals, conferences, and national meetings on these topics reflect the widespread interest and knowledge that currently exists in our academic community.

From the pioneering work of Makinodan and coworkers describing the relationship of aging and immune dysfunction to the current cellular and molecular studies of the immunology of aging of Miller, Weksler, Thoman, and others, the potential role, mechanism, and impact of aging on immunity are beginning to be clarified (Albright & Makinodan, 1966; Gutowski, Innes, & Weksler, 1986; Miller, 1989; Thoman & Weigle, 1989).

It is now evident that aging blunts the febrile response to infections (Norman, Grahn, & Yoshikawa, 1985). Approximately 25% to 30% of older adults with serious infections may fail to demonstrate fever. Recent evidence suggests that one mechanism for depressed temperature responses with age to infection may be altered responses to cytokines (e.g., interleukin [IL]-1, tumor necrosis factor, IL-6) that stimulate the hypothalamic thermoregulatory center (Miller, Yoshikawa, Castle, & Norman, 1991).

Pneumonia remains the most frequent cause of death due to an infection in older patients. Careful epidemiologic, microbiologic, and clinical studies of this infection in the geriatric population have revealed the major differences in the diagnosis, treatment, and outcome of pneumonia in older persons in comparison with younger adults (Marrie, Durant, & Yates, 1989; Verghese & Berk, 1983; Yoshikawa, 1991).

Urinary tract infection is the most common bacterial infection in aging adults and is the most frequent cause of gram-negative bacillary sepsis in this population. However, most older adults with bacteriuria are asymptomatic (Boscia, Abrutyn, & Kaye, 1987). Institutionalized elderly patients often have long-term bladder catheters, which invariably result in chronic bacteriuria (Warren, 1991). A significant number of these catheterized patients will experience acute pyelonephritis (Warren, Muncie, & Hall-Craggs, 1988). Moreover, institutionalized older patients without catheters but with chronic asymptomatic bacteriuria and local inflammatory and immune responses will have reduced survival rates (Nicolle, Brunka, McIntyre, et al., 1992).

The epidemiology, pathogenesis, clinical manifestations, and prognosis of tuberculosis in aging adults have been well described in several studies and reports (Powell & Farer, 1980; Van den Brande, Vijgen, & Demedts, 1991; Yoshikawa, 1992). In addition, good information is available on the problem of tuberculosis in nursing homes among elderly patients (Stead, Lofgren, Warren, et al., 1985), and the impact of aging on radiographic changes of the lungs and skin test response to tuberculosis (Yoshikawa, 1992).

It is now known that infective endocarditis is becoming a disease of old age. Many reports from hospitals with many infective endocarditis cases indicate that nearly 50% of such infections occur in older adults (Cantrell & Yoshikawa, 1983). The age-related differences in etiology, clinical manifestations, therapeutic outcome, and prevention of infective endocarditis have been well described (Friedlander & Yoshikawa, 1990; Terpenning, Buggy, & Kauffman, 1987).

Intraabdominal sepsis is a diagnosis that may be overlooked in frail older patients. Elderly patients are more likely to have atypical presentation, delays in definitive surgery, complicating chronic diseases, and postoperative complications (Norman & Yoshikawa, 1984). Heretofore, both patients and clinicians failed to recognize that appendicitis does occur in older adults and that most deaths related to this infection are found in the geriatric patient (Norman & Yoshikawa, 1988). Bactobilia is a common occurrence in gallbladders of older patients undergoing elective cholecystectomy (Norman & Yoshikawa, 1984). The importance of prophylactic antibiotics and role of laparoscopic surgery for cholecystectomy in elderly patients have been reported (Hill & Meakins, 1992).

The epidemiology and clinical characteristics of infections in elderly nursing home patients are now well described (Verghese & Berk, 1990). It is clear that pneumonia, urinary tract infection, and skin/soft tissue infections constitute 75% of all nursing home infections (Muder, Brennan, Wagner, et al., 1992; Yoshikawa, 1989). The importance and potential consequences of MRSA in long-term care facilities are being reported with greater frequency (Bradley, Terpenning, Ramsey, et al., 1991). The establishment and benefits of infection control programs in nursing homes and other extended care facilities are beginning to be realized as the number of older adults in these facilities increases (Smith, Daly, & Roccaforte, 1991).

The impact of age on antibiotic pharmacokinetics and pharmacodynamics is becoming better understood with careful pharmacologic studies in humans (Ljungberg & Nillson-Ehle, 1987). Clinical trials of antimicrobial therapy in infected older adults have permitted a clearer definition of which antibiotics may be most appropriate for this population (Yoshikawa, 1990). Similarly, data are becoming available on which drugs are particularly toxic or injurious to older adults (Appel, 1990).

PROSPECTS

Although much has been accomplished toward our understanding of the problem of aging, immunity, and infection, there remains a large knowledge gap in this clinical arena. This information deficit includes the epidemiology of certain infections in the geriatric population, impact of age on pathogenetic mechanisms, improved diagnostic tools for infections, better therapeutic interventions for life-threatening infections, and effective preventive measures against infectious diseases.

The following are some areas, problems, or issues that need further investigation and clarification in the domain of aging, immunity, and infection.

- Determine the true prevalence of human immunodeficiency virus (HIV) infection in older adults from different socioeconomic backgrounds.
- Assess the frequency, morbidity, and mortality of common fungal infections such as candidosis.
- Demonstrate a quantitative correlation between aging-related immune dysfunction and predisposition to infections.
- Provide a clearer definition of the impact of aging on the functions of secretory immunity; neutrophil and macrophage phagocytosis; complement, natural killer cells; and host defense in relation to infections.
- Elucidate the impact of active infection in an older person on immune function, phagocytosis, and other host defense mechanisms.

- Develop a reliable, simple, accurate, and inexpensive clinical test to assess the status of an older person's host defense mechanism (e.g., immune function and phagocytosis).
- Develop a simple, accurate, and noninvasive method to determine the microbial etiology of pneumonia.
- Define the pathogenetic mechanism of chronic asymptomatic bacteriuria in older adults.
- Establish criteria or tests to determine if and when catheter-related bacteriuria is simply colonization or responsible for true infection.
- Develop a more rapid, accurate, and inexpensive method to diagnose *active* tuberculosis.
- Develop methods to determine the etiologic pathogens in an infected pressure sore.
- Establish optimal doses, routes, and duration of antimicrobial therapy for older patients with pneumonia, urinary tract infection, sepsis, infected pressure sores, and intraabdominal infections.
- Investigate newer therapeutic approaches to reduce the mortality of gram-negative bacillary sepsis in elderly patients (e.g., antitumor necrosis factor therapy).
- Research innovative methods to eliminate or reduce bacterial colonization of chronic bladder catheters.
- Clarify the role or need for prophylactic antibiotics for older patients with prosthetic devices (e.g., joint prothesis) who undergo invasive procedures in a prospective clinical study.
- Establish shorter and more intensive chemoprophylactic regimens against tuberculous infection in older adults.
- Develop influenza vaccines or vaccine strategies that will improve the protective efficacy of influenza immunization in older adults.
- Determine interventions that will prevent postherpetic neuralgia in elderly persons following a bout of herpes zoster.

What are the prospects of finding practical solutions to these problems? From a technologic perspective, the necessary tools, skills, and expertise are *currently* available to realize meaningful solutions in the immediate future. The sophistication achieved already in the field of molecular and cell biology is enormous. Some of these advances have been applied to clinical medicine such as deoxyribonucleic acid (DNA) probe and hybridization, polymerase chain reaction, and identification of a variety of cytokines. Moreover, such diagnostic tools as magnetic resonance imaging (MRI), single photon–emitting computer tomography (SPECT), positron emission tomography (PET), and Doppler echocardiography, and such therapeutic interventions as monoclonal antibodies, laser, and laproscopic surgery provide mechanisms to pursue answers to many of the previously mentioned concerns.

However, what is seriously lacking in attaining these solutions are two items: clinical investigators and funding. The field of geriatrics and geronotology has been rapidly growing during the past decade. Nevertheless, the discipline of aging has not attracted sufficient numbers of well-trained physician clinical investigators. Furthermore, those investigators with expertise and interest in aging and infections as well as aging and immunity are even fewer in number. Second, research funding in general has been increasingly difficult to obtain for most investigators. This is further compounded by a national priority for funding research related to HIV infection, and in the field of aging, the priority has been Alzheimer's disease and other dementias.

What might be solutions to the investigator and funding issues are beyond the cope of this chapter. Nevertheless, it is encouraging and satisfying that so much has already been accomplished by a small but dedicated group of clinicians and investigators interested in aging, immunity, and infection. It is hoped that we can maintain such a high level of commitment and excellence as we face the problem of infection in a rapidly growing aging population.

REFERENCES

Albright, J. F., & Makinodan, T. (1966). Growth and senescence of antibody-forming cells. *Journal of Cell Physiology, 67*(Supplement 1), 185–206.

Appel, G. B. (1990). Aminoglycoside nephrotoxicity. *American Journal of Medicine, 88* (Suppl. 3C), 3C-16S–3C-20S.

Bibel, D. J. (1988). Elie Metchnikoff's bacillus of long life. *ASM News, 54,* 661–665.

Boscia, J. A., Abrutyn, E., & Kaye, D. (1987). Asymptomatic bacteriuria in elderly persons: Treat or not treat? *Annals of Internal Medicine, 106,* 764–765.

Bradley, S. F., Terpenning, M. S., Ramsey, M. A., Zarins, L. T., Jorgensen, K. A., Sottile, W. S., et al. (1991). Methicillin-resistant *Staphylococcus aureus* colonization and infection in a long-term care facility. *Annals Internal Medicine, 115,* 417–422.

Brock, T. D. (1975). *Milestones in microbiology* (pp. 132–140). Washington, DC: American Society for Microbiology.

Cantrell, M., & Yoshikawa, T. T. (1983). Aging and infective endocarditis. *Journal of the American Geriatrics Society, 31,* 216–222.

Friedlander, A. H., & Yoshikawa, T. T. (1990). Pathogenesis, management, and prevention of infective endocarditis in the elderly dental patient. *Oral Surgery, Oral Medicine, Oral Pathology, 69,* 177–181.

Gutowski, J. R., Innes, J. B., Weksler, M. E., et al. (1986). Impaired nuclear responses to cytoplasmic signals in lymphocytes from elderly humans with depressed proliferative responses. *Journal of Clinical Investigation, 78,* 40–43.

Hill, A. B., & Meakins, J. L. (1992). Peritonitis. In T. T. Yoshikawa (Ed.), *Clinics in geriatric medicine* (pp. 869–887). Philadelphia, WB Saunders.

Ljungberg, B., Nillson-Ehle, I. (1987). Pharmacokinetics of antimicrobial agents in the elderly. *Reviews of Infectious Diseases, 9*, 250–264.

Lyons, A. S., & Petrucelli, R. J., II. (1978). *Medicine: An illustrated history.* New York, Harry N. Abrams.

Marrie, T. J., Durant, H., & Yates, L. (1989). Community-acquired pneumonia requiring hospitalization: 5-year prospective study. *Reviews of Infectious Diseases, 11*, 586–599.

Miller, D., Yoshikawa, T. T., Castle, S. C., & Norman, D. (1991). Effect of age on fever response to recombinant tumor necrosis factor alpha in a murine model. *Journal of Gerontology, 46*, M176–M179.

Miller, R. A. (1989). The cell biology of aging: Immunological models. *Journal of Gerontology, 44*, B4–B8.

Muder, R. R., Brannan, C., Wagner, M. M., et al. (1992). Bacteremia in a long-term care facility: A five-year prospective study of 163 consecutive cases. *Clinics of Infectious Diseases, 14*, 647–654.

Nicolle, L. E., Brunka, J., McIntyre, M., et al. (1992). Asymptomatic bacteriuria, urine antibody, and survival in the institutionalized elderly. *Journal of the American Geriatrics Society, 40*, 607–613.

Norman, D. C., Grahn, D., & Yoshikawa, T. T. (1985). Fever and aging. *Journal of the American Geriatrics Society, 33*, 859–863.

Norman, D. C., & Yoshikawa, T. T. (1984). Intraabdominal infection: Diagnosis and treatment in the elderly patient. *Gerontology, 30*, 327–338.

Norman, D. C., & Yoshikawa, T. T. (1988). Acute appendicitis in the elderly. In J. L. Meakins & J. C. McClaran (Eds.), *Surgical care of the elderly* (pp. 386–391). Chicago: Year Book Medical.

Powell, K. E., & Farer, L. S. (1980). The rising age of the tuberculous patient. *Journal of Infectious Diseases, 142*, 946–948.

Silverstein, A. M. (1989). *A history of immunology* (pp. 1–23). San Diego: Academic Press.

Smith, D. W., Daly, P. B., & Roccaforte, J. S. (1991). Current status of nosocomial infection control in extended care facilities. *American Journal of Medicine, 91* (Suppl. 3B), 3B-281S–3B-285S.

Stead, W., Lofgren, J. P., Warren, E., & Thomas, C. (1985). Tuberculosis as an endemic and nosocomial infection among the elderly in nursing homes. *New England Journal of Medicine, 312*, 1483–1487.

Terpenning, M. S., Buggy, B. P., & Kauffman, C. A. (1987). Infective endocarditis: Clinical features in young and elderly patients. *American Journal of Medicine, 83*, 626–634.

Thoman, M. L., & Weigle, W. O. (1989). The cellular and subcellular bases of immunosenescence. *Advances in Immunology, 46*, 221–261.

U.S. Senate Special Committee on Aging, American Association of Retired Persons, Federal Council on Aging, et al. (1991). *Aging America: Trends and projections.* Washington, D.C., Government Printing Office.

Van den Brande, P., Vijgen, J., & Demedts, M. (1991). Clinical spectrum of pulmonary tuberculosis in older patients: Comparison with younger patients. *Journal of Gerontology, 46*, M204–M209.

Verghese, A., & Berk, S. L. (1983). Bacterial pneumonia in the elderly. *Medicine* (Baltimore), *62*, 271–285.

Verghese, A., & Berk, S. L. (Eds.), (1990). *Infections in nursing homes and long-term care facilities*. Basel, Switzerland, Karger.

Warren, J. W. (1991). The catheter and urinary tract infection. *Medical Clinics of North America, 75*, 481–493.

Warren, J. W., Muncie, H. L., Jr., Hall-Craggs, M. (1988). Acute pyelonephritis associated with the bacteriuria of long-term catheterization: A prospective clinico-pathological study. *Journal of Infectious Diseases, 158*, 1341–1346.

Yoshikawa, T. T. (1981). Important infections in elderly persons. *Western Journal of Medicine, 135*, 441–445.

Yoshikawa, T. T. (1983). Geriatric infectious diseases: An emerging problem. *Journal of the American Geriatrics Society, 31*, 34–39.

Yoshikawa, T. T. (1989). Pneumonia, UTI and decubiti in the nursing home: Optimal management. *Geriatrics, 44*, 32–43.

Yoshikawa, T. T. (1990). Antimicrobial therapy for the elderly patient. *Journal of the American Geriatrics Society, 38*, 1353–1372.

Yoshikawa, T. T. (1991). Treatment of nursing home-acquired pneumonia. *Journal of the American Geriatrics Society, 39*, 1040–1041.

Yoshikawa, T. T. (1992). Tuberculosis in aging adults. *Journal of the American Geriatrics Society, 40*, 178–187.

Yoshikawa, T. T., & Norman, D. C. (1987). *Aging and clinical practice: Infectious diseases: Diagnosis and treatment* (pp. 3–7). New York: Igaku-Shoin Medical.

PART I

Aging and Host Defenses: From Bedside to Bench

Tuberculosis in Elderly Persons

2

William W. Stead

It is remarkable how common tuberculosis is in the aged, particularly in institutions.—William Osler, *Textbook of Medicine* (1892)

Before the advent of infection by HIV, TB was close to the end of its epidemic curve in the industrially developed world. Earlier in this century, almost everyone in these same countries was infected before age 30, although only about 5% developed the disease. It inflicted a great mortality among children and young adults and morbidity among survivors. Today's octogenarians represent long-term survivors of that cohort and about 15% to 25% of them show a positive tuberculin skin test indicating they still harbor viable tubercle bacilli. So it should be no surprise that the TB attack rate is higher among the elderly than any other segment of our population.

Because of their great ability to persist in healed lesions, *Mycobacterium tuberculosis* may remain viable within a healthy host for many years (Stead, 1967). A reaction of 10 mm or more to five units of purified protein derivative of tuberculin (PPD-t) generally indicates that viable bacilli are still present that are capable of causing active tuberculosis if circumstances permit (e.g., failing health, insulin-dependent diabetes mellitus, prolonged corticosteroid therapy, or deterioration of the immune system with age). Probably the most prominent one of this group to develop and die of TB was the late Eleanor Roosevelt, who died of recrudescent TB with miliary dissemination at age 76 from an infection she had contracted in her late teens.

Elderly tuberculin nonreactors who are healthy are at almost no risk of developing TB *unless exposed*. About 90% of TB cases among the elderly today are due to recrudescence of ancient infection in the survivors of infection much earlier in life (Stead & Dutt, 1989; Stead & Lofgren, 1983). Healthy elderly tuberculin reactors have a risk of about 0.2% per year of developing active TB, which is the highest of any group except for HIV-infected persons. Those who develop active clinical TB at home usually have little chance of infecting others. This is due to the extremely great age gap between octogenarians and their great-grandchildren, which makes for minimal close contact. This is one of the principal reasons that the incidence of TB had been falling steadily by about 5% per year until HIV infection put in its appearance.

Studies in the 1930s showed that 80% of Americans had been infected by the tubercle bacillus by the age of 30 (Rich, 1951). Most healthy older persons eventually outlive all residual bacilli (Stead & To, 1987a). This is a mixed blessing: They are not at risk of recrudescence of old infection, but they no longer have the considerable protection against becoming infected again in the event of an exposure. This protection seems to persist as long as their T cells are capable of prompt recognition of and reaction to tuberculin (Stead & To, 1987a). Residents of nursing homes are, on the average, older and less healthy than their cohorts living in separate homes. Recrudescence of TB is not uncommon in either group. The difference is that in nursing homes, nonreactors are at risk of becoming infected whenever an old reactor develops active TB. Not only is the roommate at risk but also anyone breathing the air in any room on the same ventilation circuit. Thus, in a nursing home, active TB cases comprise a mixture of recrudescence of ancient infection and new infection acquired in the nursing home, giving a case rate about 4 times greater than in elderly persons living in private homes (Stead, 1989).

When a new infection is established in an elderly person there is a considerable chance of its developing into clinical TB (8% in women; 12% in men), if not treated preventively (Stead, To, Harrison, et al., 1987b). The presentation of the disease is then likely to be quite atypical, presenting as pneumonia, bronchitis, or even congestive heart failure, perhaps with a pleural effusion (Khan, Novat, Bachus, et al., 1977; Stead, Kirby, Schlueter, et al., 1968), without apical infiltration and cavitation.

The TB case rate observed among older persons is influenced by several factors. It varies directly with the prevalence of the infection in the same cohort in earlier years, and with the diligence with which the infection is

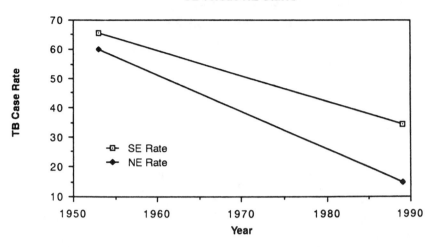

FIGURE 2.1   Comparison of TB case rates (cases/100,000 persons) in persons of
25 to 44 years in 1953 and about 40 years later when they are older than age 65.
Although the starting rates are similar, the decline in the case rate in the northeastern states is much steeper than that in the southeastern states.

sought by physicians caring for elderly persons. Figure 2.1 illustrates the
first point that in the early 1950s, the TB case rate in the 25- to 44-year age
group in the northeastern states was 60.0/100,000. Forty years later, now
that they are largely older than age 65, their care rate averages
14.7/100,000 (Centers for Disease Control, 1992; Stead, 1991). In 10 southeastern states, where in the 1950s the case rate in the 25- to 44-year age
group was 65.4, it has fallen only to 34.6 today. The great difference in the
decline in the case rate in these two sections of the country suggests that
different factors were operative in the two geographic sections in the en-
suing 40 years.

   With the decline in incidence of TB in this country, physicians may fail
to consider TB in a timely manner. Figure 2.2 shows that in 1987 to 1990
the TB case rate for adults younger than age 65 years was identical in Arkansas and in our six surrounding states (Missouri, Oklahoma, Texas,
Louisiana, Mississippi, and Tennessee). However, the case rate among
older persons in Arkansas is nearly twice that in the surrounding states
(Stead, 1991). Rather than a greater incidence of TB in Arkansas, this suggests a difference in the diligence with which TB is looked for among the
elderly.

AGE	ARKANSAS	SURROUNDING STATES	x^2	P
20-64	9.9	10.0	0.1	N.S.
65+	50.8	28.5	160.0	<.0001

FIGURE 2.2   Annual tuberculosis case rates in adults in Arkansas versus those in six surrounding states* measured in cases per 100,000[†] for 1987 to 1989. The rates for persons under age 65 are identical, whereas those among the elderly are much higher in Arkansas, where search for TB in the elderly is perhaps more diligent.

*LA, MS, MO, OK, TN, TX
[†]Data from Centers for Disease Control

TUBERCULIN SKIN TEST IN THE ELDERLY

Conventional teaching has it that a positive tuberculin skin test persists for life in the same way the antibody-mediated immunity to measles does. In the case of measles, however, the virus is all killed as the clinical illness abates, leaving only the antibodies to persist for life. In TB the T-cell–mediated positive skin test appears to be dependent on continued presence of tubercle bacilli. The corollary of this is that as long as the skin test remains positive, it indicates two things: the cell-mediated immune system is intact, and viable tubercle bacilli probably are still present. Our studies (Stead & To, 1987a) suggest that, although the test often does remain positive for years after an infection, it may become negative after several decades, even in immunocompetent persons, as shown by reactivity to other antigens of delayed hypersensitivity. Although the mechanism of immunity is separate from that causing the skin test response, our data suggest that protection against reinfection lasts only as long as the skin test remains positive.

Our experience confirms the observation that persons with a positive tuberculin skin test have a significantly longer average survival than nonreactors, because the reaction itself also signifies immune competence. However, the down side of a positive tuberculin test is that it indicates that the risk of developing TB is 150 fold greater than in persons whose skin test is negative (3% vs. 0.02%) (Stead & To, 1987a). Thus, when an elderly person is being examined initially or at the time of admission to a nursing home, it is a good practice to perform a tuberculin skin test to have it on record and to get a chest radiograph on reactors to check for active disease.

WHAT IS A POSITIVE TUBERCULIN SKIN TEST?

For elderly persons the old standard of 10 mm or more of induration 48 to 72 hours after intradermal injection of 5 units of PPD-t is still valid. Recent recommendations that define 5 mm as positive apply to persons with HIV infection, but our studies show that elderly persons who are reasonably healthy react about as well as much younger healthy persons, thus making 10 mm the appropriate cut point in the elderly.

In about 5% of elderly persons there is the phenomenon of waning of tuberculin reactivity, which may require repeating the test in 1 to 3 weeks to detect a positive reaction. If the test is positive so shortly after the negative one, it is clearly a "booster positive" and not a conversion. The significance of such a booster reaction is about the same as a positive on the first test, merely indicating a *potential* for recrudescence of old infection but not calling for preventive therapy. If, however, the second test is put off until 6 months or 1 year later, it is impossible to distinguish a positive test from a conversion, thus possibly triggering an unnecessary course of preventive therapy. This is the reason we urge that new residents be tested by the two-step method if the first test does not produce a reaction of at least 10 mm.

There is a new and improved method that should be used in reading the tuberculin skin test, the "ball-point pen" technique described by Sokal (1975). Using a ball-point or felt-tipped pen with the skin tightened by gently squeezing the forearm from the dorsal side, one approaches any detectable reaction first from above with the pen held leaning away from the test site at 45 degrees from the horizontal until the smooth motion of the pen is stopped by increased skin thickness caused by local infiltration by cells and edema. The same procedure is repeated from the distal side. The size of the induration than can be measured as the distance in millimeters between the proximal ends of the two ink marks. Measuring the transverse diameter is not satisfactory because the progress of the pen may be interrupted by irregularities caused by ligaments and muscle bundles beneath the skin.

WHICH OF THE ELDERLY ARE AT RISK OF TB?

Although the TB *case rate* is much higher among nursing home residents than among usually more healthy elderly persons in general, it is important to remember that 80% of all TB cases in the elderly arise among the 95%

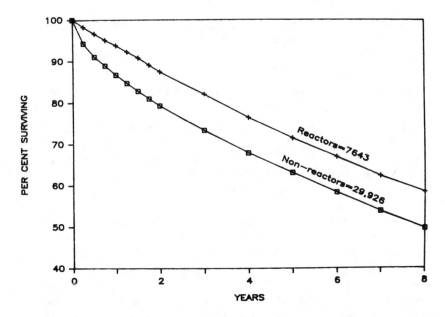

FIGURE 2.3   Survival of nonreactors to tuberculin in comparison with tuber-
culin-positive home residents. Although nonreactors suffer rapid initial loss,
those surviving 6 to 12 months show their immunocompetence by surviving
equally well from that time on.

who live at home and are largely caused by recrudescence of old infection
(Stead, 1989). About 20% of the cases arise among the 5% who live in nursing homes, and constitute a mixture of old and recently acquired infections.

Only 5% to 10% of elderly persons who fail to react to tuberculin are truly
anergic. Figure 2.3 shows that tuberculin-negative nursing home residents
show a high death rate (of 5% to 10%) in the first few months. However,
those who survive for 6 to 12 months are clearly immunocompetent as
shown by the fact that beyond that time they then survive about as well as
those whose immunocompetence is shown by the reaction to tuberculin
(Stead & To, 1987a).

A positive skin test indicates that the individual still harbors viable tubercle bacilli from the past that may still produce clinical tuberculosis as
health declines in old age. Thus, even if the initial chest radiograph shows
no evidence of TB, each positive skin test reading should be recorded in the
permanent medical record and preferably also posted on the front of the
chart. This expedites prompt study of sputum for acid fast bacilli whenev-

er a tuberculin reactor develops bronchitis or pneumonia, or begins to lose strength and weight.

LATER RETESTING OF NONREACTORS IN NURSING HOMES

Whenever there is suspicion of spread of TB in a nursing home, all previously nonreactive persons who may have been exposed should be retested, again using 5 units of PPD-t intradermally. If results of testing of each resident by the two-step technique had been recorded at the time of entry, it is easy to identify residents who are newly infected by an increase of 15 mm or more in the reaction to 5 units of PPD-t (Centers for Disease Control, 1990; Stead & To, 1987a). The reason we suggest defining a conversion among older persons as 15 mm or more increase is to avoid treating elderly people with only a late booster reaction with isoniazid (INH). Without the prior test results for comparison, one can only guess that large reactions *may* signify new infections, because a reaction resulting from a new infection is generally larger than one resulting from an ancient, dormant infection. It is much better to have knowledge that a definite conversion to positive has occurred, which is why we urge two-step testing on admission to nursing homes where exposure is common.

Once an exposure to tuberculosis in a nursing home is suspected, all nonreactors should be retested with PPD-t about 6 to 8 weeks after the end of the exposure to find new converters. All tuberculin reactors (whether old or conversions) should have chest radiographs to look for the source case and to make sure that TB is not already apparent among skin test converters. All with scarring or current pulmonary infiltration should have two to three sputum specimens submitted for smear and culture for tuberculosis. In addition, all tuberculin negative persons with a chronic cough should be radiographed to find the occasional anergic person with active TB.

TREATMENT CONSIDERATIONS IN THE ELDERLY

Therapy for Active Tuberculosis

Tuberculin reactors with chest radiographs showing lesions suspicious for TB should be studied bacteriologically. If the sputum smear reveals acid fast bacilli, it is advisable to begin therapy for active TB at once. When there is clinical suspicion of TB and the skin test is positive but three sputum smears are negative, it is generally advisable to begin therapy without awaiting confirmation of the diagnosis. If a culture is eventually reported positive, the diagnosis is confirmed. But if the cultures are negative, and the patient is tolerating the medication satisfactorily, we generally suggest completing the course of therapy as given subsequently.

Where active TB is suspected, therapy with a single drug is not satisfactory because of the likelihood of developing bacterial resistance to that drug and spreading it around the nursing home. The combination of rifampin (RIF) and INH is generally recommended, because both drugs are bactericidal for all but 1 in 10^6 organisms, making the chance of developing drug resistance extremely small. The regimen we have found most satisfactory is two combination capsules of RIF and INH (Rifamate) with pyridoxine 50 mg daily for 1 month, followed by two Rifamate capsules and two 300 mg tablets of INH at one time twice a week to completion of the course. This is generally 9 months for smear-positive cases (Dutt & Stead, 1982).

The addition of pirazinamide (PZA) or ethambutol (EMB), as recommended by the Centers for Disease Control for younger patients, is rarely indicated in the elderly. In this group the disease is usually the result of reactivation of an ancient infection originally acquired before the advent of antituberculous drugs. Daily therapy may be used, of course, but gives no better results than our largely twice-weekly regimen.

For the last 12 years we have found that it is safe to reduce the length of therapy when there is evidence on at least three examinations that the population of organisms is small. Thus, when three sputum smears are negative, but the cultures later are reported as positive, we stop therapy at 6 months (Dutt, Moers, & Stead, 1990). If three smears *and* cultures are negative, active TB still may be present but with a very small population of organisms. Some physicians discontinue treatment as soon as negative cultures are reported. However, we have seen several relapses after only 1 or 2 months of therapy for such cases and prefer to complete an adequate course of therapy, which is 4 months where three smears and cultures of sputum are negative initially (Dutt, Moers, & Stead, 1989).

MONITORING FOR DRUG TOXICITY

Before any antituberculous drugs are given, a blood specimen should be submitted for the usual liver function tests (LFTs) to rule out serious hepatic disease and to serve as a baseline to which later tests may be compared if symptoms suggestive of drug toxicity develop.

The nurse in charge of each patient who is receiving antituberculous drugs should be acquainted with their most significant side effects so that toxicity may be detected before irreparable harm is done. We do not recommend monthly LFTs, because they are commonly abnormal in the absence of clinical evidence of toxicity and lead to more confusion than enlightment.

If the patient shows anorexia, nausea, or vomiting, *the drugs should be withheld* and blood submitted promptly for LFTs. If not elevated, the drugs are probably not the cause of the symptoms, and medication can be restarted, beginning cautiously with a half dose after symptoms have subsided. If the transaminase is elevated beyond 500 units/L, INH should not be given further. However, if the transaminase is only modestly elevated, it generally is safe to rechallenge the patient with a half dose of INH for a few days after clinical and biochemical recovery. If this one is tolerated, it should be stopped and the same procedure repeated with RIF. If that is tolerated, we generally restart the combination, Rifamate, in a half dose for 2 to 3 days before continuing with the full dose. Although this process requires 10 to 14 days to complete, this lost time is not serious because of the slowness with which tubercle bacilli multiply.

We find that more than half the patients who have shown toxicity can be treated to completion if handled in this manner. If the combination of INH and RIF is not tolerated, another drug should be substituted for the offender and therapy completed. When the transaminase exceeds 500 units, however, therapy must be changed. In this situation EMB combined with PZA may be substituted for INH. In smear-positive cases we prefer streptomycin over EMB to combine with PZA, because it is bactericidal and will still permit the use of short-course therapy.

An occasional patient does not tolerate the twice-weekly regimen. In these instances we return to the daily regimen of 2 Rifamate capsules each morning to complete the course of therapy.

PREVENTIVE THERAPY

It would be nice if there were a method to prevent relapse of old infection in the elderly. However, studies have shown that the use of preventive therapy with INH for old reactors is a greater risk to an elderly patient than is the development of active tuberculosis (Stead et al., 1987). Moreover, INH toxicity can be fatal, whereas a recrudescence of an old infection rarely is.

Conversely, if the evidence is clear that a new infection has occurred (an increase of 15 mm or more over two previously negative skin tests) it indicates a significant risk of tuberculosis (8% in women; 12% in men). This is a strong indication for preventive therapy with INH, even in older people. A dose of 300 mg/day for 6 to 9 months is highly protective against TB (Stead et al., 1987).

When properly supervised, such therapy is quite safe. However, we observed an incidence of nonfatal toxic hepatitis of 4.5% in about 2000 elderly persons so treated (Stead et al., 1987). Careful clinical monitoring for toxic side effects of the drug is imperative, but monthly LFTs add little. The most common symptoms of toxic side effect are anorexia and nausea, followed by vomiting. At that point the drug should be withheld and blood drawn for LFTs. If the transaminase is elevated to 500 units/L or more, the drug should not be tried further. Conversely, if it is modestly elevated, it is appropriate to rechallenge the patient with 150 mg INH (one $^1/_2$ tablet) for 3 days (if tolerated) and then continue with full dose under careful observation. More than 50% of patients tolerate continuation of therapy if managed in this way.

It is generally advisable to give pyridoxine in a dose of 25 to 50 mg daily in elderly persons to prevent neurologic and hematologic side effects of INH.

Our study of the effect of INH preventive therapy on the long-term survival of about 2,000 elderly persons who were treated with INH for a year as a preventive against development of TB show no deleterious effect. Actually those who were treated showed a slightly longer survival (Stead et al., 1987).

EXTRAPULMONARY TUBERCULOSIS

Elderly persons who were infected in earlier years are also at risk of developing TB in other organs, with or without pulmonary TB. Tuberculous meningitis and miliary TB were most common among young children when TB was common earlier in this century, whereas the highest incidence of both of these dreaded forms of the infection today is among the elderly.

Extrapulmonary forms of TB commonly go unsuspected, because the clinical picture is so nonspecific, and radiographic abnormalities are not as readily found as in the lung. The most common manifestations are loss of weight and low-grade fever. Headache may signal early meningitis, while painless hematuria suggests renal involvement. In the case of Eleanor Roosevelt, chronic dissemination of infection followed long-term cortisone therapy, and her bone marrow was interpreted as showing aplastic anemia. A clue to infection was apparently missed in that she was febrile, which would not fit that diagnosis.

A recent report describes a tuberculous skin ulcer in an 85-year-old woman, which set off a very considerable outbreak of new infections among a hospital staff. We have recently seen an elderly nursing home resident in whom *M. tuberculosis* appears to be the pathogen in a decubitus ulcer over the sacrum. This patient is thought to account for a continuing series of tuberculin skin test conversions among the residents and staff of the nursing home.

Generally all extrapulmonary tuberculosis lesions heal quite satisfactorily on the same regimen (INH and RIF) that is described previously for pulmonary TB (Dutt & Stead, 1989). It used to be necessary to continue therapy for 18 to 24 months for all extrapulmonary lesions, whereas it has been shown that ordinary short-course chemotherapy using INH and RIF is quite adequate. However, if there is an accumulation of pus or necrosis because of TB, surgical principles of drainage must prevail along with appropriate chemotherapy for TB.

SUMMARY

TB is still common among elderly persons and is all too often overlooked. Those at risk can usually be detected by the tuberculin skin test. A chest radiograph should be made on all reactors to be sure that active tuberculosis is not already present. Therapy with INH and RIF is quite safe and effective for active TB in elderly persons.

In elderly persons, preventive therapy with INH generally is indicated only when tuberculin skin test conversion signals a newly acquired infection. This is most likely to occur in a nursing home where exposure to active TB is not uncommon. Such therapy can be given safely if the patient is watched clinically for development of hepatic toxicity, and the drug stopped promptly if nausea and vomiting occur. Monthly liver function studies often lead to confusion and may cause unnecessary cessation of therapy.

REFERENCES

Centers for Disease Control. (1990). Prevention and control of tuberculosis in facilities providing long-term care to the elderly. *Morbidity and Mortality Weekly Report, 39*, RR-10.

Centers for Disease Control (1992). *Tuberculosis in the United States, 1987–89* (HHS Publication). Washington, DC: Government Printing Office.

Dutt, A. K., Moers, D. J., & Stead, W. W. (1989). Smear- and culture-negative pulmonary tuberculosis: Four-month short course chemotherapy. *American Review of Respiratory Diseases, 139*, 867–870.

Dutt, A. K., Moers, D. J., & Stead, W. W. (1990). Smear-negative, culture-positive tuberculosis: Six-month chemotherapy with isoniazid and rifampin. *American Review of Respiratory Diseases, 141*, 1232–1235.

Dutt, A. K., & Stead, W. W. (1982). Medical perspective: Present chemotherapy for tuberculosis. *Journal of Infectious Diseases, 146*, 698–704.

Dutt, A. K., & Stead, W. W. (1989). Treatment of extrapulmonary tuberculosis. *Seminars in Respiratory Infection, 4,* 226–231.

Khan, M. A., Novat, D. M., Bachus, B., Whitcomb, M. E., Brody, J. S., & Snider, G. L. (1977). Clinical and roentgenographic spectrum of pulmonary tuberculosis in the adult. *American Journal of Medicine, 62,* 31–38.

Rich, A. R. (1951). *The pathogenesis of tuberculosis* (2nd ed., p. 110). Springfield, IL: Charles C Thomas.

Sokal, J. E. (1975). Measurement of delayed skin test response. *New England Journal of Medicine, 293,* 501–502.

Stead, W. W. (1967). Pathogenesis of a first episode of chronic pulmonary tuberculosis in man: Recrudescence of residuals of the primary infection or exogenous reinfection. *American Review of Respiratory Diseases, 95,* 729–745.

Stead, W. W. (1989). Special problems in tuberculosis: Tuberculosis in the elderly. *Clinics in Chest Medicine, 10,* 397–405.

Stead, W. W. (1991). Tuberculosis in the elderly. *Annual Review of Medicine, 42,* 267–276.

Stead, W. W., & Dutt, A. K. (1989). Tuberculosis in the elderly. *Seminars in Respiratory Infection, 4,* 189–197.

Stead, W. W., Kerby, G. R., Schlueter, D. P., & Jordahl, C. W. (1968). The clinical spectrum of primary tuberculosis in adults: Confusion with reinfection in the pathogenesis of chronic tuberculosis. *Annals of Internal Medicine, 68,* 731–745.

Stead, W. W., & Lofgren, J. P. (1983). Medical perspective: Does the risk of tuberculosis increase in old age? *Journal of Infectious Diseases, 147,* 951–955.

Stead, W. W., & To, T. (1987a). The significance of the tuberculin skin test in elderly persons. *Annals of Internal Medicine, 107,* 837–842.

Stead, W. W., To, T., Harrison, R. W., & Abraham, J. H. (1987b). Benefit-risk considerations in preventive treatment for tuberculosis in elderly persons. *Annals of Internal Medicine, 107,* 843–845.

Senescence of Cellular Immunity to Tuberculosis Infection in the Mouse

3

Some Radical Departures From Previous Thinking

Ian M. Orme

TB remains a problem of global proportions with an estimated 8 to 10 million new cases and 3 to 4 million deaths per year worldwide (Murray, Styblo, & Rouillon, 1990). Within the United States, however, a survey of lay opinion just a few years ago might have led one to suppose that TB had "disappeared." During the last year or so, reports in the popular press have alerted the public to epidemiologic data revealing not only that TB is "back" but that, for the first time since records were begun in the United States in the mid-1950s, the incidence of TB has begun to rise significantly (Fox, 1990). The cause of this is clearly multifactorial, involving the spread of the acquired immunodeficiency syndrome (AIDS), particularly with

27

drug users; as a result of immigration patterns; and as a reflection of a rise in the numbers of the homeless.

Although one cannot ascribe the recent rise in the TB rate to the increasing size of the elderly population in this country, the fact remains that TB is still relatively common within this population. Indeed, the overall decline in the rate of TB infection that has been observed in the United States during the past several decades disguises a demographic shift from a disease that once afflicted young people disproportionally to one that today is more often a problem within the elderly (Powell & Farer, 1980).

In this regard, there are pressing justifications why we must continue to study and understand the immunopathology, detection, and treatment of TB in the elderly. The first reason is simply because the elderly, that is, those older than 65 years of age, are the fastest growing segment of our overall population. The second reason is that tuberculin surveys performed in the 1930s showed that at least 80% of the population by 30 years of age had come into contact with the tuberculosis bacterium. What percentage of these people may subsequently undergo latent recrudescence of disease is difficult to estimate from current Centers for Disease Control figures, but it may be as high as 20% of people older than age 80 (Stead & Lofgren, 1983).

During the past several years we have attempted to provide a basic scientific explanation for the increased susceptibility of the elderly to TB infection, using as a model inbred mice that are infected with *Mycobacterium tuberculosis* at various times during their life-span. This approach has revealed new information regarding the acquired cellular response to tuberculosis, both in young and old animals.

ACQUIRED CELLULAR RESPONSE IN YOUNG MICE TO *MYCOBACTERIUM TUBERCULOSIS* INFECTION

Following intravenous inoculation of mice with a moderate (sublethal) dose of the virulent Erdman strain of *M. tuberculosis*, the bacterial infection proceeds in a triphasic manner (Orme, 1987a). The first phase lasts 10 to 15 days and is characterized by rapid proliferation of the organism. The second, which begins at this point and lasts until about day 50 of the infection, is characterized by progressive mycobacterial elimination and is followed in turn by a tertiary phase in which a low-grade chronic disease ensues, with small numbers of acid-fast bacilli evident within well-formed granulomas.

Figure 3.1 indicates that the T-cell response during this period is highly complex, and consists of waves of different T-cell subsets, each with a certain kinetics of emergence and loss. We have shown that the early phase of immunity to live infection is mediated by T cells expressing the CD4 marker (Orme, 1987a). This CD4 population comprises cells that may be operationally divided into two separate functional subsets. The first is the *protective T-cell population*, so-called because its original identification was based on its ability to protect irradiated recipients from a challenge infection following adoptive transfer (Orme & Collins, 1983). In addition to protective activity, we have now identified this cell as the source of interferon (IFN)-γ secretion during the early stages of the infection (Orme, Miller, Roberts, et al., 1992); IFN-γ is a key cytokine that presumably mediates the cessation of bacterial growth, and the onset of bacterial elimination (Nathan, Murray, Wiebe, et al., 1983). During this process, the protective T-cell population is undergoing a period of differentiation including conversion from a CD45RB$^+$ phenotype to CD45RB$^-$ (Griffin & Orme, unpublished data).

By culturing CD4 cells in vitro and determining IFN-γ secretion, we have found that the key target antigens of such cells are primarily represented within the culture filtrate fraction of *M. tuberculosi* and constitute a pool of secreted or export proteins of the bacillus (Orme et al., 1992). We have hypothesized that infected macrophages pinocytose these materials from vacuoles containing bacteria and present these antigens to class II–restricted CD4 cells (Orme, 1991; Orme et al., 1991).

The second functional subset of CD4 cells mediates delayed-type hypersensitivity (DTH). DTH effector T cells also react strongly to culture filtrate proteins containing secreted/export proteins of *M. tuberculosis* (Orme et al., 1992), but they also appear to recognize constitutive cell wall antigens, which protective T cells do not (Orme, 1988a). Attempts to distinguish between the two-cell populations remain difficult because both populations are CD4 and arise with similar kinetics in mice given the live infection.

Approximately 3 weeks into the experimental infection, a sizable population of T cells bearing the $\gamma\delta$ T-cell receptor can be found in target organs (Griffin, Harshan, Born, et al., 1991). The role of these cells is unclear. Their contribution may be critical to the overall cellular response (Janis, Kaufman, Schwartz, et al., 1989) or, alternatively, they simply may be "inflammatory" T cells that nonspecifically accumulate at sites of infection. Their target antigens are also a matter of controversy. Some reports suggest that they recognize nonprotein antigens (Pfeffer, Schoel, Gulle, et al., 1990). Others suggest that the hsp60 stress protein of *M. tuberculosis* is a major target (Born, Hall, Dallas, et al., 1990; Born, Happ, Dallas, et al., 1990; O'Brien, Fu, Cranfill, et al., 1992). Our (unpublished) data are consistent with the latter observation and are supportive of the idea that these cells lyse heavily infected (probably dead) macrophages that they recognize by virtue of both microbial and autologous stress proteins expressed on the infected

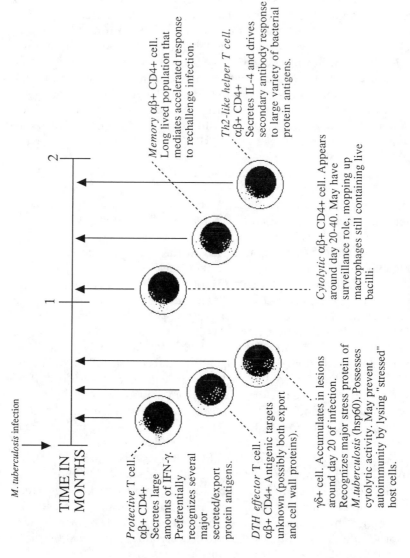

M. tuberculosis infection

TIME IN
MONTHS

Protective T cell.
αβ+ CD4+
Secretes large
amounts of IFN-γ.
Preferentially
recognizes several
major
secreted/export
protein antigens.

DTH effector T cell.
αβ+ CD4+ Antigenic targets
unknown (possibly both export
and cell wall proteins).

γδ+ cell. Accumulates in lesions
around day 20 of infection.
Recognizes major stress protein of
M.tuberculosis (hsp60). Possesses
cytolytic activity. May prevent
autoimmunity by lysing "stressed"
host cells.

Memory αβ+ CD4+ cell.
Long lived population that
mediates accelerated response
to rechallenge infection.

Th2-like helper T cell.
αβ+ CD4+
Secretes IL-4 and drives
secondary antibody response
to large variety of bacterial
protein antigens.

Cytolytic αβ+ CD4+ cell. Appears
around day 20-40. May have
surveillance role, mopping up
macrophages still containing live
bacilli.

FIGURE 3.1

cell surface. By doing so, the γδ cells guard against an αβ T-cell response to such antigens that could potentially give rise to autoimmunity (van Eden, Hogervorst, van der Zee, et al., 1989). In addition, γδ cells show evidence of apoptosis following such interactions (Janssen, Wesselborg, Heckl-Ostreicher, et al., 1991) and hence have no anamnestic response (Griffin et al., 1991).

As the infection is contained and slowly cleared, a CD4 cytolytic T-cell population can be observed (Orme et al., 1992). This cell subset also appears preferentiallly to recognize secreted/export proteins and probably functions as a surveillance mechanism responsible for eliminating remaining macrophages that still harbor live bacilli. It should be noted that lysis is unlikely to cause dissemination of the infection because this event would tend to occur within granulomas that are fully formed by this time.

A further CD4 population mediates immunologic memory to TB infection (Orme, 1988b). Although protective T cells are dividing and short-lived, memory CD4 cells are not affected by antimitotic agents, and can be detected in mice that had been infected then treated with isoniazid chemotherapy up to a year later. Regrettably, little else is known about these cells, despite the fact that it is this population that is the central target of vaccination strategies.

Finally, recent data have shown that a late-emerging CD4 T-cell population that secretes IL-4 can be identified approximately 2 months after initiation of infection, at a time when a substantial antibody response to mycobacterial proteins begins to emerge. We therefore regard this cell as a Th2-type helper T cell that is involved in mediating this antibody response.

BASIS OF INCREASED SUSCEPTIBILITY OF OLD MICE TO TUBERCULOSIS INFECTION

B6D2F1 hybrid mice live approximately 26 to 30 months. As they pass the 22- to 24-month stage there is an appreciable age-related decline in their

---

FIGURE 3.1   The evolution of acquired cellular immunity in an experimental murine model of *M. tuberculosis* infection. During the initial course of the infection evidence has accumulated to suggest that possibly as many as six T cell subsets may be involved, based on functional activity and cell surface marker expression criteria. Whether each represents a discrete subset, or arises as a result of differentiation from one or two primary effector populations remains unknown. The reader should also bear in mind that other populations, such as CD8+ cells and natural killer cells, may also be involved in the eviential expression of specific resistance.

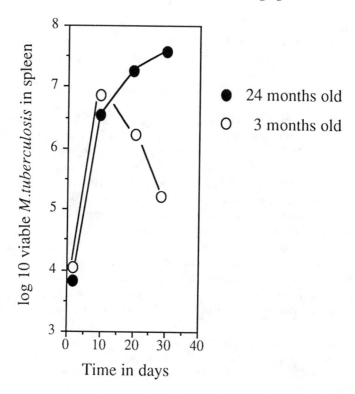

FIGURE 3.2   Growth of *M. tuberculosis* strain Erdman in the spleens of young and old mice.

ability to resist infection with *M. tuberculosis* strain Erdman. The standard inoculum of these bacilli is slowly cleared in young mice as described earlier, whereas in 24-month-old mice the infection continues to grow progressively (see Figure 3.2), with the animals dying of the infection by day 60 (Orme, 1987b).

Based on these observations, and based on the observation that mice given aerosol infections when 3 months of age began to die from recrudescent TB when approximately 2 years old (Orme, 1988c), we hypothesized that old mice underwent an age-related decline in their ability to generate protective T cells capable of containing the progressively growing infection. This was further supported by the observation that CD4 cells harvested from infected 24-month-old mice on days 10 or 20 of the infection failed to adoptively protect irradiated young mice from a challenge inoculum (Orme, 1987b). Thus, it appeared that the old animals completely lacked the ability to mount a protective T-cell response.

Recent data, however, have suggested an alternative explanation. We had previously disregarded later time points (day 20 plus) because by then the infected old animals had very large bacterial loads in target organs and were seemingly immunoincompetent. However, we serendipitously included CD4 cells harvested on day 30 in an experiment designed to compare the kinetics of IFN-γ secreting CD4 cells in young and old mice. What we found (see Figure 3.3) was surprising, in that on day 30 of the infection, old mice possessed T cells that secreted as much IFN-γ as "young"

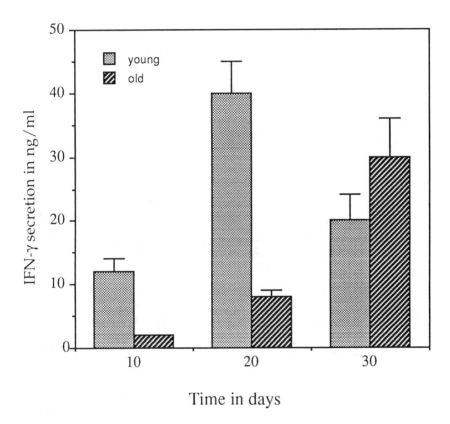

FIGURE 3.3   Evidence that the emergence of IFN-γ secreting CD4 T cells is delayed in old mice compared with young animals but eventually reaches similar peak levels. CD4 cells were harvested from infected mice at times shown and overlaid on bone marrow–derived macrophages pulsed 24 hours earlier with mycobacterial culture filtrate proteins. After a further 72 hours of incubation supernatants were assayed for the presence of IFN-γ by sandwich enzyme-linked immunosorbent assay (ELISA).

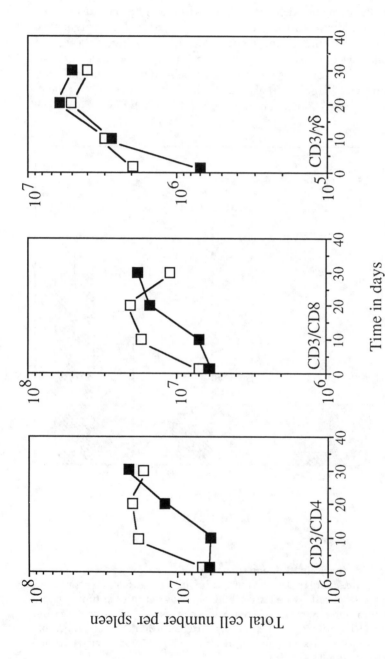

FIGURE 3.4   Evidence that "old" CD3 cells in general accumulate more slowly in the spleens of mice infected with *M. tuberculosis*. Numbers of cells was determined by flow cytometric analysis.

CD4 cells harvested on day 10 of the infection. It was therefore apparent that old mice are capable of generating protective cells, although the kinetics of this response was delayed compared with that seen in younger animals. Unfortunately for the aged animals, the bacterial load was approaching lethal levels by the time such cells had emerged.

Subsequent data have now indicated that the apparent lack of such cells may reflect their reduced capacity to focus quickly at sites of bacterial implantation where acquired immunity needs to be efficiently expressed. As shown in Figure 3.4, CD3 cells in general accumulate more slowly in the spleens of infected mice. An explanation for this slower pattern of accumulation was revealed by flow cytometric analysis, in which we observed defective expression in old mice of homing markers that allow T cells to leave the blood and enter into inflamed tissues (Shimizu, Newman, Tanaka, et al., 1992). Specifically, the L-selectin and CD11a molecules, which interact with complementary ligands on the surface of inflamed blood vessel endothelial cells (see Figure 3.5), were poorly expressed on cells present in the spleens of infected aged mice, and only reached levels comparable with those seen on young mice only by days 20 to 30 of the infection (see Figure 3.6). These data suggest that increased susceptibility of old mice to TB reflects a reduced capacity to focus mediator cells at sites of infection as a result of poor expression of critical cell homing molecules.

PROSPECTS FOR ELDERLY MICE: CAN RESISTANCE BE INCREASED?

At a time when our central hypothesis proposed a *lack* of protective T cells in old mice, we held little hope that this important class of response could be restored. Now in light of the finding that such cells do exist, we are more optimistic that their response can be improved. The central issue appears to be finding ways in which the expression of L-selectin, CD11a, and other homing markers can be up-regulated in "old" T cells, and then to test whether this, indeed, increases antimicrobial resistance. Approaches to achieve this might include immunotherapy, such as cytokines, or monoclonal antibodies directed against other cell surface molecules to trigger the T cell to up-regulate these homing molecules.

PROSPECTS FOR ELDERLY PERSONS: ARE THINGS LIKELY TO GET BETTER OR GET WORSE?

Recrudescence of latent TB is believed to occur in elderly humans who contracted the infection at a much earlier age, but who at that time did not pres-

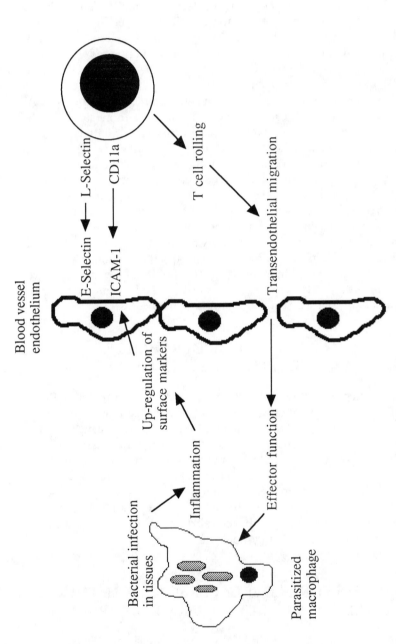

FIGURE 3.5 Present evidence suggests that "homing" molecules such as L-selectin and CD11a on the surface of T cells interact with complementary ligands on inflamed blood vessel endothelia, which enables them to extravasate into sites of tissue inflammation. Once sensitized T cells reach the site of a TB infection, either in the tissues or within lymphoid organs, then they will secrete cytokines that will give rise to macrophage activation and granuloma formation.

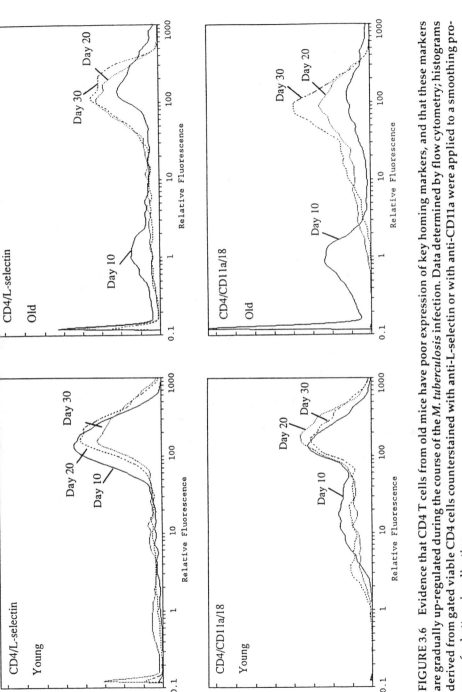

FIGURE 3.6 Evidence that CD4 T cells from old mice have poor expression of key homing markers, and that these markers are gradually up-regulated during the course of the *M. tuberculosis* infection. Data determined by flow cytometry; histograms derived from gated viable CD4 cells counterstained with anti-L-selectin or with anti-CD11a were applied to a smoothing program for better visualization.

ent with active disease. Because the incidence of TB dropped dramatically in the United States after the advent of chemotherapy and improved diagnosis in the middle of this century, it is logical to predict that the numbers of current elderly people who are at risk of endogenous reactivation of disease, although still significant, will continue to decline in parallel with the percentage of the population who were born before the 1940s to 1950s. It is also recognized that elderly people are more susceptible to exogenous infection, as illustrated by various nursing home outbreaks. However, this risk also declines as the incidence of total TB cases decreases.

Unfortunately the incidence of TB in the United States has increased by 11.8% in the last few years, and this is reflected by rises in other developed countries, for example, by 33% in Switzerland and 28% in Italy (Bloom, 1992). Also, the emergence of drug-resistant strains of *M. tuberculosis* has rendered conventional chemotherapeutic regimens almost impotent.

What are the potential consequences for the elderly population given these circumstances? A worse-case scenario could involve health professionals who are HIV positive and infected with TB having contact with elderly people. Under such conditions, elderly individuals would be at very substantial risk. There is no doubt that the TB field is in crisis, be it prevention, treatment, diagnosis, or, for that matter, resources for basic research. How this will impact on the older members of our population in the near future remains to be seen.

ACKNOWLEDGMENT

This work was supported by USPHS Grant AG127288 and AG06946.

REFERENCES

Bloom, B. R. (1992). Back to a frightening future. *Nature, 358*, 538–539.

Born, W., Hall, L., Dallas, A., Boymel, J., Shinnick, T., Young, D., Brennan, P., & O'Brien, R. (1990). Recognition of a peptide antigen by heat shock reactive γδ T lymphocytes. *Science, 249*, 67–69.

Born, W., Happ, M. P., Dallas, A., Reardon, C., Kubo, R., Shinnick, T., Brennan, P., & O'Brien, R. (1990). Recognition of heat shock proteins and γδ cell function. *Immunology Today, 11*, 40–43.

Fox, J. L. (1990). TB: A grim disease of numbers. *ASM [American Society of Microbiology] News, 56*, 363–365.

Griffin, J. P., Harshan, K. V., Born, W. K., & Orme, I. M. (1991). Kinetics of accumulation of γδ receptor-bearing T lymphocytes in mice infected with live mycobacteria. *Infection and Immunity, 59*, 4263–4265.

Janis, E. M., Kaufmann, S. H. E., Schwartz, R. H., & Pardoll, D. M. (1989). Activation of γδ T cells in the primary immune response to *Mycobacterium tuberculosis*. *Science, 244*, 713–716,

Janssen, O., Wesselborg, S., Heckl-Ostreicher, B., Pechhold, K., Bender, A., Schondelmaier, S., Moldenhauer, G., & Kabelitz, D. (1991). T cell receptor/CD3 signalling induces death by apoptosis in human T cell receptor γδ+ T cells. *Journal of Immunology, 146*, 35–39.

Murray, C. J. L., Styblo, K., & Rouillon, A. (1990). Tuberculosis in developing countries: Burden, intervention, and cost. *Bulletin of the International Union for Tuberculosis and Lung Disease, 65*, 6–24.

Nathan, C. F., Murray, H. W., Wiebe, M. E., & Rubin, B. Y. (1983). Identification of interferon-γ as the lymphokine that activates human macrophage oxidative metabolism and antimicrobial activity. *Journal of Experimental Medicine, 158*, 670–689.

O'Brien, R. L., Fu, Y., Cranfill, R., Dallas, D., Ellis, C., Reardon, C., Lang, J., Carding, S. R., Kubo, R., & Born, W. (1992). Heat shock protein Hsp60-reactive γδ cells: A large diversified T-lymphocyte subset with highly focused specificity. *Proceedings of the National Academy of Science USA, 89*, 4348–4352.

Orme, I. M. (1987a). The kinetics of emergence and loss of mediator T lymphocytes acquired in response to infection with *Mycobacterium tuberculosis*. *Journal of Immunology, 138*, 293–298.

Orme, I. M. (1987b). Aging and immunity to tuberculosis: Increased susceptibility of old mice reflects a decreased capacity to generate mediator T lymphocytes. *Journal of Immunology, 138*, 4414–4418.

Orme, I. M. (1988a). The immune response to the cell wall of *Mycobacterium bovis* BCG. *Clinics in Experimental Immunology, 71*, 388–393.

Orme, I. M. (1988b). Characteristics and specificity of acquired immunologic memory to *Mycobacterium tuberculosis* infection. *Journal of Immunology, 140*, 3589–3593.

Orme, I. M. (1988c). A mouse model of the recrudescence of latent tuberculosis in the elderly. *American Review of Respiratory Diseases, 137*, 716–718.

Orme, I. M. (1991). Processing and presentation of mycobacterial antigens: Implications for the development of a new improved vaccine for tuberculosis control. *Tubercle, 72*, 250–252.

Orme, I. M., & Collins, F. M. (1983). Protection against *Mycobacterium tuberculosis* infection by adoptive immunotherapy. *Journal of Experimental Medicine, 158*, 74–83.

Orme, I. M., Lee, B. Y., Appelberg, R., Miller, E. S., Chi, D., Griffin, J. P., & Roberts, A. D. (1991). T cell response in acquired protective immunity to *Mycobacterium tuberculosis* infection. *Bulletin of the International Union for Tuberculosis and Lung Disease, 66*, 7–13.

Orme, I. M., Miller, E. S. Roberts, A. D., Furney, S. K., Griffin, J. P., Dobos, K. M., Chi, D., Rivoire, B., & Brennan, P. J. (1992). T lymphocytes mediating protection and cellular cytolysis during the course of *Mycobacterium tuberculosis* infection. *Journal of Immunology, 148*, 189–196.

Pfeffer, K., Schoel, B., Gulle, H., Kaufmann, S. H. E., & Wagner, H. (1990). Primary responses of human T cells to mycobacteria: A frequent set of γδ T cells are

 `   stimulated by protease-resistant ligands. *European Journal of Immunology, 20,* 1175–1179.

Powell, K. E., & Farer, L. S. (1980). The rising age of the tuberculosis patient: A sign of success and failure. *Journal of Infectious Diseases, 142,* 946–948.

Shimizu, Y., Newman, W., Tanaka, Y., & Shaw, S. (1992). Lymphocyte interactions with endothelial cells. *Immunology Today, 13,* 106–112.

Stead, W. W., & Lofgren, J. P. (1983). Does the risk of tuberculosis increase in old age? *Journal of Infectious Diseases, 147,* 951–955.

van Eden, W., Hogervorst, E. J. M., van der Zee, R., van Embden, J. D. A., Hensen, E. J., & Cohen, I. R. (1989). The mycobacterial 65kD heat-shock protein and auto-immune arthritis. *Rheumatology International, 9,* 187–191.

Immunity to Influenza in the Elderly

4

Douglas C. Powers

Lower respiratory infections and influenza combined are the fourth leading cause of mortality in the geriatric population, accounting for approximately 5% of all deaths in this age group. A typical influenza A virus epidemic in the United States will be associated with hundreds of thousands of excess hospitalizations and tens of thousands of excess deaths, up to 90% of which occur in persons older than the age of 65 years (Barker & Mullooly, 1980a). Epidemiologic data demonstrate that age-related differences in the medical impact of an influenza epidemic vary according to the clinical outcome being measured. Attack rates for upper respiratory infection, or "influenza-like illness," peak in school or preschool-age children and then decline among successively older groups (Glezen, 1982; National Center for Health Statistics, 1985). Conversely, the incidence of serious illness, usually characterized by lower respiratory complications and the need for hospitalization, increases with age among adults, and this trend is even more dramatic when examining mortality rates (Eickhoff, Sherman, & Serfling, 1961; Glezen, 1982). All persons aged 65 and older are therefore targeted to receive annual immunization with commercially available inactivated influenza virus vaccine (Immunization Practices Advisory Committee, 1992).

It is generally assumed that the susceptibility of older adults to severe disease and life-threatening complications following infection is at least in part attributable to the senescence of influenza-specific immunity. Immunologic effector mechanisms of host defense against influenza can be divided into two broad categories: humoral and cellular (Ada & Jones, 1986). Humoral immunity refers to antibodies that are produced by B lymphocytes and that specifically recognize and neutralize influenza viruses. Although antibodies are usually measured in the bloodstream, it is generally assumed that they must be present locally (i.e., at mucosal surfaces) to be protective. The respiratory tract, which is the portal of entry for influenza viruses, may be thought of as anatomically compartmentalized according to the predominant class of immunoglobulins that are locally present. Antibodies are mainly of the IgA class in the upper respiratory tract, where they are produced locally within the submucosae and actively transported to the lumen in their dimeric secretory IgA (SIgA) form. In contrast, most of the antibodies in the lower respiratory tract are of the IgG class, and are thought to be derived from the serum by passive transudation (Wagner, Clements, Reimer, et al., 1987). The concentration of local IgG antibodies would therefore be expected to be proportional to serum titers. Antibodies act in a prophylactic fashion and serve primarily to prevent infection from occurring. As might be expected from the foregoing, and as has been documented in studies with both animals and humans, SIgA is the primary mediator of protection against upper respiratory influenza infection, whereas passively derived local IgG is probably more important in preventing lower respiratory infection and viral pneumonia (Clements, Betts, Tierney, et al., 1986; Clements, O'Donnell, Levine, et al., 1983; Liew, Russell, Appleyar, et al., 1984; Ramphal, Cogliano, Shands, et al., 1979; Renegar & Small, 1991).

Cellular, or cell-mediated, immunity to viruses may comprise several mechanisms, including antibody-dependent cell-mediated cytotoxicity and natural killer cell activity, although the role of these processes in vivo has not been well established for influenza. The best studied mechanism of cell-mediated immunity to influenza involves CTL, which are primarily $CD8^+$ T cells that lyse infected host cells, which they recognize by virtue of viral antigens expressed on the cell surface in combination with class I major histocompatibility complex (MHC) molecules (Ada & Jones, 1986; Townsend & McMichael, 1985). Unlike antibodies, whose main function is to prevent infection, CTL are more important for viral clearance and host recovery once infection has occurred (Ada & Jones, 1986; McMichael, Gotch, Noble, et al., 1983; Reiss & Schulman, 1980; Taylor & Askonas, 1986; Yap, Ada, & McKenzie, 1978).

The target antigens for most influenza-specific CTL are internal viral proteins, particularly nucleoprotein, which is found in the viral core complexed to genomic ribonucleic acid (RNA) (Gotch, McMichael, Smith, et al., 1987; Townsend & McMichael, 1985; Yewdell, Bennink, Smith., et al., 1985). Core proteins are antigenically highly conserved between variants of a given influenza type (i.e., A or B), so that most CTL are type-specific but broadly cross-reactive between strains or even subtypes within a type (Biddison, Shaw, & Nelson, 1979). In contrast, the major target antigens for antibodies are the hemagglutinin (HA) and neuraminidase (NA) glyco-proteins that project outward from the surface of the bilipid membrane en-velope of the virus. From the viewpoint of developing a vaccine capable of eliciting durable immunity, a particular problem is that the envelope gly-coproteins are highly variable and undergo frequent antigenic changes. Antibody against HA is generally neutralizing, presumably preventing in-fection by interfering with virus attachment to host cells or possibly by in-terfering with the fusion event subsequent to endocytosis. Point mutations in the gene(s) coding for HA or NA can cause structural changes at the mo-lecular level, which make the mutant viruses less susceptible to immuno-logic recognition and neutralization by antibodies that are present in a population that has been previously exposed to related strains (Wilson & Cox, 1990). There is thus a continuous process of natural immunoselection driven by human antibodies that accounts for antigenic variation or "drift" among influenza A and B viruses, and that results in the annual emergence of new strains with epidemic potential.

Much less frequently, influenza A viruses undergo major antigenic changes, or "shifts," probably as the result of HA/NA genetic reassort-ment within a host cell that has presumably been coinfected by two or possibly more different subtypes. Influenza A variants arising by this mechanism have pandemic potential because of their antigenic novelty, such as occurred with the sudden appearance in 1957 of H2N2 viruses, and with their subsequent replacement in 1968 by the H3N2 subtype. H1N1 variants, which had been the prevailing influenza A subtype throughout the first half of the century, reemerged in the late 1970s and have since been cocirculating with H3N2 as well as B type viruses. For this reason, current day vaccines are trivalent and contain two type A (H1N1 and H3N2) and one type B component. An interesting phenomenon related to humoral im-munity is that the antibodies in a given individual that are secondarily stimulated by repeat infection or by vaccination tend to be cross-reactive with antigenic determinants that were present on the virus with which the person had their original priming infection (Francis, Davenport, & Hen-nessy, 1953; Noble, Kaye, Kendal, et al., 1977).

My laboratory first became interested in the issue of the susceptibility of the elderly to influenza infection while conducting trials of intranasally ad-ministered live attenuated cold-adapted reassortant viruses in this age group. Cold-adapted reassortant viruses are promising vaccine candi-dates with proven immunogenicity and efficacy in infants and children

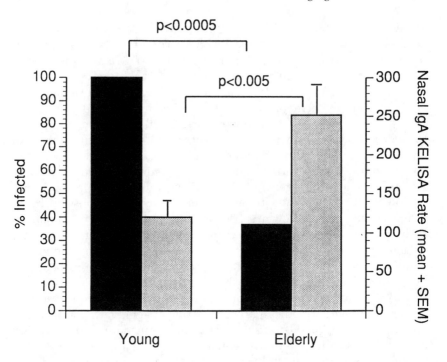

FIGURE 4.1 Inverse relationship between susceptibility to infection with intranasally administered live attenuated cold-adapted influenza A/Kawasa-
ki/86 (H1N1) reassortant virus (black bars) and prevaccination levels of local
(nasal) IgA antibody to the virus (hatched bars) in 20 young and 14 elderly subjects. Data derived from Powers et al. [1992]. Reduced infectivity of cold-
adapted influenza A H1N1 viruses in the elderly: Correlation with serum and
local antibodies. *Journal of the American Geriatrics Society,* 40:163–167.

and to a lesser extent in young adults, but we found that they were poorly
immunogenic in healthy elderly volunteers (Powers, Sears, Murphy, et al.,
1989; Powers, Fries, Murphy, et al., 1991). To highlight the differences between age groups further, we retested serum and nasal wash specimens
from young and elderly subjects who had all been inoculated with the
same dose of the same virus, and who all had very low or undetectable pre-
immunization serum levels of HAI antibody to the vaccine strain (Powers,
Murphy, Fries, et al., 1992). As seen in Figure 4.1, there was a dramatically
lower rate of infection in the elderly compared with the younger subjects.
Furthermore, the levels of SIgA antibody to the vaccine virus that were detected in nasal wash specimens by kinetic ELISA were significantly higher
in the elderly and were inversely correlated with susceptibility to infection

with the vaccine virus. We believe that our data are consistent with the previously mentioned epidemiologic observations suggesting that the elderly as a population are relatively resistant to upper respiratory tract infection, probably as the result of durable mucosal immunity acquired from earlier, and possibly repeated, natural infection(s).

To investigate the basis for the increased susceptibility of elderly adults to serious complications following influenza infection, we have been studying the senescence of cellular immunity to influenza and have focused specifically on CTL activity. The rationale for this work derives from previous reports demonstrating that (a) immune senescence is largely accounted for by T-cell dysfunction (Thoman & Weigle, 1989); (b) CTL are the primary immunologic mediator of influenza virus clearance and host recovery (Ada & Jones, 1986; McMichael et al., 1983; Reiss & Schulman, 1980; Taylor & Askonas, 1986; Yap et al., 1978); and (c) CTL responses following influenza infection are impaired in old versus young mice (Bender, Johnson, & Small, 1991; Effros & Walford, 1983). At the time of this writing, there are very little published data examining the effect of age on influenza-specific T-cell immunity in humans. One group reported that inactivated virus antigen-induced proliferative responses of purified T lymphocytes from healthy old donors were significantly lower than those of cells from young donors (Schwab, Russo, & Weksler, 1990). Others have observed an age-related decline in vitro IFN or IL-2 secretion by peripheral blood lymphocytes in the presence of virus antigen (Abb, Abb, & Deinhardt, 1984; McElhaney, Beattie, Devine, et al., 1990; McElhaney, Meneilly, Beattie, et al., 1992).

To examine the effect of age on CTL activity, we have employed conventional laboratory methods, using peripheral blood mononuclear cell effectors that are stimulated in vitro with virus-infected autologous cells and then assayed for lytic activity against infected autologous target cells by a ^{51}chromium release assay. For the experiments summarized in this chapter, influenza A H1N1 virus was used for in vitro stimulation and the percent specific lysis (%SL) was measured at an effector to target cell ratio of 50:1. We have consistently found that influenza A virus-specific CTL activity declines with advancing age (Powers, 1993; Powers & Belshe, 1993). Representative data are depicted in Figure 4.2A. As expected, cytologic effectors were completely cross-reactive between influenza A subtypes but did not lyse influenza B-infected autologous targets (see Figure 4.2B). Furthermore, the cytotoxicity appeared to be MHC class I–restricted, because low levels of lysis were seen against influenza A–infected allogeneic targets with which effectors were completely class I mismatched, and higher levels were observed against partially class I–matched targets. These findings have been further substantiated by more recent work in our laboratory in which immunomagnetic cell separation methods were used to

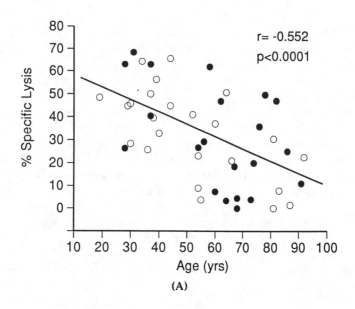

(A)

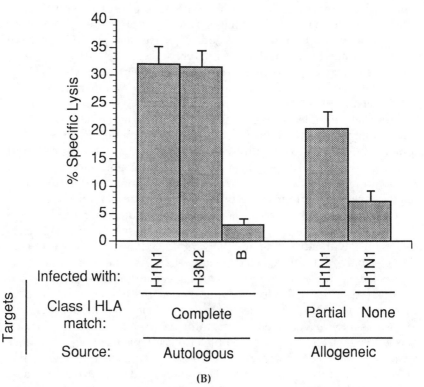

(B)

demonstrate that CD8$^+$ T cells were primarily responsible for the lytic activity measurable in bulk cultures (Powers, 1994).

We found no apparent relationship between individual levels of %SL and a history of vaccination within the preceding 12 months, suggesting that the effect of vaccination on CTL memory is relatively short-lived. To address this question further, a vaccine study was conducted with 47 healthy adult volunteers ranging in age from 19 to 96 and stratified according to age as < 40 (young), 40 to 64 (middle-aged), and ≥ 65 (elderly) years. Comparable numbers of persons in each of the three subject groups had received influenza vaccine during the preceding year, as well as during the preceding 5 years. All subjects were immunized intramuscularly with a standard dose of trivalent subvirion vaccine containing influenza A/Taiwan/1/86 (H1N1), A/Shanghai/6/89 (H3N2) and B/Yamagata/16/88 components. Blood and nasal wash specimens were obtained from just before vaccination and then 2 and 12 weeks later.

CTL responses to vaccination are summarized in Table 4.1. By 2 weeks postvaccination there was a significant enhancement of mean %SL against both H1N1 and H3N2-infected targets in all age groups. Compared with younger adults, the elderly had significantly lower baseline and peak-postvaccination levels of cytolytic activity, although the magnitude of the vaccine-induced rise in mean %SL was comparable among age groups. An unexpected finding was that there were age-associated differences in the duration of the CTL response. By 12 weeks postvaccination, the mean %SL had returned to prevaccination levels in both young and middle-aged volunteers but remained significantly elevated in the elderly ($p < .05$, Wilcoxon signed ranks test). To examine the duration of the CTL response in the latter group, we obtained from the elderly volunteers an additional whole blood specimen at approximately 16 weeks postvaccination, by which time the mean %SL of autologous influenza A virus-infected cells had declined to baseline levels. As can be seen, mean %SL of influenza B-infected targets was generally negligible. Mean %SL of influenza A-infected class I

FIGURE 4.2   (A) Influenza A virus-specific CTL activity in healthy seropositive adults with (●) or without (○) a history of inactivated influenza virus vaccination within the previous 12 months. Cytolytic effectors were assayed against infected autologous targets following 1 week of in vitro stimulation with influenza A (H1N1) virus. Each point represents one individual. (B) Effector cells from each individual were tested against autologous targets infected with A (H1N1), A (H3N2), or B virus, or against A (H1N1)-infected allogeneic targets with which they had partial or complete HLA class I mismatch. Data represent the mean (+SEM) %SL of all subjects shown in A.

TABLE 4.1 Effect of Aging and Vaccination on Cell Recovery and Cytotoxicity[a] of In Vitro Influenza A (H1N1) Virus-Stimulated PBMC Effectors Obtained From Adult Volunteers Immunized With Trivalent Inactivated Subvirion Vaccine Containing A/Taiwan (H1N1), A/Shanghai (H3N2), and B/Yamagata Components.

Vaccinee age (yrs)	No. in group	No. weeks postvaccination	No. viable cells recovered per culture (mean ± SEM x 10⁴)	% Specific lysis (mean ± SEM) of autologous target cells infected with designated influenza virus			% Specific lysis (mean ± SEM) of influenza A (H1N1)-infected allogeneic targets with designated degree of class 1 HLA match	
				A(H1N1)	A(H3N2)	B	None	Partial
<40	15	0	12.3 ± 1.5[b]	47.4 ± 3.9[d]	36.9 ± 3.9[*]	2.9 ± 1.5	6.0 ± 2.1	15.4 ± 2.1
		2	22.7 ± 4.2[c]	52.3 ± 5.0[*]	59.9 ± 4.1[*A]	4.7 ± 1.9	10.3 ± 1.8	29.8 ± 5.0
		12	10.8 ± 0.8	34.7 ± 3.1	36.6 ± 3.4	6.7 ± 1.4	13.4 ± 1.5	23.9 ± 4.4
40-64	15	0	10.1 ± 1.2[b]	32.2 ± 5.2[d]	36.4 ± 5.5[b]	1.6 ± 0.7	7.3 ± 2.0	32.0 ± 4.5
		2	15.1 ± 1.4[c]	41.9 ± 5.2	50.7 ± 4.0[iJ]	4.2 ± 1.7	4.7 ± 1.7	34.0 ± 5.0
		12	10.4 ± 1.2	28.3 ± 3.9	35.1 ± 4.6	4.9 ± 1.7	7.7 ± 2.3	33.8 ± 6.3
≥65	17	0	6.5 ± 0.7[b]	18.7 ± 4.1[d]	19.0 ± 4.4[d]	3.4 ± 2.1	5.0 ± 2.1	20.8 ± 5.3
		2	10.5 ± 1.5[c]	31.6 ± 6.4[*]	36.3 ± 7.9[iJ]	1.4 ± 0.9	9.9 ± 3.5	19.0 ± 6.8
		12	10.7 ± 1.0	26.8 ± 4.4[*]	33.8 ± 5.0[*]	4.3 ± 1.1	4.0 ± 1.6	18.3 ± 3.5
		14-16	9.7 ± 0.6	16.2 ± 4.6	18.6 ± 5.4	1.7 ± 0.8	0.3 ± 0.1	8.3 ± 1.8

a: Effector to target ratio 50:1
b: p <.005, comparing mean cell recovery per bulk culture between age groups (ANOVA)
c: p <.01, comparing mean cell recovery per bulk culture between age groups (ANOVA)
d: p <.002, comparing mean percent specific lysis between age groups (ANOVA)
e,f: p <.05, comparing mean percent specific lysis between age groups (ANOVA)

g: p <.05, compared with prevaccination value for respective age group and target cell type (Wilcoxon signed ranks test)
h: p <.01, compared with prevaccination value for respective age group and target cell type (Wilcoxon signed ranks test)
i: p <.005, compared with prevaccination value for respective age group and target cell type (Wilcoxon signed ranks test)

NOTE: These data were previously published in The Journal of Infectious Diseases, 1993, 167:584–592. © 1993 by The University of Chicago.

HLA-mismatched targets was also low, usually < 10%, and did not change appreciably following vaccination.

Table 4.2 summarizes the serologic responses to vaccination, measured both by hemagglutination inhibition and immunoglobulin class-specific ELISA using purified HA antigen. It was particularly noteworthy, and fortuitous from the viewpoint of data analysis, that the prevaccination antibody titers were remarkably well matched between the three age groups, probably as a reflection of their comparable vaccination histories. As can be seen, there was a very consistent and generally significant decline with aging in the mean-fold increase of antibody titers following vaccination. Between 2 and 12 weeks following immunization, mean antibody titers fell only slightly if at all, and there were no differences between age groups regarding the rate of decline. Age-related differences in rates of antibody response, which is conventionally defined as a fourfold or greater rise in titer from prevaccination to postvaccination, paralleled the mean-fold changes in antibody titers, and were consistently lowest in the elderly vaccinees.

Parenteral immunization elicited a local IgG HA-specific antibody response to all three vaccine component strains that was measurable by ELISA in nasal wash specimens (Table 4.3). As with serum antibodies, the proportion of vaccinees who achieved at least a fourfold response was consistently reduced with aging. In contrast to local IgG antibody responses, there were no appreciable changes in mean titers of nasal wash IgA HA antibodies following immunization, and the frequency of fourfold or greater titer rises was generally ≤ 20%.

The accumulated experience from efficacy studies to date suggests that in older adult populations influenza vaccines are more effective at reducing the risk of severe complications than they are at preventing nonhospitalizing illness (Arden, Patriarca, & Kendal, 1986; Barker & Mullooly, 1980b; Foster, Talsma, Furumoto-Dawson, et al., 1992; Patriarca, Weber, Parker, et al., 1985; Strassburg, Greenland, Sorvillo, et al., 1986). We believe, as has been suggested by others, that the reduced efficacy of conventional parenterally administered vaccines in preventing upper respiratory influenza is probably attributable to their inability to elicit secretory IgA antibodies in the upper airways. In contrast, vaccine-induced passively derived local IgG antibody and CTL may both contribute to the proven efficacy of vaccination against serious illness, although the relative contributions of these two mechanisms in mediating protection against or recovery from lower respiratory infection and subsequent life-threatening complications remain to be established. There is convincing evidence that vaccinated individuals are not well protected when there is a major antigenic difference between the vaccine component strain and the circulating wild-type virus (Barker & Mullooly, 1980b; Eickhoff & Meiklejohn, 1969). This observation, along with the relatively short duration of CTL responses to

TABLE 4.2 Serum Antibody Responses to Trivalent Inactivated Subvirion Vaccine Containing Influenza A/Taiwan (H1N1), A/Shanghai (H3N2), and B/Yamagata Components in Seropositive Adults of Varying Age

Antigen	Vaccinee age in years (No. in group)	HAI No. weeks postvaccination			HAI Response rate (%)	ELISA IgG HA No. weeks postvaccination			ELISA IgG HA Response rate (%)	ELISA IgA HA No. weeks postvaccination			ELISA IgA HA Response rate (%)
		0	2	12		0	2	12		0	2	12	
A/Taiwan (H1N1)	<40 (15)	5.5 ± 1.1	8.7 ± 0.6	8.8 ± 0.6	53	12.5 ± 0.5	14.1 ± 0.4[d]	13.8 ± 0.5	73[h]	6.0 ± 0.9	8.5 ± 0.7	7.7 ± 0.8	67
	40-64 (15)	5.5 ± 0.9	8.0 ± 0.5	7.6 ± 0.5	40	12.2 ± 0.6	13.4 ± 0.4[d]	13.0 ± 0.3	47[h]	6.8 ± 0.5	9.6 ± 0.7	8.6 ± 0.7	73
	≥65 (17)	5.9 ± 0.6	7.2 ± 0.5	7.1 ± 0.5	29	12.8 ± 0.3	13.2 ± 0.3[d]	13.1 ± 0.3	18[a]	7.4 ± 0.7	8.8 ± 0.7	8.0 ± 0.6	65
A/Shanghai (H3N2)	<40 (15)	5.5 ± 0.3	7.7 ± 0.4[b]	7.4 ± 0.4	53	11.8 ± 0.6	14.2 ± 0.5[e]	14.1 ± 0.3	67	5.6 ± 0.3	7.6 ± 0.6[f]	6.9 ± 0.6	67
	40-64 (15)	5.3 ± 0.4	8.3 ± 0.5[c]	7.9 ± 0.6	53	11.4 ± 0.5	13.7 ± 0.4[e]	13.3 ± 0.3	67	5.8 ± 0.4	9.6 ± 1.0[f]	8.2 ± 0.8	80
	≥65 (17)	6.1 ± 0.3	7.2 ± 0.4[b]	6.8 ± 0.4	29	12.8 ± 0.3	13.5 ± 0.3[e]	13.4 ± 0.3	41	7.1 ± 0.5	8.2 ± 0.6[f]	7.5 ± 0.5	53
B/Yamagata	<40 (15)	6.7 ± 0.6	9.9 ± 0.3[c]	9.1 ± 0.3	73	12.4 ± 0.5	14.1 ± 0.5	13.7 ± 0.5	73	8.0 ± 0.5	10.5 ± 0.5[g]	9.0 ± 0.5	67[i]
	40-60 (15)	6.6 ± 0.7	9.5 ± 0.3[c]	8.7 ± 0.4	73	12.9 ± 0.5	14.4 ± 0.3	14.4 ± 0.3	53	7.6 ± 0.5	10.2 ± 0.7[g]	8.5 ± 0.5	80[i]
	≥65 (17)	6.6 ± 0.3	8.2 ± 0.3[c]	7.7 ± 0.3	59	12.4 ± 0.3	13.2 ± 0.3	13.2 ± 0.4	47	7.4 ± 0.3	8.2 ± 0.3[g]	7.9 ± 0.4	35[i]

Serum titers (reciprocal mean $\log_2$ ± SEM) at specified times and vaccine response[a] rate of designated antibody

a: A significant antibody response was defined as a fourfold or greater rise in titer between the prevaccination specimen and either of the two postvaccination specimens

b,c,d,e,f: $p < 0.05$, comparing mean-fold rises in antibody titers between age groups by ANOVA

g: $p < 0.01$ comparing mean-fold rises in antibody titers between age groups by ANOVA

h: $p < .01$, comparing proportions of antibody responses between age groups by Chi square

i: $p < .02$, comparing of proportions of antibody responses between age groups by Chi square

NOTE: These data were previously published in The Journal of Infectious Diseases, 1993, 167:584–592. © 1993 by The University of Chicago.

TABLE 4.3 Nasal Wash Antibody Responses to Parenterally Administered Trivalent Inactivated Subvirion Vaccine Containing Influenza A/Taiwan (H1N1), A/Shanghai (H3N2), and B/Yamagata Components in Seropositive Adults of Varying Age

		Nasal wash titers (reciprocal mean log$_2$ ± SEM) at specified times and vaccine response[a] rate of designated antibody							
		ELISA IgG HA				ELISA IgA HA			
		No. weeks postvaccination			Response rate (%)	No. weeks postvaccination			Response rate (%)
Antigen	Vaccinee age in years (No. in group[b])	0	2	12		0	2	12	
A/Taiwan (H1N1)	<40 (15)	1.1 ± 0.3	2.5 ± 0.4	2.8 ± 0.3	60[c]	5.4 ± 0.4	5.3 ± 0.3	4.7 ± 0.4	13
	40-64 (15)	2.6 ± 0.4	3.1 ± 0.4	2.5 ± 0.4	27[c]	5.2 ± 0.4	5.2 ± 0.4	5.0 ± 0.4	7
	≥65 (15)	1.7 ± 0.5	2.6 ± 0.5	2.3 ± 0.4	20[c]	6.1 ± 0.4	5.6 ± 0.5	4.7 ± 0.5	13
A/Shanghai (H3N2)	<40 (15)	0.9 ± 0.3	2.7 ± 0.4	2.9 ± 0.4	53	3.3 ± 0.5	3.8 ± 0.4	2.6 ± 0.5	20
	40-64 (15)	1.6 ± 0.4	3.3 ± 0.5	2.8 ± 0.5	47	3.0 ± 0.6	3.6 ± 0.7	3.4 ± 0.6	20
	≥65 (15)	1.3 ± 0.4	2.3 ± 0.4	2.0 ± 0.4	27	4.1 ± 0.4	4.1 ± 0.5	3.1 ± 0.5	0
B/Yamagata	<40 (15)	0.9 ± 0.2	2.2 ± 0.3	1.8 ± 0.3	33	1.5 ± 0.5	2.5 ± 0.5	2.2 ± 0.4	27
	40-64 (15)	1.7 ± 0.3	2.6 ± 0.3	2.0 ± 0.2	20	2.0 ± 0.5	1.8 ± 0.5	1.9 ± 0.5	7
	≥65 (15)	1.3 ± 0.5	1.9 ± 0.3	1.6 ± 0.4	13	2.4 ± 0.4	2.1 ± 0.4	2.2 ± 0.3	7

a: A significant antibody response was defined as a fourfold or greater rise in the titer between the prevaccination specimen and either of the two postvaccination specimens

b: Nasal wash specimens could not be obtained from 2 of the 17 elderly vaccinees

c: $p < .05$, comparing proportions of antibody responses between age groups by Chi square

NOTE: These data were previously published in The Journal of Infectious Diseases, 1993, 167:584-592. © 1993 by The University of Chicago.

vaccination documented in studies to date (Ennis, Rook, Hua, et al., 1981; Grose & Belshe, 1990; McMichael, Gotch, Cullen, et al., 1981; Powers & Belshe, 1993), suggests that the overall contribution of cross-reactive CTL to immunity induced by vaccination is relatively minor compared with that provided by the more durable humoral response. Our results nevertheless suggest that T-cell effector mechanisms may be an important component of vaccine-induced protection in high-risk older adult populations, whose cellular immunity to influenza is likely to have otherwise waned.

REFERENCES

Abb, J., Abb, H., & Deinhardt, F. (1984). Age-related decline of human interferon alpha and interferon gamma production. *Blut, 48,* 285–289.

Ada, G. L., & Jones, P. D. (1986). The immune response to influenza infection. *Current Topics in Microbiology and Immunology, 128,* 1–54.

Arden, N. H., Patriarca, P. A., & Kendal, A. P. (1986). Experiences in the use and efficacy of inactivated influenza vaccine in nursing homes. In A. P. Kendal & P. A. Patriarca (Eds.), *Options for the Control of Influenza.* New York: Alan R. Liss.

Barker, W. H., & Mullooly, J. P. (1980a). Impact of epidemic type A influenza in a defined adult population. *American Journal of Epidemiology, 112,* 798–813.

Barker, W. H., & Mullooly, J. P. (1980b). Influenza vaccination of elderly persons: Reduction in pneumonia and influenza hospitalizations and deaths. *Journal of the American Medical Association, 244,* 2547–2549.

Bender, B. S., Johnson, M. P., & Small, P. A. (1991). Influenza in senescent mice: Impaired cytotoxic T-lymphocyte activity is correlated with prolonged infection. *Immunology, 72,* 514–519.

Biddison, W. E., Shaw, S., & Nelson, D. L. (1979). Virus specificity of human influenza virus-immune cytotoxic T cells. *Journal of Immunology, 122,* 660–664.

Clements, M. L., Betts, R. F., Tierney, E. L., & Murphy, B. R. (1986). Serum and nasal wash antibodies associated with resistance to experimental challenge with influenza A wild-type virus. *Journal of Clinical Microbiology, 24,* 157–160.

Clements, M. L., O'Donnell, S., Levine, M. M., Chanock, R. M., & Murphy, B. R. (1983). Dose response of A/Alaska/6/77 (H3N2) cold-adapted reassortant vaccine virus in adult volunteers: Role of local antibody in resistance to infection with vaccine virus. *Infection and Immunity, 40,* 1044–1051.

Effros, R. B., & Walford, R. L. (1983). The immune response of aged mice to influenza: Diminished T-cell proliferation, interleukin 2 production and cytotoxicity. *Cellular Immunology, 81,* 298–305.

Eickhoff, T. C., & Meiklejohn, G. (1969). Protection against Hong Kong influenza by adjuvant vaccine containing A2/Ann Arbor/67. *Bulletin of the World Health Organization, 41,* 562–563.

Eickhoff, T. C., Sherman, I. L., & Serfling, R. E. (1961). Observations on excess mortality associated with epidemic influenza. *Journal of the American Medical Association, 176,* 776–782.

Ennis, F. A., Rook, A. H., Hua, Q. Y., Schild, G. C., Riley, D., Pratt, R., & Potter, C. W.

(1981). HLA-restricted virus-specific T-lymphocyte responses to live and inactivated influenza vaccines. *Lancet, 2,* 887–891.

Foster, D. A., Talsma, A., Furumoto-Dawson, A., Ohmit, S. E., Margulies, J. R., Arden, N. H., & Monto, A. S. (1992). Influenza vaccine effectiveness in preventing hospitalization for pneumonia in the elderly. *American Journal of Epidemiology, 136,* 296–307.

Francis, T., Jr., Davenport, F. M., & Hennessy, A. V. (1953). Serological recapitulation of human infection with different strains of influenza virus. *Transactions of the Association of American Physicians, 66,* 231–239.

Glezen, W. P. (1982). Serious morbidity and mortality associated with influenza epidemics. *Epidemiologic Reviews, 4,* 25–44.

Gorse, G. J., & Belshe, R. B. (1990). Enhancement of anti-influenza A virus cytotoxicity following influenza A virus vaccination in older, chronically ill patients. *Journal of Clinical Microbiology, 28,* 2539–2550.

Gotch, F., McMichael, A., Smith, G., & Moss, B. (1987). Identification of viral molecules recognized by influenza-specific human cytotoxic T lymphocytes. *Journal of Experimental Medicine, 165,* 408–416.

Immunization Practices Advisory Committee. (1992). Prevention and control of influenza. *Morbidity and Mortality Weekly Report, 41,* 1–17.

Liew, F. Y., Russell, S. M., Appleyar, G., Brand, C. M., & Beale, J. (1984). Cross protection in mice infected with influenza A virus by the respiratory route is correlated with local IgA antibody rather than serum antibody or cytotoxic T cell reactivity. *European Journal of Immunology, 14,* 350–356.

McElhaney, J. E., Beattie, B. L., Devine, R., Grynoch, R., Toth, E. L., & Bleackley, R. C. (1990). Age-related decline in interleukin 2 production in response to influenza vaccine. *Journal of the American Geriatrics Society, 38,* 652–658.

McElhaney, J. E., Meneilly, G. S., Beattie, B. L., Helgason, C. D., Lee, S. F., Devine, R. D. O., & Bleackley, R. C. (1992). The effect of influenza vaccination on IL2 production in healthy elderly: Implications for current vaccination practices. *Journal of Gerontology, 47,* M3–8.

McMichael, A. J., Gotch, F., Cullen, P., Askonas, B. A., & Webster, W. G. (1981). The human cytotoxic T cell response to influenza A vaccination. *Clinical and Experimental Immunology, 43,* 276–284.

McMichael, A. J., Gotch, F. M., Noble, G. R., & Beare, P. A. S. (1983). Cytotoxic T-cell immunity to influenza. *New England Journal of Medicine, 309,* 13–17.

National Center for Health Statistics. (1985). Current estimates from the National Health Interview Survey, United States, 1982. *Vital and Health Statistics* (Series 10, No. 150, DHHS Publication No. [PHS] 85-1578). Public Health Service. Washington, DC: U.S. Government Printing Office.

Noble, G. R., Kaye, H. S., Kendal, A. P., & Dowdle, W. R. (1977). Age-related heterologous antibody responses to influenza virus vaccination. *Journal of Infectious Diseases, 136,* S686–692.

Patriarca, P. A., Weber, J. A., Parker, R. A., Hall, W. N., Kendal, A. P., Bregman, D. J., & Schonberger, L. B. (1985). Efficacy of influenza vaccine in nursing homes, reduction in illness and complications during an influenza A (H3N2) epidemic. *Journal of the American Medical Association, 253,* 1136–1139.

Powers, D. C. (1993). Influenza A virus-specific cytotoxic T lymphocyte activity declines with advancing age. *Journal of the American Geriatrics Society, 41*, 1–5.

Powers, D. C., & Belshe, R. B. (1993). Effect of age on cytotoxic T lymphocyte memory as well as serum and local antibody responses to inactivated influenza virus vaccine. *Journal of Infectious Diseases, 167*, 584–592.

Powers, D. C., Fries, L. F., Murphy, B. R., Thumar, B., & Clements, M. L. (1991). In elderly persons live attenuated influenza A virus vaccines do not offer an advantage over inactivated virus vaccine in inducing serum or secretory antibodies or local immunologic memory. *Journal of Clinical Microbiology, 29*, 498–505.

Powers, D. C., Murphy, B. R., Fries, L. F., Adler, W. H., & Clements, M. L. (1992). Reduced infectivity of cold-adapted influenza A H1N1 viruses in the elderly: Correlation with serum and local antibodies. *Journal of the American Geriatrics Society, 40*, 163–167.

Powers, D. C., Sears, S. D., Murphy, B. R., Thumar, B., & Clements, M. L. (1989). Systemic and local antibody responses in elderly subjects given live or inactivated influenza A virus vaccines. *Journal of Clinical Microbiology, 27*, 2666–2671.

Powers, D. C. (1994). Increased immunogenicity of inactivated influenza virus vaccine containing purified surface antigen compared to whole virus in elderly women. *Clinical and Diagnostic Laboratory Immunology, 1*, 16–20.

Ramphal, R., Cogliano, R. C., Shands, J. W., Jr., & Small, P. A., Jr. (1979). Serum antibody prevents lethal murine influenza pneumonitis but not tracheitis. *Infection and Immunity, 25*, 992–997.

Reiss, C. S., & Schulman, J. L. (1980). Cellular immune responses of mice to influenza virus infection. *Cellular Immunology, 56*, 502–509.

Renegar, K. B., & Small, P. A., Jr. (1991). Immunoglobulin A mediation of murine nasal anti-influenza virus immunity. *Journal of Virology, 65*, 2146–2148.

Schwab, R., Russo, C., & Weksler, M. E. (1990). Loss of MHC-restricted T cell recognition of influenza antigens in aging. *Aging: Immunology and Infectious Disease, 2*, 111–116.

Strassburg, M. A., Greenland, S., Sorvillo, F. J., Lieb, L. E., & Habel, L. A. (1986). Influenza in the elderly: Report of an outbreak and a review of vaccine effectiveness reports. *Vaccine, 4*, 38–44.

Taylor, P. M., & Askonas, B. A. (1986). Influenza nucleoprotein specific cytotoxic T cell clones are protective *in vivo*. *Immunology, 58*, 417–420.

Thoman, M. L., & Weigle, W. O. (1989). The cellular and subcellular bases of immunosenescence. *Advances in Immunology, 46*, 221–226.

Townsend, A. R. M., & McMichael, A. J. (1985). Specificity of cytotoxic T lymphocytes stimulated with influenza virus. Studies in mice and humans. *Progress in Allergy, 36*, 10–43.

Wagner, D. K., Clements, M. L., Reimer, C. R., Snyder, M., Nelson, D. L., & Murphy, B. R. (1987). Analysis of immunoglobulin G antibody responses after administration of live and inactivated influenza A vaccine indicates that nasal wash immunoglobulin G is a transudate from serum. *Journal of Clinical Microbiology, 25*, 559–562.

Wilson, I. A., & Cox, N. J. (1990). Structural basis of immune recognition of influenza virus hemagglutinin. *Annual Reviews of Immunology, 8,* 737–771.
Yap, K. L., Ada, G. L., & McKenzie, I. F. C. (1978). Transfer of specific cytotoxic T lymphocytes protects mice inoculated with influenza virus. *Nature, 273,* 238–239.
Yewdell, J. W., Bennink, J. R., Smith, G. L., & Moss, B. (1985). Influenza A virus nucleoprotein is a major target antigen for cross-reactive and anti-influenza A virus cytotoxic T lymphocytes. *Proceedings of the National Academy of Sciences of the United States of America, 82,* 1785–1789.

Influenza in Aged Mice

5

Bradley S. Bender

HOST DEFENSE AGAINST INFLUENZA

Influenza infection is a disease of both upper airways (ciliated epithelium), or rhinotracheitis, and lower airways (alveoli), or pneumonia. The major role of antibody is in the *prevention* of disease. Even though serum antibody (primarily antihemagglutinin but also antineuraminidase) has been known for decades to prevent viral pneumonia (Loosli, Hamre, & Berlin, 1953), it has only more recently been shown that passive administration of antiinfluenza serum to virgin mice prevents pneumonia but not rhinotracheitis (Ramphal, Cogliana, Shands, et al., 1979). Further, intravenously administered IgA against influenza has been shown to be specifically transported into the nasal secretions and protect the murine nasopharynx against influenza infection (Renegar & Small, 1991a, b).

The classic role for cellular immunity is in the *recovery* from disease (Lin & Askonas, 1981; Lukacher, Braciale, & Braciale, 1984; Wells, Ennis, & Albrecht, 1981; Yap, Ada, & McKenzie, 1978). This was best shown with nude (athymic) mice, which do not recover from an influenza infection unless their immunity is enhanced with the adoptive transfer of antiinfluenza CTLs (Wells et al., 1981). In contrast, administration of antiinfluenza antibody to nude mice will stop viral shedding only as long as antibody is present (Kris, Yetter, Cogliano, et al., 1988). In immunologically normal mice, serum IgG antibody speeds recovery of influenza infection but is not by it-self able to effect recovery (Kris, Asofsky, Evans, et al., 1985).

The belief that CTLs are the only method of recovery has been chal-lenged by more recent studies. Mice transgenic for β_2-microglobulin dele-tion (and therefore lacking CD8[+] CTLs) can recover from an influenza infection (Eichelberger, Allan, Zijlstra, et al., 1991) though at a substantially slower rate (Bender, Croghan, Zhang, et al., 1992). Further, severe com-bined immunodeficiency (SCID) mice infected with influenza and given a "cocktail" of IgA, IgG, and IgM can permanently clear the virus from their respiratory tract (Scherle, Palladino, & Gerhard, 1992). Mazanec, Kaetzel, Lamm, et al. (1992) showed in tissue culture that IgA can neutralize virus intracellularly. Hence, IgA could be an important backup host defense mechanism in clearing the respiratory tract of viruses.

Another important aspect of cellular immunity against influenza A is the concept of homotypic and heterotypic immunity. Even though serum antibodies are highly specific and show negligible cross reaction, there is significant cross-reaction of CTL activity between different serotypes of in-fluenza A (heterotypic immunity). The reason for this was shown in a se-ries of elegant experiments using recombinant DNA technology: heterotypic immunity is generated by CTLs that recognize other viral pro-teins, primarily nucleoprotein (NP) (Andrew, Coupar, Boyle, et al., 1987; Yewdell, Bennick, Smith, et al., 1985). In contrast, CTLs against different subtypes of hemagglutinin or neuraminidase do not cross-react.

Heterotypic immunity is extremely important for host defense when an antigenic shift occurs, as these individuals will have no antibody protec-tion. Yetter, Lehrer, Ramphal, et al. (1980) demonstrated in mice that heter-otypic immunity also serves an important protective role. Following influenza infection of the nose of virgin mice, the virus spreads to the tra-chea in 3 days and to the lung in 5 days. The heterotypic immunity of mice previously infected with a different influenza A serotype, however, was capable of preventing the spread of influenza from the nose to the lung, that is, it prevented viral pneumonia (Yetter et al., 1980).

HOST DEFENSE IN AGING

There is abundant clinical evidence that elderly persons have impaired im-mune responsiveness, impaired delayed-type hypersensitivity reactions, increased incidence of certain tumors, and increased frequency and severi-ty of many infections (Adler & Nagel, 1985; Gottesman, 1987; Yoshikawa & Norman, 1987). More recently, we have begun to understand the biologic basis for these observations. The primary defect lies in the T lymphocyte, related to the marked thymic atrophy postmaturity. Aged mice have been shown to have impaired mixed lymphocyte reactions, decline in cytotoxic activity against allogeneic stimulators, reduced proliferative responses, and lower IL-2 production (Adler & Nagel, 1985; Goidl, 1987; Gottesman, 1987). Impaired antibody responses exist, but this is most likely because of a defect in collaborative T-cell help (Bender, 1985).

Influenza has a significant impact on the health of the elderly; influenza and pneumonia are the fourth leading cause of death of persons older than age 65 in the United States (Brody & Brock, 1985). We believe that much of this increased severity is attributable to the decline in cell-mediated immunity in aging (Adler & Nagel, 1985; Goidl, 1987; Gottesman, 1987; Yoshikawa & Norman, 1987).

Homotypic Immunity

Based on previously published data on the decline in antiinfluenza cellular immunity in aging (Effros & Walford, 1983a, 1983b) and the role of CTL in the recovery from influenza infection (Lin & Askonas, 1981; Lukacher et al., 1984; Wells et al., 1981; Yap et al., 1978), we hypothesized that, following infection with influenza, aged mice would have significant impairment in the generation of CTL activity and that this would correlate with persistent viral shedding from their lungs (Bender, Johnson, & Small, 1991). To test this, young and aged mice were anesthetized and infected intranasally with H3N2 influenza virus, thus infecting the total respiratory tract. Mice were sacrificed and assayed for viral shedding from their lungs, splenic CTL activity, and serum IgG anti-H3 antibody titers.

As shown in Table 5.1, young mice responded in a homogeneous fashion. They developed maximal splenic CTL activity of $61 \pm 2\%$ by days 11 to 13, and all except one mouse cleared virus from the lung by day 7. The aged mice were relatively heterogeneous in their response. The splenic CTL activity of old mice peaked at $47 \pm 5\%$ and lagged 5 to 7 days behind the young mice. Of the aged mice, 42% were still shedding virus at days 7 and 8, and shedding persisted for up to 13 days in some mice. There was a strong correlation in both young and aged mice between the presence of virus in the lungs and decreased splenic CTL activity ($\chi^2 = 7.92, p < .005$). Aged mice also had lower pulmonary CTL activity. No significant differences were found in serum anti-H3 antibody.

Heterotypic Immunity

The preceding studies were done with virgin mice. In the real world, however, essentially all elders have been previously infected with influenza in childhood. Because influenza A viruses go through periodic antigenic shifts, the influenza virus a person is infected with when old has different surface antigens than that he was infected with when young. Bender, Tall-

TABLE 5.1 Results of Influenza A/Port Chalmers/1/73 (H3N2) Infection in Virgin Young and Aged BALB/c Mice

	Days Following Infection			
	3-5	7-9	11-13	19
Secondary Splenic CTL Activity[1]				
Young	2 ± 1[2]	33 ± 2	56 ± 3	61 ± 1
Aged	0 ± 0	14 ± 4	20 ± 5	47 ± 2
Pulmonary Viral Shedding[3]				
Young	2.1 ± 0.6 (4/4)[4]	-0.7 ± 0.3 (1/12)	-1 ± 0 (0/17)	-1 ± 0 (0/5)
Aged	2.5 ± 0.5 (4/4)	1.2 ± 0.4 (5/12)	-0.5 ± 0.2 (5/16)	-1 ± 0 (0/5)
Serum Anti-H3 Titer[5]				
Young	4 ± 0	14 ± 5	13 ± 14	ND[6]
Aged	2 ± 0	31 ± 12	25 ± 6	ND
Primary Pulmonary CTL Activity[1]				
Young	26 ± 3	10 ± 1	ND	ND
Aged	18 ± 5	4 ± 2	ND	ND

[1]%^{51}Cr release at effector:target ratio of 10:1
[2]Mean ± SE
[3]Log$_{10}$ of 50% egg infectious doses
[4]Numbers in parentheses are numbers of mice shedding virus/total numbers of mice tested
[5]ELISA titer expressed as a percentage of high titer sera from animals convalescent from influenza
[6]ND = Not determined

man and Small (1990b) and Effros and Walford (1983a) have shown that there is decreased in vitro heterotypic CTL activity in aged mice. The question was whether the decreased heterotypic CTL activity of aged mice would correlate with the spread of a different influenza serotype from the nose to the lungs. Young and aged mice previously infected with H3N2 were given H1N1 intranasally while awake. As discussed previously, this limits the initial infection to the nose (Yetter et al., 1980).

The data in Table 5.2 show several interesting findings. First, young mice cleared virus more rapidly than aged mice (compare day 9 of group 1 vs. group 2). Second, young and aged virgin mice could not prevent the spread of virus from the nose to the lung, i.e., they were susceptible to viral pneumonia. The virus also spread more rapidly to the lungs of the older mice (day 5). Third, heterotypic immune young mice were almost completely protected from viral pneumonia and recovered very quickly (group 3 vs. group 1). Fourth, heterotypic immunity in aged mice provided incomplete protection against viral pneumonia: on days 5 to 9, only 1 out of 15 mice in group 3 had virus detected in their lungs versus 7 out of 17 mice in group 4 ($p < .05$). These mice also had prolonged respiratory tract infection (1 of 15 vs. 10 of 17 noses infected on days 5 to 9 ($p < .01$). However, heterotypic immunity in old mice does hasten recovery compared with virgin old mice (compare group 4 vs. group 2). The mouse in group 4 still shedding virus from its lungs on day 9 had CTL activity of 28% compared with 58% to 67% for the other mice in group 4. Thus, compared with heterotypic immune young mice, heterotypic immune aged mice had an increased propensity to develop viral pneumonia, and this increased severity of disease correlated with decreased antiinfluenza CTL activity.

The data from the preceding studies on homotypic and heterotypic immunity are quite consistent with clinical observations on influenza. Elderly persons have more severe illness (chiefly, pulmonary involvement) following an influenza infection. Fry (1959) reported on the frequency of respiratory involvement in 849 patients with clinically diagnosed influenza who were seen in a general medical practice. The rate of pulmonary complications (lobar pneumonia, segmental pneumonia, and acute bronchitis) varied from a low of 4% in patients aged 10 to 39 years to 73% in persons older than 70. Similarly, Bennett (1973) studied 333 patients who were hospitalized with culture-proven influenza. He found 6% of patients aged 20 to 49 had pneumonia compared with 51% of persons aged 60 to 80 years. Moreover, influenza has a longer duration of illness in the elderly (Mathur, Bentley, Hall, et al., 1981). Wyde, Six, Ambrose, et al. (1989) have also shown that following dual influenza and bacterial infection, aged mice also have a delay in bacterial clearance.

TABLE 5.2   Viral Shedding From the Nose and Lungs of Heterotypic Immune Young and Aged BALB/c Mice

Day Following Infection

GROUP	1			3		5		7		9			15		
	N^1	L	CTL	N	L	N	L	N	L	N	L	CTL	N	L	CTL
1. Virgin young	$3/4^2$	0/5	0±0	5/5	1/5	5/5	1/5	4/5	3/5	1/5	0/5	46±5	0/5	0/5	61±1
2. Virgin old	5/5	1/5	0±0	5/6	2/6	6/6	3/6	6/6	5/6	5/6	3/6	17±6	0/5	0/5	38±8
3. Heterotypic young	4/5	0/5	61±1	2/4	0/4	0/5	1/5	1/4	0/5	0/5	0/5	69±1	0/5	0/5	66±2
4. Heterotypic old	4/5	0/5	27±10	6/6	1/4	5/6	4/6	3/5	1/5	2/6	1/6	56±6	0/5	0/5	33±5

¹N=nose, L=lung, CTL=splenic CTL activity (mean ± SE)
²Number infected/Total

Vaccines and Aging

We hypothesized that following influenza vaccination, aged mice would have decreased antiinfluenza CTL activity compared with young mice. To test this hypothesis, separate groups of mice were given either an intraperitoneal injection of an inactivated H1N1 vaccine or intradermal scarification with recombinant vaccinia viruses that expressed either H1 hemagglutinin or nucleoprotein (Flexner, Hügin, & Moss, 1987). As positive controls, mice were infected intranasally with H1N1. The animals were sacrificed 8 weeks later, and splenic CTL activity and serum antibody measured. We found that CTL activity was significantly lower in the aged animals for all three vaccines. There was a trend to lower antiinfluenza antibody titers in the older animals, but this was not statistically significant (Bender, Johnson, Flexner, et al., 1990a).

Mitogen-stimulated peripheral blood lymphocytes from aged humans and mice produce less IL-2 than cells from young donors, and the addition of IL-2 can improve the cellular immune function of mice (Thoman & Weigle, 1985). We therefore tested our "Ponce de Leon" hypothesis, which is whether vaccination with a double recombinant that expressed both viral proteins, and IL-2 could rejuvenate either CTL or serum IgG antiinfluenza response. Again we found that CTL activity was lower in aged animals than in young animals and that there were no differences in serum IgG antibody between young and aged mice. Further, no significant augmentation was seen in either mean CTL activity or antibody response in the mice that received the IL-2–expressing recombinant vaccine (Bender, Croghan, Zhang, & Small, 1992; Bender, Johnson, Flexner, Moss, & Small, 1990).

Though there was no demonstrable increase in either CTL activity or antibody response in the mice that received the IL-2–containing recombinant vaccines, this does not rule out decreased IL-2 production as a significant cause of immunodeficiency in aging animals, as an alternative method of delivering IL-2 may be more effective. For example, Mbawuike, Wyde, & Anderson (1990) studied the effect of administering IL-2 in liposomes. They found that the IL-2 liposomes significantly enhanced serum neutralizing antibody titers in influenza-vaccinated young and aged mice. Further, this increased response correlated with improved protection from live virus challenge. No effect of the IL-2 liposomes was seen on splenic antiinfluenza CTL activity.

In summary, our data show that aged mice have lower pulmonary and splenic CTL activity than young mice, and this correlates with prolonged and more severe disease. We postulate that a primary reason for the increased mortality owing to influenza in the elderly is their lower antiinfluenza CTL activity (Powers, 1993).

REFERENCES

Adler, W. H., & Nagel, J. E. (1985). Clinical immunology. In R. Andres, E. L. Bierman, & W. H. Hazzard (Eds.), *Principles of geriatric medicine and gerontology* (pp. 413–423). New York: McGraw-Hill.

Andrew, M. E., Coupar, B. E. H., Boyle, D. B., & Ada, G. L. (1987). The roles of influenza virus hemagglutinin and nucleoprotein in protection: Analysis using vaccinia virus recombinants. *Scandinavian Journal of Immunology, 25,* 21–28.

Bender, B. S. (1985). B lymphocyte function in aging. In M. Rothstein (Ed.), *Review of biological research in aging* (Vol. 2, pp. 143–154). New York: Alan R. Liss.

Bender, B. S., Croghan, T., Zhang, L., & Small, P. A., Jr. (1992). Transgenic mice lacking class I major histocompatibility complex-restricted T-cells have delayed viral clearance and increased mortality after influenza virus challenge. *Journal of Experimental Medicine, 175,* 1143–1145.

Bender, B. S., Johnson, M. P., Flexner, C., Moss, B., & Small, P. A., Jr. (1990). Cytotoxic-T-lymphocyte activity induced by influenza vaccination in young and aged mice. In F. Brown, R. M. Chanock, H. S. Ginsberg, & R. A. Lerner (Eds.), *Modern approaches to new vaccines including prevention of AIDS* (pp. 69–73). Cold Spring Harbor: Cold Spring Harbor Laboratory Press.

Bender, B. S., Johnson, M. P., & Small, P. A. (1991). Influenza in senescent mice: Impaired cytotoxic T-lymphocyte activity is correlated with prolonged infection. *Immunology, 72,* 514–519.

Bender, B. S., Tallman, E., & Small, P. A., Jr. (1990). Influenza pneumonia and splenic cytotoxic T-lymphocyte activity in aged and young heterotypic immune mice following challenge with a different influenza A serotype. *Clinical Research, 38,* 394A.

Bennett, N. M. (1973). Diagnosis of influenza. *Medical Journal of Australia, 1* (Special Suppl.), 19–22.

Brody, J. A., & Brock, D. B. (1985). Epidemiologic and statistical characteristics of this United States elderly population. In C. E. Finch & E. L. Schneider (Eds.), *Handbook of the biology of aging* (2nd ed., pp. 3–26). New York: Van Nostrand Reinhold.

Effros, R. B., & Walford, R. L. (1983a). Diminished T-cell response to influenza virus in aged mice. *Immunology, 49,* 387–392.

Effros, R. B., & Walford, R. L. (1983b). The immune response of aged mice to influenza: Diminished T-cell proliferation, interleukin-2 production and cytotoxicity. *Cellular Immunology, 81,* 298–305.

Eichelberger, M., Allan, W., Zijlstra, M., Jaenisch, R., & Doherty, P. C. (1991). Clearance of influenza virus respiratory infection in mice lacking class I major histocompatibility complex-restricted CD8$^+$ T cells. *Journal of Experimental Medicine, 174,* 875–880.

Flexner, C., Hügin, A., & Moss, B. (1987). Prevention of vaccinia virus infection in immunodeficient mice by vector-directed IL-2 expression. *Nature, 330,* 259–262.

Fry, J. (1959). Influenza, 1959: The story of an epidemic. *British Medical Journal, 2,* 135–138.

Goidl, E. A. (1987). *Aging and the immune response*. New York: Marcel Dekker.

Gottesman, S. R. S. (1987). Changes in T-cell-mediated immunity with age: An update. In M. Rothstein (Ed.), *Review of biological research in aging* (Vol. 3, pp. 95–127). Alan R. Liss.

Kris, R. M., Asofsky, R., Evans, C. B., & Small, P. A., Jr. (1985). Protection and recovery in influenza virus infected mice immunosuppressed with anti-IgM. *Journal of Immunology, 134*, 1230–1235.

Kris, R. M., Yetter, R. A., Cogliano, R., Ramphal, R., & Small, P. A., Jr. (1988). Influenza virus infection: Serum antibody causes temporary recovery of the upper respiratory tract and lung of nude mice. *Immunology, 63*, 349–353.

Lin, Y., & Askonas, B. A. (1981). Biological properties of an influenza A virus-specific killer T cell clone. *Journal of Experimental Medicine, 154*, 225.

Loosli, C. G., Hamre, D., Berlin, B. S. (1953). Airborne influenza virus A infections in immunized animals. *Transactions of the Association of American Physiology, 66*, 222–230.

Lukacher, A. E., Braciale, V. L., & Braciale, T. J. (1984). In vivo effector function of influenza virus–specific cytotoxic T-lymphocyte clones is highly specific. *Journal of Experimental Medicine, 160*, 814–826.

Mathur, U., Bentley, D. W., Hall, C. B., Roth, F. K., & Douglas, R. G., Jr. (1981). Influenza A/Brazil/78 (H1N1) infection in the elderly. *American Review of Respiratory Diseases, 123*, 633–635.

Mazanec, M. B., Kaetzel, C. S., Lamm, M. E., Fletcher, D., & Nedrud, J. G. (1992). Intracellular neutralization of virus by immunoglobulin A antibodies. *Proceedings National Academy of Sciences, 89*, 6901–6905.

Mbawuike, I. N., Wyde, P. R., & Anderson, P. M. (1990). Enhancement of the protective efficacy of inactivated influenza A virus vaccine in aged mice by IL-2 liposomes. *Vaccine, 8*, 347–352.

Powers, D. C. (1993). Immunity to influenza in the elderly. In D. C. Powers, J. E. Morley & R. M. Coe (Eds.), *Aging, immunity, and infection*. New York: Springer.

Ramphal, R., Cogliano, R. C., Shands, J. W., Jr., & Small, P. A., Jr. (1979). Serum antibody prevents murine influenza pneumonia but not influenza tracheitis. *Infection & Immunology, 25*, 992–997.

Renegar, K. B., & Small, P. A., Jr. (1991a). Immunoglobulin A mediation of murine nasal anti-influenza virus immunity. *Journal of Virology, 65*, 2146–2148.

Reneger, K. B., & Small, P. A., Jr. (1991b). Passive transfer of local immunity to influenza virus infection by IgA antibody. *Journal of Immunology, 146*, 1972–1978.

Scherle, P. A., Palladino, G., & Gerhard, W. (1992). Mice can recover from pulmonary influenza virus infection in the absence of class I-restricted cytotoxic T cells. *Journal of Immunology, 148*, 212–217.

Thoman, M. L., & Weigle, W. O. (1985). Reconstitution of in vivo cell-mediated lympholysis responses in aged mice with interleukin 2. *Journal of Immunology, 134*, 949–952.

Wells, M. A., Ennis, F. A., & Albrecht, P. (1981). Recovery from a viral respiratory infection: II. Passive transfer of immune spleen cells to mice with influenza pneumonia. *Journal of Immunology, 126*, 1042–1046.

Wyde, P. R., Six, H. R., Ambrose, M. W., & Throop, B. J. (1989). Influenza virus infection and bacterial clearance in young adult and aged mice. *Journal of Gerontology, 44*, B118–124.

Yap, K. C., Ada, G. L., & McKenzie, I. F. C. (1978). Transfer of specific cytotoxic T-lymphocytes protects mice inoculated with influenza virus. *Nature, 273*, 238–239.

Yetter, R. A., Lehrer, S., Ramphal, R., & Small, P. A., Jr. (1980). Outcome of influenza infection: Effect of site of initial infection and heterotypic immunity. *Infection & Immunology, 29*, 654–662.

Yewdell, J. W., Bennick, J. R., Smith, G. L., & Moss, B. (1985). Influenza A virus nucleoprotein is a major target antigen of cross-reactive anti-influenza A virus cytotoxic T-lymphocytes. *Proceedings of the National Academy of Science, 82*, 1785–1789.

Yoshikawa, T. T. (1987). Epidemiology of infectious diseases in the geriatric population. In T. T. Yoshikawa & D. C. Norman (Eds.), *Aging and clinical practice. Infectious diseases* (pp. 3–7). New York: Igaku-Shoin Medical Publishers, Inc.

Immune Deficiency 6
of Aging

William H. Adler, Lijun Song,
Rajesh K. Chopra, Richard A. Winchurch,
Kimberly S. Waggie, and James E. Nagel

The relationship between immune function and aging can be pursued both in experimental animal models and in human populations. However, a problem in comparing results from humans with those obtained from animal models is that in animal studies the primary cellular populations used for the assays are spleen or lymph node lymphocytes, whereas human studies almost universally use peripheral blood lymphocytes (PBL) as their course of experimental material. The differences between peripheral blood and splenic white cell function appear most commonly when agents or conditions are used that cause a sequestration of circulating white cells. Splenic and lymph node populations also contain a much higher percentage of accessory and B cells than are found in peripheral blood.

Because concurrent illness can affect the results of many immune function assays, the selection of study subjects is another important consideration. As with many age-related physiologic changes, it is difficult to establish that diminished immune function is not the result of medical conditions that often accompany aging. The human populations that have been used to study immune function and aging range between rigorously screened superhealthy individuals through nursing home populations to uncategorized outpatients.

In terms of study design, longitudinal studies have advantages over cross-sectional studies, but they also have disadvantages. Because many tests of immune function rely on biologic reagents, it is difficult to precisely repeat the same assay over a long time. Also, because the field of immunology is progressing at an exponential rate, there are constantly new reagents and assay systems being developed that give better and more precise information. Cross-sectional studies have their difficulties because the old and young populations may differ in their genetic or gender representations (such as using young male students and comparing them with elderly nursing home residents who are generally predominantly female). It is also sometimes difficult to demarcate the young from the old because various assays show age-related changes at different times during the lifespan.

A good example of this sort of difficulty can be seen with the data on NK cell function. A comparison of young and old men in the levels of NK activity of their peripheral blood lymphocytes shows no appreciable difference. However, middle-aged individuals show a lower degree of NK activity than seen in either the young or the old. Therefore, a comparison of NK activity between the young and middle-aged cohorts would show a decline, whereas a comparison of middle age to old would show an increase in NK function (Nagel, Collins, & Adler, 1981). Further, examination of NK activity throughout the age spectrum suggests that higher NK function provides a survival benefit leading to the elimination of middle-aged individuals who have low NK activity and yielding a group of survivors who have higher NK activity. Therefore in examining age and immune function, the results of many studies may not agree.

The results reported here consist of work from both human studies and murine models. Most of the data on humans is from studies of volunteers participating in the Baltimore Longitudinal Study of Aging (BLSA). These individuals are a well-characterized group of healthy ambulatory men and women from approximately ages 20 to 95 years. They visit the Gerontology Research Center (GRC) for 3 days every 2 years where they receive a complete physical, history, and a variety of physiologic and psychological tests. We have excluded individuals taking medications that could influence lymphocyte function from the data (although they are not excluded from the BLSA). In some cases additional information was obtained from nursing home residents who had various debilitating illnesses or conditions. This group contributed the data on the levels of inflammatory factors in ill elderly individuals. The mouse model consisted of C57BL/6J male mice obtained from Jackson Laboratories at 6 weeks of age and kept in the GRC aging animal colony.

MORBIDITY AND MORTALITY
ASSOCIATED WITH INFECTIOUS DISEASES
IN THE ELDERLY

In general, for both bacterial and viral infectious illnesses there is an age-related increase in both morbidity and mortality. This can be seen in the studies of Finland and Barnes (1977) at Boston City Hospital investigating people with bacterial meningitis in two periods: one before the availability of antibiotics and the other after widespread antibiotic use. These authors showed that from the teenage years on, in the group treated with antibiotics there was an increase in mortality. There was almost a 3-fold increase in mortality comparing the teenage group to individuals in the fourth decade of life. Mortality was the highest (about 80%) in persons older than 60 years of age and differed little from that seen in individuals who did not receive antibiotic therapy. Therefore, with age there is an increase in mortality, and the older age groups respond poorly to antibiotic therapy. Influenza infections display a similar pattern. Although patients with influenza who are under 5 years of age or older than age 70 have almost identical hospitalization rates, individuals older than 70 years of age have a 35-fold increase in mortality compared with children (Couch, Kasel, Glezen, et al., 1986). These studies show that even with appropriate hospital care influenza is a much more serious illness in the elderly. HIV infection also has an age-related pattern in its rate of progression. HIV infected patients older than age 40 years progress from a symptom-free period to AIDS in a much shorter time. During an 8-year follow-up after infection with HIV, the percentage of individuals older than age 35 who develop AIDS is more than 3 times that of infected teenagers (Goedert, Kessler, Aledort, et al., 1989). Related to the increase in infectious disease problems in the elderly is a decline in their ability to respond to immunization. One study involving armed forces officers showed that the antibody response to hepatitis B vaccine in 30-year-olds was about half of the level seen in 20-year-olds (D'Amelio, Matricardi, Nisini, et al., 1989). A Polish study of tetanus immunity showed a lessening of protective levels in individuals older than age 40 (Galazka & Kardymowicz, 1989). Further, it was shown that young women make more antibody than young men, but this was reversed in the older age group. We have found in the BLSA population that older men have higher levels of antitetanus antibodies. This may relate to gender-associated changes in circulating memory cells where older women have fewer memory T cells than older men and conversely greater numbers of naive T cells. Gender differences and the effects of sex hormones on immune function are also important considerations in the description of age-related changes in immune activity (Schuurs & Verheul, 1990).

GENETIC INFLUENCES ON IMMUNE FUNCTION

There are at least two studies that dramatically demonstrate the influence of genetics on host resistance to disease. One study of 2,000 adopted children compared their cause of death with that of their biologic or adoptive parents and found that if a biologic parent had died from an infection there was a fivefold to sixfold increase in the risk of the biologic child also dying from an infection. There was no such increase in risk associated with the parent and adopted child relationship (Sørensen, Nielsen, Andersen, et al., 1988). In a strain of mouse in which there is an identified segregation of a gene that controls immune function, the mice carrying the immune response gene make normal levels of antibody when challenged with an antigen, whereas the deficient mice make very little antibody. By selective breeding it is possible to form F1, F2, backcross high, and backcross low responder individuals, each of which have their own level of antibody synthesis ranging between the upper and lower limits of the high and low responders. The life-span of the animals is directly related to their ability to make antibody with the high responders living the longest. The usual cause of death in this strain of mouse is an infectious disease or cancer so it is not surprising that the ability to respond to an antigen would be linked to survival (Covelli, Mouton, Di Majo, et al., 1989). From these data on infectious diseases and genetic influences on immune function, it is possible to hypothesize that the immune deficiency of aging is an important factor in the ability of the older host to interact favorably with the environment. It is important then to determine the scope of this immune deficiency, and the possible ways to maintain immune function or restore that function in the elderly individual.

T-CELL FUNCTION IN THE AGING HOST

It is well established that the main component of the immune system responsible for the immune dysfunction of aging is the T-cell system. Because T-cell activation is intimately involved in maintaining immunocompetence, a disparate variety of clinical findings result from impairment of different components in the T-cell activation pathway (Arnaiz-Villena, Timón, Rodríguez-Gallego, et al., 1992). The concept that the T-cell system is defective in aging could probably be predicted by what has been known for several decades concerning the age-related involution of the thymus and the crucial role the thymus plays in the generation of immunocompetent T lymphocytes. The role of the human thymus was initially demonstrated by the study of children born without this gland. These children had a lymphopenia together with a lack of cell-mediated immunity and an inability to make antibody. Subsequent experiments showed that trafficking of immature lymphocytes through the thymus results in their differentiation into immunocompetent T cells.

The proliferative ability of a T-cell population declines with age because of the increasing presence of nonfunctional cells in that population (Nagel, Chopra, Powers, et al., 1989). The decline in DNA synthesis (proliferative ability), shown in Table 6.1, is associated with a decrement in IL-2 production and IL-2 receptor expression, but only when certain triggering agents such as phytohemagglutin (PHA) are used to stimulate the cells (Nagel, Chopra, Chrest, et al., 1988). Although these studies did not differentiate between the possible causes for the lack of function, they did suggest that perhaps the genes responsible for promoting a proliferative response were defective in their expression. However, further studies have shown that this is not the case (also shown in Table 6.1). Using a different stimulus of phorbal myristate acetate (PMA) in the presence of a calcium ionophore, it is possible to induce levels of proliferation, IL-2 synthesis, IL-2R expression, and mRNA levels for IL-2 and IL-2–receptor (IL-2R) for cells from elderly donors that are no different from the levels seen when using cells from young donors (Chopra, Holbrook, Powers, et al., 1989).

The most frequently used assay of T-cell function involves the in vitro addition of a stimulatory substance (mitogen) to the T cells to induce them to proliferate. This proliferative response is dependent on many factors including the expression of a membrane receptor for the stimulant, the transduction of the membrane signal to the cytoplasm and nucleus, the expression of genes responsible for the elaboration of growth factors and their receptors, the expression of genes responsible for the progression of the cell through the cell cycle, and the general ability of the cells to survive in culture. An alteration in only one component usually results in either a lack of or a decrease in proliferation. Direct protein kinase C (PKC) activation through PMA, increasing intracellular calcium via ionophores such as ionomycin or A23187, or direct G-protein activation produce the same levels of proliferation, IL-2 synthesis, and IL-2R expression in cells from young and old (Chopra et al., 1989). By using a stimulant that avoids the activation of a membrane component and the cytoplasmic transduction pathway, it is possible to activate T cells from the elderly to a level seen among the young. It now appears that the defect in T-cell function responsible for the decline in proliferative ability seen with aging resides in the cell membrane and the activation pathways that transduce membrane signals into nuclear events.

To examine this hypothesis further, the effects of two different but closely related activation agents were compared. Using monoclonal antibodies with cell membrane receptors, it is possible to examine the integrity of two activation pathways. The two antibodies are anti-CD3, which has a speci-

TABLE 6.1   Effect of Different Stimulants on Peripheral Blood Lymphocytes

PHA Stimulation of Peripheral Blood Lymphocytes

	Young	Old	p
Age	28.7	74.4	
IL-2 mRNA	1852	685	< .01
IL-2R mRNA	4860	3002	< .01
%IL-2R+ cells	73	50.6	< .001
IL-2 produced (units/ml.)	14.9	8.3	< .05
[^{3}H] thymidine incorporation (cpm)	136,000	72,450	< .001

PMA + A23187 Stimulation of Peripheral Blood Lymphocytes

	Young	Old	p
Age	30.6	72.5	
IL-2 mRNA	8.75	10.6	NS
IL-2R mRNA	1.9	1.7	NS
%IL-2R+ cells	79.7	75.7	NS
IL-2 produced (units/ml.)	2333	1914	NS
[^{3}H] thymidine incorporation (cpm)	158,722	127,389	NS

ficity against the T-cell antigen receptor complex, and anti-CD2, which has a specificity to the sheep red blood cell (SRBC) receptor on the T-cell membrane. These two receptors are closely associated on the cell membrane and participate in the response of T cells to an antigenic signal. Using an anti-CD3 antibody as the activation agent and T cells from the elderly humans, it could be seen that the cells from the elderly donors proliferate less well and secrete less IL-2 than do the cells from young donors (see Table 6.2). However, using the anti-CD2 antibody as the activation agent resulted in no age-related deficit in proliferative ability. IL–2 production was minimal in cultures of cells from either young or old donors stimulated with the anti-CD2 antibody (Song, Nagel, Chrest, et al., 1992). Therefore, a membrane activation signal that does not result in IL-2 production is able to induce the same proliferative ability in cells from young and old donors. These results continue to suggest that a major defect in the cells from the elderly may reside in the activation pathway specific for the promotion of the IL-2 gene. However, this does not explain many of the other features of the immune response in the elderly.

INFLAMMATORY FACTORS AND AGING

Although much has been made of the lack of IL-2 production, proliferative ability, and antibody production in the aging individual, there are other changes occurring that are not associated with an age-related lack or decrement of function. Factors are released in the body that are associated with the inflammatory response and in many cases the levels of these factors, either in a steady state or after an activation event, are found to be elevated in older animals and humans. The first report of this finding concerned the factor gamma interferon (IFN-γ) which was found to be secreted by concanavalin A (Con A)–stimulated spleen cells from two different strains of 24-month-old mice at levels 4 to 10 times greater than that seen using spleen cells from young mice (see Figure 6.1) (Heine & Adler, 1977). This finding was reported in various experimental models, and in one model it was strongly suggested that the cells from the old mice were not able to respond to some of the effects of the IFN-γ. In those studies, the cells from the old mice were able after in vitro Con A stimulation to lyse tumor cell targets at levels 3 to 4 times those seen when using the cells from young mice (Saxena, Saxena, & Adler, 1988). The cytolytic activity of cells from the young mice could be augmented by adding an anti–IFN-γ antibody to the reaction culture. In contrast, the cells from the old mice showed no effect of the antibody although the cultures of these cells contained large amounts of IFN-γ.

Other factors that have been found to be elevated in older persons or in culture supernatants of cells from old donors are transforming growth factor (TGF)-β and IL-6 (see Figures 6.2 and 6.3). Serum levels of tumor necrosis factor (TNF)-α were found to be markedly elevated in debilitated nursing home patients (see Figure 6.4). This finding did not depend on the diagnosis of the patient but was related to the presence of decubiti. The patients were also thin and cachectic. Elevated TNF-α levels are found in endotoxin treated animals and have been associated with the presence of

TABLE 6.2 T-Cell Response to Anti-CD3 and Anti-CD2 Stimulation

	anti-CD2			anti-CD3		
	Young	Old	p	Young	Old	p
[³H] thymidine incorporation (cpm)	69,000	62,000	NS	97,000	68,000	<.05
IL-2R mRNA	.278	.240	NS	.685	.264	<.05
IL-2 produced (units/fnl.)	282	203	NS	1779	258	<.05

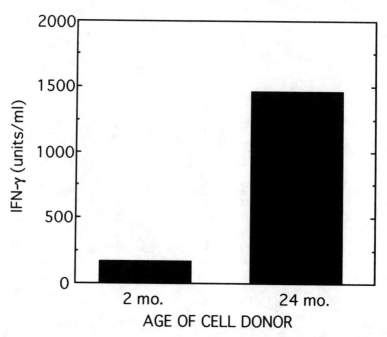

FIGURE 6.1   IFN-γ production by concanavalin A–activated mouse spleen cells.

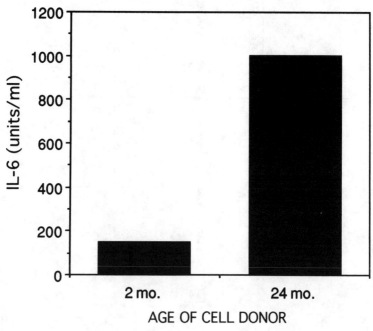

FIGURE 6.2   IL-6 production by lipopolysaccharide (LPS)-activated mouse spleen cells.

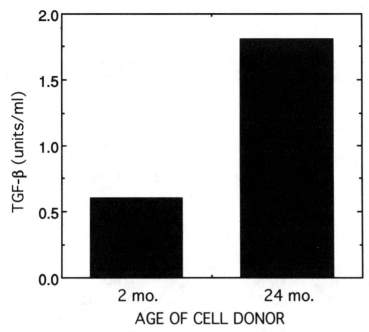

FIGURE 6.3   TGF-β production by LPS-activated mouse spleen cells.

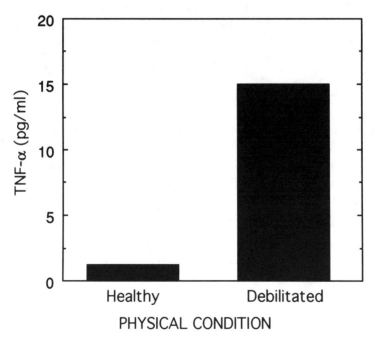

FIGURE 6.4   Serum levels of TNF-α in elderly patients.

endotoxin-induced shock. Treatment protocols that remove TNF-α from the circulation have been reported to decrease mortality because of endo-toxemia. These protocols depend on the use of anti–TNF-α antibody or sol-uble forms of the TNF-α receptor. Both TGF-β and IL-6 are also sensitive to endotoxin-driven release. TGF-β levels in spleen cell cultures increase with the age of the cell donor in both unstimulated and stimulated cultures (Zhou, Chrest, Adler, et al., 1992a). IL-6 levels in endotoxin-stimulated spleen cell cultures also increase with age but only in stimulated cultures. There are two interesting features of the IL-6 and TGF-β elevations. TGF-β, when added to spleen cell cultures from young mice, is able to inhibit markedly the induced proliferation of the cells in culture (see Figure 6.5). Antibody to TGF-β when added to cell cultures from old mice is able to augment the level of proliferation (see Figure 6.6) (Zhou, Chrest, Adler, et al., 1992b). In humans who have sustained major thermal burns, the serum level of IL-6 is inversely related to the number or percentage of circulating T cells (Guo, Dickerson, Chrest, et al., 1990). The higher the IL-6 level the fewer the circulating T cells (a somewhat paradoxic finding considering the recognized effects of IL-6 on pluripotential hematopoietic precursor cells). All of these factors have an ability to modulate the immune re-sponse, are elevated in the elderly, and can be immunosuppressive (see Table 6.3). This is another example of an imbalance in the host defense-im-mune system that is occurring with age in which some factors such as IL-2 are expressed at a lower level and others are at higher levels. Aging does not simply cause a decline in function; it causes changes that disrupt the balance.

NONIMMUNE HOST DEFENSE FUNCTIONS

NK cell function shows an interesting age related pattern of activity. This pattern suggests that high NK activity may be associated with a survival benefit. However, there are other factors that can influence NK function. Cigarette smoking, alcohol ingestion, amyl nitrite and cocaine use, and stress have all been linked to changes in NK activity. Gender also in-fluences NK activity in young people. In the young, women have lower pe-ripheral blood NK activity than do men (Bender, Chrest, & Adler, 1986). In older persons the levels of NK activity are about the same for both men and women. Therefore in an aging study there could be differences in NK activ-ity reported depending on the proportion of men and women in the young age group. In general, women show an increase in NK activity with age while men show either a slight decline or no change with age. In the popu-lation older than age 70 there seems to be an increase in NK activity that

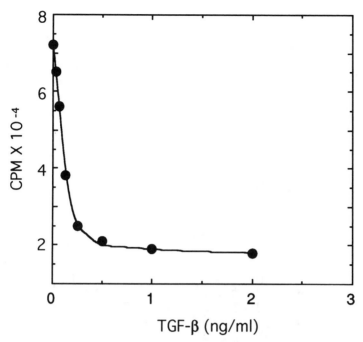

FIGURE 6.5   Effect of the addition of TGF-β on thymidine incorporation by mouse spleen cells.

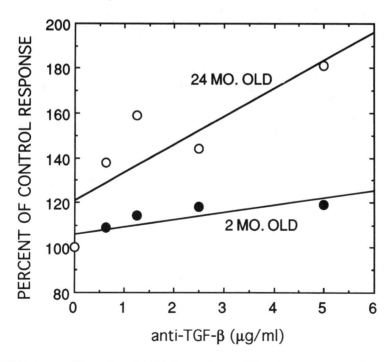

FIGURE 6.6   Effect of anti–TGF-β on the proliferative response of mouse spleen cells.

TABLE 6.3 Changes in Factor Release and Receptor Expression in Aging.

Factor	Change	Receptor	Comment
IL-2	Decrease	Decrease	Dependent on activation signal. While IL-2 added *in vitro* can augment function, it cannot completely restore levels of function to those found using cells from the young.
IL-6	Increase	?	May signal an abnormal response to inflammation
IFN-γ	Increase	Decrease	Cells from old mice appear non-responsive
TNF	Increase	?	Related to debilitation
TGF-β	Increase	?	Can inhibit proliferative responses *in vitro*

TABLE 6.4   Characteristics of Immune Function in Aging.

•Thymic involution
•Decreased antibody synthesis
•Loss of T cell function
•Increase in the appearance of auto-antibody
•Changes in lymphocyte subpopulation representations (naive and memory)
•Decreased IL-2 and IL-2R synthesis
•Increased synthesis of some inflammatory mediators
•Increased morbidity and mortality due to infectious diseases

---

may be due to a selection process if NK activity is linked to a survival benefit as has been reported.

The phagocytic ability of granulocytes has been reported to show an
age-related decline (Nagel, Han, Coon, et al., 1986). This finding does not
seem related to disease and affects the activity of about half of the circulating granulocytes in people older than the age of 70. The significance of this
finding is that while an older patient may have a normal white count, there
may be a functional granulocytopenia that can inhibit the host response to
an invading organism.

SUMMARY

There is ample clinical evidence that the elderly have more frequent episodes of infectious disease, and that the outcomes of these episodes are
more serious with a higher associated mortality. The basis for this problem
would seem to be a faltering immune system as well as a decline in nonimmune host defense mechanisms. The age-associated problem in immune
function seems to be a complex series of events that lead to an imbalance of
the various arms of the system listed in Table 6.4. The loss of T-cell function
and control mechanisms can be seen in the appearance of monoclonal immunoglobulin and autoantibody in the elderly. The loss of ability for T cells
to replenish themselves, or to undergo thymic-derived differentiation processes, leads eventually to a buildup of nonfunctional T cells in the older
person. This change is accompanied by the appearance of inappropriate
inflammatory responses and an increase in the levels of several important
cytokines. These factors can cause problems on their own with their ability
to influence metabolic and regulation pathways. A major consideration in
the evaluation of an elderly patient with an infection is that there may be
less time available to the clinician for the institution of appropriate effec-

tive therapy. The faltering host response allows fewer organisms to be able to establish an infection as well as to spread and multiply more easily in the first stages of an infection. Although the agents to replenish T cells, reconstitute immune function, or maintain immune function are not available, there is hope that management of the inflammatory factors, preventive immunizations, and appropriate antibiotic use can help to prevent illness and death in the elderly because of infectious disease.

REFERENCES

Arnaiz-Villena, A., Timón, M., Rodríguez-Gallego, C., Pérez-Blas, M., Corell, A., Maritín-Villa, J. M., & Regueiro, J. R. (1992). Human T-cell activation deficiencies. *Immunology Today, 13,* 259–265.

Bender, B. S., Chrest, F. J., & Adler, W. H. (1986). Phenotypic expression of natural killer cell associated membrane antigens and cytolytic function of peripheral blood cells from different aged humans. *Journal of Clinical and Laboratory Immunology, 21,* 31–36.

Chopra, R. K., Holbrook, N. J., Powers, D. C., McCoy, M. T., Adler, W. H., & Nagel, J. E. (1989). Interleukin 2, interleukin 2 receptor and interferon-γ synthesis and mRNA expression in phorbol myristate acetate and calcium ionophore A23187 stimulated T cells from elderly humans. *Clinical Immunology and Immunopathology, 53,* 297–308.

Couch, R. B., Kasel, J. A., Glezen, W. P., Cate, T. R., Six, H. R., Taber, L. H., Frank, A. L., Greenberg, S. B., Zahradnik, J. M., & Keitel, W. A. (1986). Influenza: Its control in persons and populations. *Journal of Infectious Diseases, 153,* 431–440.

Covelli, V., Mouton, D., Di Majo, V., Bouthillier, Y., Bangrazi, C., Mevel, J.-C., Rebessi, S., Doria, G., & Biozzi, G. (1989). Inheritance of immune responsiveness, life span, and disease incidence in interline crosses of mice selected for high or low multispecific antibody production. *Journal of Immunology, 142,* 1224–1234.

D'Amelio, R., Matricardi, P. M., Nisini, R., Le Moli, S., Fattorossi, A., Di Addario, A., & Castagliuolo, P. P. (1989). Prevalence of HBV markers in the Italian Armed Forces and HBV vaccination. *Military Medicine, 154,* 589–592.

Finland, M., & Barnes, M. W. (1977). Acute bacterial meningitis at Boston City Hospital during 12 selected years, 1935–1972. *Journal of Infectious Diseases, 136,* 400–415.

Galazka, A., & Kardymowicz, B. (1989). Tetanus incidence and immunity in Poland. *European Journal of Epidemiology, 5,* 474–480.

Goedert, J. J., Kessler, C. M., Aledort, L. M., Biggar, R. J., Andes, W. A., White II, G. C., Drummond, J. E., Vaidya, K., Mann, D. L., Eyster, M. E., Ragni, M. V., Lederman, M. M., Cohen, A. R., Bray, G. L., Rosenberg, P. S., Friedman, R. M., Hilgartner, M. W., Blattner, W. A., Kroner, B., & Gail, M. H. (1989). A prospective study of human immunodeficiency virus type 1 infection and the development of AIDS in subjects with hemophilia. *New England Journal of Medicine, 321,* 1141–1148.

Guo, Y., Dickerson, C., Chrest, F. J., Adler, W. H., Munster, A. M., & Winchurch, R.

A. (1990). Increased levels of circulating interleukin 6 in burn patients. *Clinical Immunology and Immunopathology, 54,* 361–371.

Heine, J. W., & Adler, W. H. (1977). The quantitative production of interferon by mitogen-stimulated mouse lymphocytes as a function of age and its effect on the lymphocytes proliferative response. *Journal of Immunology, 118,* 1366–1369.

Nagel, J. E., Chopra, R. K., Chrest, F. J., McCoy, M. T., Schneider, E. L., Holbrook, N. J., & Adler, W. H. (1988). Decreased proliferation, interleukin 2 synthesis, and interleukin 2 receptor expression is accompanied by decreased mRNA expression in phytohemagglutinin stimulated cells from elderly donors. *Journal of Clinical Investigation, 81,* 1096–1102.

Nagel, J. E., Chopra, R. K., Powers, D. C., & Alder, W. H. (1989). Effect of age on the human high affinity interleukin 2 receptor of phytohemagglutinin stimulated peripheral blood lymphocytes. *Clinical and Experimental Immunology, 75,* 286–291.

Nagel, J. E., Collins, G. D., & Adler, W. H. (1981). Spontaneous or natural killer cytotoxicity of K562 erythroleukemic cells in normal patients. *Cancer Research, 41,* 2284–2288.

Nagel, J. E., Han, K., Coon, P. J., Adler, W. H., & Bender, B. S. (1986). Age differences in phagocytosis by polymorphonuclear leukocytes measured by flow cytometry. *Journal of Leukocyte Biology, 39,* 399–407.

Saxena, R. K., Saxena, Q. B., & Adler, W. H. (1988). Lectin-induced cytotoxic activity in spleen cells from young and old mice: Age-related changes in types of effector cells, lymphokine production and response. *Immunology, 64,* 457–461.

Schuurs, A. H. W. M., & Verheul, H. A. M. (1990). Effects of gender and sex steroids on the immune response. *Journal of Steroid Biochemistry, 35,* 157–172.

Song, L., Nagel, J. E., Chrest, F. J., Collins, G. D., & Adler, W. H. (1992). Comparison of CD3 and CD2 activation pathways in T cells from young and elderly adults. *Aging (Milano), 4,* 307–315.

Sørensen, T. I. A., Nielsen, G. C., Andersen, P. K., & Teasdale, T. W. (1988). Genetics and environmental influences on premature death in adult adoptees. *Journal of Infectious Diseases, 318,* 727–732.

Zhou, D., Chrest, F. J., Adler, W. H., Munster, A. M., & Winchurch, R. A. (1993). Increased production of TGF-β and IL-6 by aged spleen cells. *Immunology Letters, 36,* 7–12.

Zhou, D., Chrest, F. J., Adler, W. H., Munster, A. M., & Winchurch, R. A. (1992b). Age related changes in the expression of the TGFβ receptor on the CD4+ and CD8+ subsets of T cells. *Aging: Immunology and Infectious Disease, 3,* 217–226.

Alterations in
T-Cell Heterogeneity and Responsiveness in Aging Mice

7

*Richard A. Miller, Shaokang Li, Hiren R. Patel,
Jia Shi, and Jacek M. Witkowski*

A major objective of immunogerontology is to explain the age-dependent loss in T-cell immune function in terms of underlying changes in the cellular composition of the immune system, and changes in the biochemical mechanisms by which T cells respond to activating stimuli. The demonstration that aging leads to an accumulation of memory T cells and a corresponding decline in the proportion of naive T cells (Ernst, Hobbs, Torbet, et al., 1990; Lerner, Yamada, & Miller, 1989; Nagelkerken, Hertogh-Huijbregts, Dobber, et al., 1991) now seems to explain much of the age-dependent loss in T-cell proliferation, production of IL-2, and generation of cytotoxic effector cells. As we argue, however, these do not fully account for age-related changes in composition and responsiveness *within* the naive and memory cell subsets.

Our studies showing that memory T cells accumulate in old mice and that the shift from naive to memory cell predominance has important functional implications are reviewed here briefly. Lerner et al. (1989), using antibodies to the CD44 determinant which is expressed at higher levels on memory T cells than on naive T cells, documented a dramatic increase with age in the ratio of memory to naive T cells. Memory T cells make up about 30% of the CD4 and CD8 populations of young mice but were found to comprise up to 70% of the CD4 and CD8 cells of older animals. Parallel changes were seen in spleen, lymph node, and peripheral blood T-cell pools (Lerner et al., 1989), and similar changes have also been reported in other strains of mice (Ernst et al., 1990; Nagelkerken et al., 1991) and in humans (De Paoli, Battistin, & Santini, 1988; Pilarski, Yacyshyn, Jensen, et al., 1991). By separating the CD44^{hi} from the CD44^{lo} cells, we were able to show (Lerner et al., 1989) that the age-associated increase in CD44^{hi} memory cells could account for the corresponding decline in the proportion of T cells that could respond to the mitogen Con A in assays for proliferation, IL-2 production, or IL-2–dependent expansion of cytotoxic cells.

A second line of experimentation established that memory T cells, in both young and old mice, had a biochemical abnormality that could in principle contribute to their functional hyporesponsiveness. We had previously shown that T cells from old mice were less able than young T cells to generate an intracellular calcium signal after stimulation by Con A (Miller, Jacobsen, Wiel, et al., 1987), or after exposure to the receptor-by-passing ionophore ionomycin (Miller, Philosophe, Ginnis, et al., 1989). Using four-color flow cytometric analysis we found (Philosophe & Miller, 1990) that memory T cells, from mice of any age, were more resistant to calcium signal generation than naive T cells. Statistically significant differences between naive and memory cells were seen using ionomycin for both CD4 and CD8, and using Con A or anti-CD3 antibody for CD4 cells.

Did this age-related increase in calcium-resistant T cells, mostly of the memory cell class, account for or contribute to the loss in the proportion of mitogen-reactive helper, cytotoxic, and proliferator T cells? We tested this hypothesis in two ways. In the first set of experiments (Philosophe & Miller, 1989), electronic flow sorting was used to separate those T cells that did produce an internal calcium signal within a few minutes after Con A stimulation from those that did not. The separated T cells were then tested for their ability to function in Con A–stimulated in vitro functional assays, and only those that had generated a calcium signal were found to be able to produce IL-2, or to proliferate and generate IL-2–dependent cytotoxic cells. The distinction in functional competence between calcium-resistant and calcium-nonresistant T-cell subsets was seen equally in T cells from young and old mice. A second approach used a density gradient method (Miller, Flurkey, Malloy, et al., 1991) to separate T cells based on their sensitivity to ionomycin-induced alterations in K$^+$ and water loss. T cells whose volume changed most in the presence of ionomycin were found predominantly to express the surface markers of naive cells (CD44^{lo}, CD45RB^{hi}), and these preparations of ionomycin-sensitive cells were also found to contain most of the Con A reactive helper and cytotoxic cells. This is in good agreement with the studies of electronic cell sorting for calcium signal generation. We thus concluded that naive and memory T cells of mice differed in their resistance to agents that increased internal calcium concentrations, and that this difference largely accounted for the age-related decline in calcium signal generation and in the proportion of mitogen-responsive T cells in assays of IL-2 production and response.

There was also, however, some evidence of age-related changes *within* the naive and memory subsets. Memory T cells of aged mice, for example, were significantly less likely than memory T cells of young donors to respond to Con A or the superantigen staphylococcal enterotoxin B in IL-2 production assays (Flurkey, Stadecker, & Miller, 1992). The proportion of memory T cells that could generate a calcium signal also declined with age (Philosophe & Miller, 1990) for responses of CD4 cells to Con A and anti-CD3, and for responses of CD8 cells to Con A, anti-CD3, and ionomycin. Tests for protein kinase function (described later) also revealed differences between the naive and memory T cells. It seems possible that these changes could reflect an unsuspected age-dependent shift between subsets contained within the naive and memory populations. Recent evidence from our laboratory (Witkowski & Miller, 1993) may provide a way to follow this hypothesized transition. Using the fluorochrome Rhodamine-123 to stain T cells from mice of different ages, we have found that a large proportion of the T cells from old mice, and a smaller fraction of T cells from young donors, are able to extrude R123 in a time- and temperature-dependent pumping process. The extrusion seems to be mediated by a 170 kD-plasma membrane pump known as P-glycoprotein (P-Gp) because each of five different P-Gp inhibitors was shown to be able to block the extrusion of R123 from prelabeled T cells, and because a similar age-dependent difference was demonstrable with a second P-Gp substrate, Rhodamine-6G. Interestingly, both the naive and memory T-cell populations contained both R123^{bright} and R123^{dull} T-cell subpopulations, with the proportion of R123^{dull} (i.e., P-Gp^{high}) cells increasing with age in each subset (see Figure 7.1). Thus R123 staining reveals unsuspected and age-sensitive heterogeneity within the naive and memory pools. It will be of interest to learn if there are functional differences between the R123^{bright} and R123^{dull} T cells that can help to account for the effect of aging on T-cell function.

Another line of evidence has provided some insights into the ways in which aging might lead to impairments of T-cell function independent of the naive-to-memory cell transition. Studies in young mice have shown that while naive T cells are good producers of IL-2, production of IL-4 is principally attributable to memory T cells (Akbar, Salmon, & Janossy, 1991; Sanders, Makgoba, & Shaw, 1988). Thus the accumulation of memory T

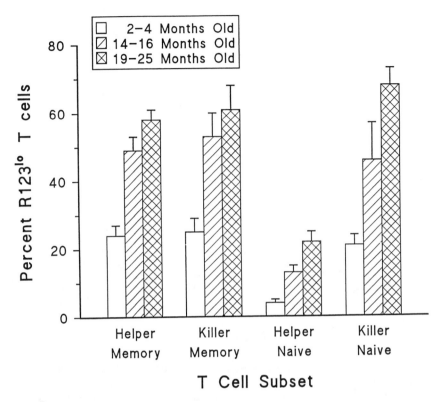

FIGURE 7.1   Age-dependent increase in the proportions of T cells exhibiting high levels of P-Glycoprotein in different subsets. P-glycoprotein function was assessed by the ability of R123-labeled cells to extrude the fluorochrome in a 30 minute incubation; R123^{lo} T cells are high in P-glycoprotein function. Cells were also stained with anti-CD44 and either anti-CD4 or anti-CD8 so that R123 levels could be assessed in each of the four indicated subsets. Bars indicate means ± standard errors of the Means for $N = 9$ young, 4 middle-aged, and 8 old mice each tested separately. Differences between young and old mice are statistically significant for each of the four subsets. See Witkowski and Miller (1993) for additional details.

cells in old mice might be expected to lead to increases in IL-4 production, but only if the memory T cells were fully functional. Indeed, several published studies (Ernst et al., 1990; Nagelkerken et al., 1991; Araneo, Dowell, Diegal, et al., 1991) have recently suggested an age-dependent increase in IL-4 production in short-term in vitro cultures, consistent with the hypothesis that the memory T cells that accumulate in old mice are immunocom-

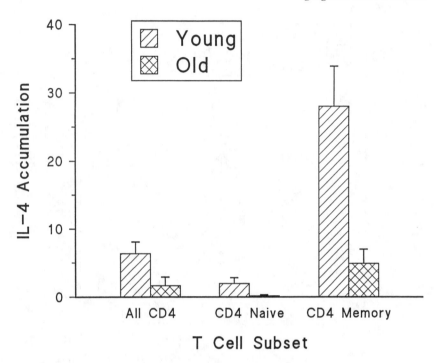

FIGURE 7.2   Age-dependent decline in IL-4 production in CD4 subsets. Each bar indicates mean ± standard errors of the means for $N = 7$ experiments. T cells were separated into subsets by negative immunomagnetic bead adherence, stimulated with immobilized anti-CD3 antibody for 2 days, and then cultured with anti-CD3 and added IL-2 for an additional 9 days, with supernatants assayed for IL-4 accumulation at days 3, 6, and 9 of the IL-2 culture interval; the values shown represent cumulative IL-4 production over the 9-day interval. The effects of age are significant in each subset, and in addition the responses of memory cells are significantly higher than those of naive or unseparated T cells (Li & Miller, unpublished data).

petent. Our own work, however, has suggested that the situation may be more complicated. Using an extended culture method (Rocken, Muller, Saurat, et al., 1991) in which T cells are first activated with anti-CD3 antibody and then allowed to produce IL-4 during a 9-day culture interval in the presence of both anti-CD3 and added IL-2, we have found a clear decline with age in the production of IL-4 by either unseparated CD4 T helper cells or by purified (CD45RB^{lo}) helper memory cells (Li & Miller, unpublished data). Figure 7.2 shows summary data from a series of seven experiments comparing unseparated, naive, and memory T cells from young and old mice. Taken together with the published reports, our data suggest that while memory T cells from old mice may be as competent as memory T cells from young donors in the initial production of IL-4 over short intervals, they may be less able to generate this lymphokine in conditions that test the ability to proliferate and differentiate in the presence of IL-2 and continued antigenic stimulation. It will be of interest to see if differences in R123 staining can discriminate among memory T cells that differ in their ability to generate IL-4 in extended cultures.

In addition to work on lymphocyte heterogeneity and lymphokine production, recent investigations have revealed age-dependent changes in several aspects of protein kinase function. Stimuli that activate resting T cells are thought to work through induction of several parallel and intersecting signal pathways. One pathway is thought to involve activation of several tyrosine-specific protein kinases (TPK) of the *src* family including the *lck* and *fyn* kinases. A second pathway requires both an increase in intracellular calcium and the activation of the serine/threonine-specific PKC; this latter pathway can be stimulated in a receptor-independent fashion by using a combination of the calcium ionophore ionomycin together with the PKC-stimulating phorbol ester PMA.

In an initial attempt to look for age effects on the protein kinase system, Patel and Miller (1991) used two-dimensional gel electrophoresis to quantitate phosphorylation rates of a number of distinct, but anonymous, substrates in T cells exposed to PMA, ionomycin, or a receptor-dependent agonist like Con A or anti-CD3 antibody. This survey identified 14 substrates that could respond to anti-CD3 antibody, and classified each of these phosphoproteins (PPN) according to its response to PMA and ionomycin alone or in combination. This battery of "indicator PPNs" was then used to compare the responsiveness of T cells from young, middle-aged, and old donors (Patel & Miller, 1992). We found that each of the PPNs that responded well to anti-CD3 in T cells from young mice was less responsive in middle aged animals and essentially unresponsive in donors 22 months of age (see Figure 7.3). Thus aging led to a progressive, synchronous, and severe decline in the phosphorylation of a wide range of anti–CD3-sensitive PPN.

Two lines of evidence suggested that this functional deficit was not due simply to a decline in the ability of the T-cell receptor/CD3 complex to transduce signals. First of all, aging led to an increase in CD3-inducible phosphorylation of three PPN substrates that did not respond appreciably in T cells from young mice (see Figure 7.3), suggesting that the anti-CD3 stimulus did generate some signals, though apparently atypical ones, in T cells from old donors. Second, defects in phosphorylation were also observed in T cells from old mice that were exposed to PMA or to ionomycin, which bypass the TCR/CD3 receptor-dependent transduction pathway.

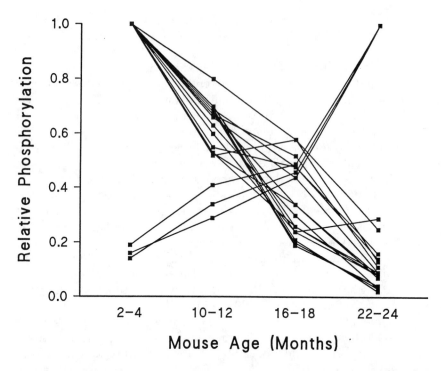

FIGURE 7.3   Progressive age-dependent changes in anti-CD3 induced phosphorylation in mouse T cells, as assessed by autoradiography of two-dimensional electrophoretic patterns of lysates in ^{32}P-labeled cells. Of the 17 PPNs
that respond vigorously (i.e., at least fivefold) in *either* old or young mice, 14 decline progressively with age, whereas the other 3 show parallel age-dependent
increases in mitogen-induced phosphorylation levels. Each point represents
the mean value of phosphorylation in three independent experiments; standard errors of the mean were < 10% of the mean value in nearly all cases, and
each line connects points corresponding to one of the 17 PPNs studied. For con-
venient comparison, each value is shown relative to its own maximum phosphorylation level. The effects of age are statistically significant for each of the
PPNs. See Patel and Miller (1992) for additional details.

Thus none of the 10 PPNs that were phosphorylated in young T cells after
ionomycin treatment were responsive in T cells from old donors. PMA induces the phosphorylation of 12 PPNs in T cells from young mice, and of
these 10 were found to be unresponsive in old mice, but the other two were
found to be fully as reactive in old as in young donors (see Figure 7.4). In
addition, the three PPNs that responded to anti-CD3 only in old T cells also
were PMA-inducible in old, but not young, T-cell populations. We con-

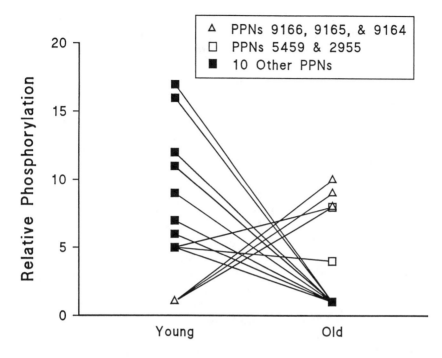

FIGURE 7.4   Protein phosphorylation in response to PMA in T cells of old and young mice. Each value represents the mean of three independent experiments, relative to phosphorylation levels of a set of 8 invariant internal reference PPNs in the same set of gels; standard errors of the mean were < 10% of the mean value in nearly all cases. Of the 15 PPNs that responded at least fivefold in *either* young or old mice, 10 responded only in young mice (filled squares), 3 responded only in old mice (triangles), and 2 responded equally well in mice of either age (open squares). See Patel and Miller (1992) for additional details.

cluded from these results that aging led to profound alterations in the pattern of internal protein kinase function, or perhaps alterations in the balance of kinase and phosphatase activity, and that a simple loss of CD3-mediated transduction could not explain the data. The PMA data suggested, moreover, that T cells from old mice did indeed retain some aspects of PKC dependent signals, but that the pattern of PKC-mediated substrate phosphorylation was grossly disordered.

Further analysis of these PPN patterns showed that the effect of aging cannot simply be attributed to the accumulation of memory T cells at the expense of naive T cells (Patel & Miller, 1992). PPN patterns from anti–CD3-stimulated CD4 T cells (both naive and memory combined) were compared with patterns from purified CD4 memory T cells. Of the nine PPNs that responded vigorously (> fivefold increase) in CD4 cells, two responded equally well in purified memory T cells from young mice but failed to respond even in unseparated T cells from old mice. This result showed that the memory T cells from old donors were deficient in at least this aspect of the earlier activation process. The other seven PPNs that responded well in unseparated CD4 populations from young mice responded much less well, or in some cases not at all, in purified memory T cells, suggesting that they were responsive only (or preferentially) in naive T cells. None of these seven responded in preparations of old CD4 cells, suggesting an age-dependent defect in the responses of the naive CD4 population. The demonstration of three PPNs that respond to anti-CD3 and to PMA *only* in T cells from old mice also shows that the PPN patterns of old mice are not simply those predicted on the assumption that old mice contain altered numbers of functionally unchanged naive and memory T cells.

Although the autoradiographic method used in the studies just described cannot discriminate between proteins phosphorylated on tyrosine and those phosphorylated on serine or threonine residues, it seems likely that most of the PPNs present in our lysates were indeed serine- or threonine-phosphorylated, because approximately 99% of protein phosphate is in the form of phosphothreonine or phosphoserine. Nonetheless, tyrosine-specific protein kinases (TPK) are thought to play critical roles in T-cell activation. For this reason, we have used antiphosphotyrosine immunoblots to study phosphotyrosine-containing PPNs (PY-PPNs) in lysates of stimulated T cells (Shi & Miller, 1992). These data showed that T cells from aging mice are deficient not only in overall patterns of PPN phosphorylation, but in the patterns of TPK function as well. Figure 7.5, for example, shows the relative phosphorylation levels of the three PY-PPNs that were found to respond consistently to anti-CD3 stimulation in young mice, using anti-PY immunoblotting to detect PY-PPNs in lysates of T cells prepared 2 minutes after addition of anti-CD3. Phosphorylation of all three mitogen-responsive PY-PPNs was found to be significantly diminished in old (compared with young) mice; middle-aged mice yielded more variable results. Lysates made at 5 and 10 minutes after stimulation also showed a statistically significant defect in the T cells from old donors for all three responsive PY-PPNs (not shown). A more limited series of experiments using antibody to the T-cell receptor, or Con A, as stimulants also showed the same pattern of age-dependent decline (Shi & Miller, 1992). Two of these PY-PPNs (p120 and p80) were found to be present in phosphorylated form at low levels in unstimulated T cells, but these baseline levels did not change with age. Nor was there any effect of age on the levels of several other PY-PPNs that failed to respond to anti-CD3 or Con A stimulation. We concluded that aging led to a decline in the ability of T cells to carry out at least some mitogen-in-

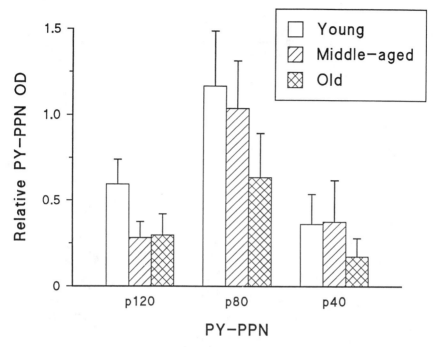

FIGURE 7.5   Age-dependent decline in anti–CD3-induced tyrosine-specific phosphorylation of three PY-PPNs, as measured by antiphosphotyrosine immunoblotting. Each bar represents the mean ± standard error of the mean for 9 to 11 independent experiments, except that only 4 to 6 determinations were made for p40. Differences between the young and old mice were statistically significant by the Friedman test. The data shown are from lysates made at 2 minutes after mitogen addition; data obtained on lysates made at 5 and 10 minutes gave similar patterns and also showed a statistically significant difference between young and old mice. See Shi and Miller (1992) for additional details.

duced tyrosine-specific protein phosphorylation, although whether these particular PY-PPNs play an important role in T-cell activation has yet to be determined.

Can the loss with age in mitogen-induced PY-PPN phosphorylation be attributed primarily to the shift from naive to memory T cells? At this point our data provide only a partial answer, in the affirmative. CD4 T cells from old and young mice were stimulated with anti-CD3, Con A, or anti–T-cell receptor antibodies, and PY-PPN levels compared with those in lysates made from purified memory CD4 cells. The data for the p80 responses are shown in Figure 7.6, and show that memory T cells, from mice of either age group, are substantially (and significantly) less able to phosphorylate p80

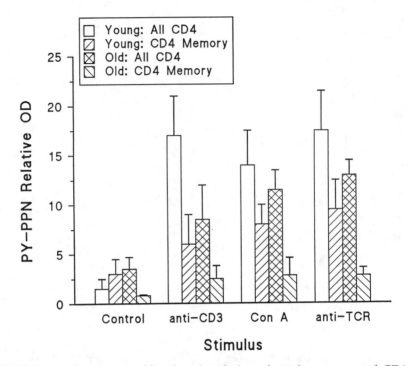

FIGURE 7.6   Tyrosine-specific phosphorylation of p80 in unseparated CD4 and in CD4 memory T cells of old and young mice in responses to anti-CD3, Con A, and anti–T-cell receptor (TCR) antibody. Each bar shows the mean ± standard error for $N = 4$ independent determinations. Memory T cells were significantly less responsive than unseparated T cells for both young and old mice. In addition, young CD4 cells were found to be significantly more responsive than CD4 cells from old donors (Shi & Miller, unpublished data).

than are unseparated CD4 cells. Thus the accumulation of memory T cells in mice accounts for the decline, with age, in p80 phosphorylation within the CD4 subset. Phosphorylation of p120 is also significantly lower in memory CD4 cells than unseparated CD4 cells of old or young mice, but the response of p120 in CD4 cells is not significantly age sensitive, perhaps because aging leads to a significant increase in the baseline level of p120 in unstimulated CD4 cells (Shi & Miller, unpublished data). Phosphorylation of p40 in responses to anti-CD3 and Con A is also lower in memory than in unseparated CD4 cells; p40 does not respond to anti–T-cell receptor antibody in mice of any age.

In summary, the shift from naive to memory T cells seems to account for some, but not all, of the effects of age on T-cell responsiveness. The decline in IL-2–producing and IL-2–responding T cells, and the defects in calcium signal generation that may account for these functional deficits, all seem to be directly linkable to memory T-cell accumulation. At least a part of the alteration in tyrosine-specific protein phosphorylation can also be tied to this developmental transition. Other changes, however, seem to be controlled independently including the accumulation of T cells with high levels of P-glycoprotein function, the decline in IL-4 production in extended, IL-2 supplemented cultures, and the major changes in the pattern of mitogen-inducible protein phosphorylation. The challenges now confronting us are to link these new phenomena into a coherent causal chain, to show how later events in the activation cascade, including gene expression, cell division, and memory cell formation are tied to the early activation defects, and then to determine which of these biochemical and developmental changes are responsible for age-dependent increases in vulnerability to infectious agents and perhaps to neoplasia as well.

ACKNOWLEDGMENTS

This research was supported by NIA grants AG03978, AG09801, and AG08808, and by an award from the American Federation for Aging Research, Inc.

REFERENCES

Akbar, A. N., Salmon, M., & Janossy, G. (1991). The synergy between naive and memory T cells during activation. *Immunology Today, 12,* 184–188.

Araneo, B. A., Dowell, T., Diegel, M., & Daynes, R. A. (1991). Dihydrotestosterone exerts a depressive influence on the production of interleukin-4 (IL-4), IL-5, and γ-interferon, but not IL-2 by activated murine T cells. *Blood, 78,* 688–699.

De Paoli, P., Battistin, S., & Santini, G. F. (1988). Age-related changes in human lymphocyte subsets: Progressive reduction of the CD4, CD45R (suppressor inducer) population. *Clinics in Immunology & Immunopathology, 48,* 290–296.

Ernst, D. N., Hobbs, M. V., Torbett, B. E., Glasebrook, A. L., Rehse, M. A., Bottomly, K., Hayakawa, K., Hardy, R. R., & Weigle, W. O. (1990). Differences in the expression profiles of CD45RB, Pgp-1, and 3G11 membrane antigens and in the patterns of lymphokine secretion by splenic CD4[+] T cells from young and aged mice. *Journal of Immunology, 145,* 1295–1302.

Flurkey, K., Stadecker, M., & Miller, R. A. (1992). Memory T lymphocyte hyporesponsiveness to non-cognate stimuli: A key factor in age-related immunodeficiency. *European Journal of Immunology, 22,* 931–935.

Lerner, A., Yamada, T., & Miller, R. A. (1989). PGP-1[hi] T lymphocytes accumulate with age in mice and respond poorly to Concanavalin A. *European Journal of Immunology, 19,* 977–982.

Miller, R. A., Flurkey, K., Molloy, M., Luby, T., & Stadecker, M. J. (1991). Differential sensitivity of virgin and memory T lymphocytes to calcium ionophores suggests a buoyant density separation method and a model for memory cell hyporesponsiveness to Con A. *Journal of Immunology, 147,* 3080–3086.

Miller, R. A., Jacobson, B., Weil, G., & Simons, E. R. (1987). Diminished calcium influx in lectin-stimulated cells from old mice. *Journal of Cellular Physiology, 132,* 337–342.

Miller, R. A., Philosophe, B., Ginis, I., Weil, G., & Jacobson, B. (1989). Defective control of cytoplasmic calcium concentration in T lymphocytes from old mice. *Journal of Cellular Physiology, 138,* 175–182.

Nagelkerken, L., Hertogh-Huijbregts, A., Dobber, R., & Drager, A. (1991). Age-related changes in lymphokine production related to a decreased number of CD45RB[hi] CD4[+] T cells. *European Journal of Immunology, 21,* 273–281.

Patel, H. R., & Miller, R. A. (1989). Age-associated changes in mitogen-induced protein phosphorylation in murine T lymphocytes. *European Journal of Immunology, 22,* 253–260.

Patel, H. R., & Miller, R. A. (1991). Analysis of protein phosphorylation patterns reveals unanticipated complexity in T lymphocyte activation pathways. *Journal of Immunology, 146,* 3332–3339.

Philosophe, B., & Miller, R. A. (1989). T lymphocyte heterogeneity in old and young mice: Functional defects in T cells selected for poor calcium signal generation. *European Journal of Immunology, 19,* 695–699.

Philosophe, B., & Miller, R. A. (1990). Diminished calcium signal generation in subsets of T lymphocytes that predominate in old mice. *Journal of Gerontology: Biological Sciences, 45,* B87–B93.

Pilarski, L. M., Yacyshyn, B. R., Jensen, G. S., Pruski, E., & Pabst, H. F. (1991). $\beta 1$ integrin (CD29) expression on human postnatal T cell subsets defined by selective CD45 isoform expression. *Journal of Immunology, 147,* 830–837.

Rocken, M., Muller, K. M., Saurat, J. H., & Hauser, C. (1991). Lectin-mediated induction of IL-4-producing CD4[+] T cells. *Journal of Immunology, 146,* 577–584.

Sanders, M. E., Makgoba, M. W., & Shaw, S. (1988). Human naive and memory T cells: Reinterpretation of helper-inducer and suppressor-inducer subsets. *Immunology Today, 9,* 195–199.

Shi, J., & Miller, R. A. (1992). Tyrosine-specific protein phosphorylation in response to anti-CD3 antibody is diminished in old mice. *Journal of Gerontology: Biological Sciences, 47,* B147–B153.

Witkowski, J. M., & Miller, R. A. (1993). Increased function of P-glycoprotein in T lymphocytes of aging mice. *Journal of Immunology, 150,* 1296–1306.

PART II

Psychoneuro-endocrine Modulation of Immunity: Implications for the Elderly

Reversibility of Age-Related Thymic Involution by Hormonal and Nutritional Interventions

8

Nicola Fabris

There is good experimental evidence to support the existence of numerous interactions among the nervous, endocrine, and immune systems. Communication between these networks is mediated by soluble mediators, such as hormones, neurotransmitters, and immune-derived cytokines, which are to a large extent shared by the different homeostatic systems. Hormones and neurotransmitters reach lymphoid organs and cells through blood circulation or through direct autonomic nervous system (ANS) connections between neural tissue and the organs of the lymphoid system itself (Bullock, 1987; Fabris, 1992a; Fabris, Macchegiani, Muzzioli, et al., 1988). The neuroendocrinimmune interactions are regulated primarily by the hypothalamus-pituitary axis via direct release of circulating hormones and neuropeptides or by indirect regulation of hormonal secretion from peripheral endocrine glands. Microanatomic studies have shown that nerve endings of the sympathetic and the parasympathetic systems innervate various organs of the immune system such as thymus, spleen, bone marrow, and lymph nodes. Furthermore, ANS-related neurosubstances such as substance P, vasoactive intestinal peptide, somatostatin, neurotensin, oxytocin, and calcitonin have been immunocytochemically identified in lymphoid organs (Felten, Felten, Carlson, et al., 1985).

The existence of signals generated within the immune system, capable of modulating neuroendocrine functions, was originally suggested by the alterations that can be induced in the neuroendocrine balance either by removal of lymphoid organs such as the thymus (Besedovsky & Sorkin, 1984; Pierpaoli, Fabris, & Sorkin, 1970) or by immune responses to antigen (Besedovsky & Del Rey, 1992). The discovery that most of these effects can be mimicked by various immune-derived factors, including thymic peptides and lymphokines, suggests a biochemical basis for those findings (Bernton, Beach, Holaday, et al., 1987; Spangelo, Judd, Ross, et al., 1987). The observation that lymphoid and accessory cells may synthesize and secrete neurohormonal factors, such as adrenocorticotropic hormone (ACTH), growth hormone (GH), thyrotropic-stimulating hormone (TSH), prolactin (PRL), gonadotropins, and endogenous opioid (Blalock, 1988) has implicated these as additional humoral signals shared by the immune and the neuroendocrine systems.

Despite increased understanding of these kinds of interconnections, little effort has been made to investigate the more classical neuroendocrinologic pathways. Hormones, neurotransmitters, and immune cytokines may exert developmental actions, related to the structural and functional organization of target organ or cell (Bernton et al., 1987; Fabris et al., 1988) and can also regulate the actual performance of mature cells, such as those required to counteract stressful conditions (Fabris, 1991). The findings related to neuroendocrinimmune interactions responsible for developmental steps should, therefore, be clearly distinguished from those related to emergency events in fully matured systems. The stimuli required to activate a given pathway as well as the end effects may differ according to the functional demand of the organism.

These considerations have suggested at least two levels of neuroendocrinimmune interaction (Fabris et al., 1988). The first level concerns the relationship between the neuroendocrine system and the thymus (see Figure 8.1A), which is the site of stem cell differentiation into mature T lymphocytes. An understanding of this relationship must consider the fact that the thymus produces various hormones that regulate T-cell differentiation (Zatz & Goldstein, 1985). The second level of interaction is at

IMMUNE-NEUROENDOCRINE PATHWAYS

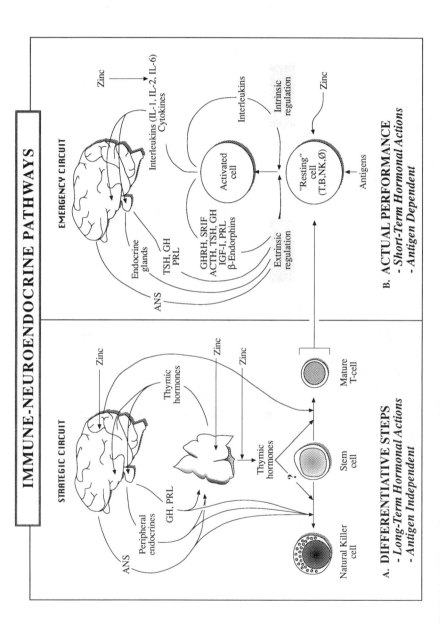

STRATEGIC CIRCUIT

EMERGENCY CIRCUIT

Zinc

Interleukins (IL-1, IL-2, IL-6)
Cytokines

Endocrine glands

TSH, GH
PRL

Interleukins

Intrinsic regulation

ANS

Activated cell

GHRH, SRIF
ACTH, TSH, GH
IGF-I, PRL
β-Endorphins

Extrinsic regulation

"Resting" cell
(T,B,NK,Ø)

Zinc

Antigens

Zinc

Thymic hormones

Zinc

Peripheral endocrines

GH, PRL

Thymic hormones

Mature T-cell

Stem cell

Natural Killer cell

A. DIFFERENTIATIVE STEPS
 - *Long-Term Hormonal Actions*
 - *Antigen Independent*

B. ACTUAL PERFORMANCE
 - *Short-Term Hormonal Actions*
 - *Antigen Dependent*

FIGURE 8.1 Schematic representation of the two major pathways of neuroendocrine-immune. (A) Strategic circuit. (B) Emergency circuit. See text for explanation.

the periphery (see Figure 8.1B) between neuroendocrine signals and the humoral products, which are secreted by immune cells during specific reactions to various antigens (Besedovsky & Del Rey, 1992; Spangelo et al., 1987).

The rationale for discriminating these two levels is based on several considerations. The first level of interaction is primarily involved in maturation of both immune and neuroendocrine systems, which occurs independently of antigenic stimulation. In fact, neuroendocrine-thymus interactions are observable even in animals maintained under germ-free conditions. The second level of interaction requires the presence of fully differentiated immune cells and the occurrence of a specific antigenic or stress-mediated hormonal stimulus. The main role played by these interactions appears to be homeostatic (i.e., that of maintaining the normal neuroendocrine immune balance when suddenly altered by a stressful cognitive or noncognitive event) (Blalock, 1988).

This chapter summarizes the data available on the "strategic" circuit and the evidence supporting the hypothesis that such a circuit does not undergo intrinsic and irreversible processes with advanced age or, in any case, that a certain degree of restorability of the age-related alterations does exist.

THYMUS–NEUROENDOCRINE INTERACTIONS

The thymus is a complex organ that is the site of T-lymphocyte differentiation. The cellular components of the thymus are quite diversified, according to the function accomplished (Kendall, 1991). In addition to T cells at various stages of maturation, the thymus contains epithelial cells capable of producing thymic peptides (Savino & Dardenne, 1984) that regulate T-cell maturation as well as neuropeptides whose significance is still to be defined (Geenen, Legrus, Franchimont, et al., 1986). These epithelial cells contain various peptides, such as thymopoietin, thymosin α_1, α_7, and β_4, and thymulin (Savino & Dardenne, 1984). This last peptide requires binding to zinc ions to be biologically active (Dardenne, Plau, Nabama, et al., 1982). The zinc-unbound peptide, in addition to being inactive, prevents the active form from exerting its action on the specific targets, thus suggesting that zinc bioavailability may be of relevance for thymic hormone (Fabris, Mocchegiani, Amadio, et al., 1984). Thymic epithelial cells express receptors for prolactin (Dardenne, Savino, Gagnerault, et al., 1989), growth hormone (GH) (Ban, Gagnerault, Jammes, et al., 1991), glucocorticoids (Dardenne, Itoh, & Homo-Delarche, 1986), and progesterone (Kendall, Fitzpatric, Greenstein, et al., 1990).

Functional Evidence

Initial evidence of thymus–neuroendocrine interaction was based on the discovery that a congenital mutation affecting pituitary dwarf mice causes concomitant alterations in the thymus and in the thymus-dependent immune system (Fabris, Pierpaoli, & Sorkin, 1971, 1972). Thymic involution in these animals results in defective T-cell dependent function as indicated by prolonged allogeneic skin-graft survival, depressed capability of spleen cells to induce graft-versus-host reactions, and reduced humoral antibody response to thymus-dependent antigens (Fabris, 1993).

These findings have been recently confirmed in a strain of dwarf dogs (Weimaraner dogs), which show retarded growth, small thymus, absence of thymus cortex, and deficient lymphocyte mitogen responses (Roth, Laeberle, Grier, et al., 1980). All these immunologic defects can be corrected by GH treatment (Roth, Lamax, Alszulev, et al., 1984).

Some thymic factors are secreted into the blood stream and the circulating level of at least one of them (i.e., the factuer thymique serique [FTS], more recently called thymulin in its zinc-bound form [Dardenne et al., 1982]) correlates with thymic functional activity. This discovery has offered a new technical approach to evaluate thymus-neuroendocrine interactions both in animal and humans.

It has been demonstrated that congenital hypopituitarism, experimentally induced diabetes, and thyroidectomy all cause a rapid reduction of plasma thymulin levels, whereas removal of the gonads or of the adrenals does not induce any significant change. Reconstitution experiments by substituting specific hormonal therapy have demonstrated that the circulating level of thymulin returns to normal levels within a few days after the beginning of the hormonal treatment (Fabris & Mocchegiani, 1985).

In humans, many endocrinopathies are associated with alterations of circulating thymulin (see Figure 8.2). For example, congenital hypopituitarism (Fabris, Mocchegiani, Muzzioli, et al., 1983; Mocchegiani, Paolucci, Basalmo, et al., 1990a) and hypothyroidism (Fabris, Mocchegiani, Mariotti, et al., 1986) following thyroidectomy are both associated with reduced thymulin level. By contrast, hyperthyroidism resulting from diffuse nodular goiter (particularly common in old individuals) is associated with higher levels of thymulin than is typically seen at this age (Fabris et al., 1986).

It has been recently demonstrated that the low thymulin levels seen with hypopituitarism significantly recover following GH injection (Mosshegiani et al., 1990a). In these studies no correlation was found between GH and thymulin levels, although a positive correlation was found between insulin-like growth factor (IGF-1) and thymulin blood concentrations, suggesting that GH probably acts on the thymus through somatomedins.

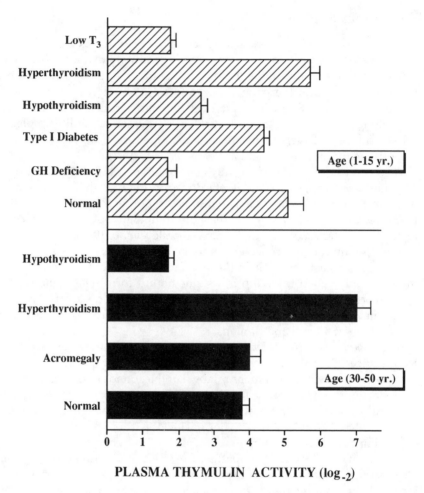

FIGURE 8.2 Alterations of plasma thymulin concentrations in various human disendocrinopathies.

In conditions characterized by hypersecretion of GH, such as acromegaly, thymulin blood levels are modestly increased (Travaglini, Mocchegiani, Demin, et al., 1992; Travaglini, Mocchegiani, Togni, et al., 1990). Patients suffering from prolactin-secreting tumors, conversely, have thymulin levels either reduced or in the lower range of normal values when compared with age-matched controls (see Figure 8.2).

Insulin is another hormone that may regulate thymic function, because low thymulin blood levels have been observed in type 1 juvenile diabetes.

This defect, however, does not depend on thymic failure but rather on reduced zinc ion availability, resulting in incomplete saturation (and biologic activation) of thymulin (Mocchegiani, Boemi, Fumelli, et al., 1989).

ROLE OF NUTRITIONAL ELEMENTS

The frequent association between malnutrition, infectious disease, and aging has provoked several experimental and clinical studies designed to analyze the effect of single nutrients on immune function (Chandra, 1985, 1989). Several single nutrients relevant to immune function have been identified, including trace elements (Underwood, 1977), vitamins (Bendich, 1988), and amino acids (Daly, Reynolds, Siga, et al., 1990), although their effects on thymus functions have remained unclear. Recent evidence suggests a specific role for zinc and arginine. In animals, zinc-deficient diet causes atrophy of the thymus and lymph nodes, and is associated with impaired cell-mediated immunity (Iwata, Incefy, Tanaha, et al., 1979). In humans, zinc deficiency causes underdevelopment of the thymus and reduced thymic endocrine activity (Chandra, 1985; McClain, 1985). Patients with Down's syndrome, who suffer from marginal zinc deficiency, have low levels of plasma thymic hormone that can be corrected with zinc supplementation (Fabris, Mocchegiani, Muzzioli, et al., 1991). As mentioned earlier, zinc-unbound thymulin is not only biologically inactive but competes with the active form for the binding to the specific target (Dardenne et al., 1982; Fabris et al., 1984).

Regarding the effect of arginine on the immune system, a good body of evidence has been accumulated since the first observation of its role in the recovery of wound healing capacity in experimentally injured rats (Returra, Barbul, et al., 1978). Subsequent studies demonstrated that arginine supplementation was able to prevent posttraumatic atrophy of the thymus and the associated reduced response of peripheral lymphocytes to T-cell mitogens (Barbul, Returra, Levinson, et al., 1980; Barbul, Wasserkrug, Seifter, et al., 1983) and that the same supplementation was able to increase thymic weight and cellularity even in otherwise normal rats (Daly et al., 1990).

PLASTICITY OF THYMUS–NEUROENDOCRINE INTERACTIONS DURING AGING

The thymus attains its maximum size at puberty, after which it undergoes a progressive involution characterized by a decrease in weight because of the depletion of cortical lymphocytes and by an infiltration of fat (Gold-

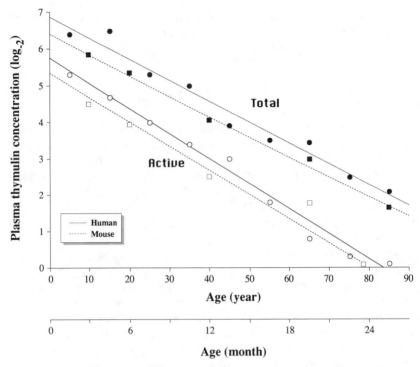

FIGURE 8.3   Age-dependent decline of plasma concentrations of total (active and inactive), and of active thymulin in mice and humans.

stein & McKay, 1969). Fat cells are most abundant in the cortex and differentiate in situ during involution. Thymocytes decrease in number, and of those present many are pycnotic in old age (Simpson, Gray, Michie, et al., 1975). Epithelial cells also decrease in number during aging and show cystic changes and reduction of intracellular granules (Meleg-Smith & Ossa-Gomez, 1981; Simpson et al., 1975; Steinmann, Klaus, & Mullerhermelink, 1985).

In both animals and humans the plasma level of thymulin declines progressively from birth to old age and is virtually undetectable over 60 years of age in humans. According to a recent and more precise determination of thymulin, which takes into account marginal zinc deficiency present with advancing age (Fabris et al., 1984), the decline of thymulin levels is less pronounced than that previously reported. Even in very old age, significant residual production of thymulin is observable (see Figure 8.3). The age-associated decline of thymic endocrine activity, which parallels the anatomic involution of the thymus, seems to be one of the major causes for the peripheral immune deterioration observed with senescence (Zatz & Goldstein, 1985).

In the neuroendocrine system, several age-associated alterations have been documented. These include reduced activity of hypothalamic neurosecretory cells, increased hypothalamic threshold level to negative feedback mechanisms, abnormalities in nearly all endocrine glands (particularly the pituitary-adrenal axis and thyroid hormone secretion), and reduced peripheral sensitivity to the stimulation of hormones and neurotransmitters (Meites, Boya, & Takahashi, 1986).

THYMUS REJUVENATION IN OLD AGE BY HORMONAL OR NUTRITIONAL TREATMENTS

Because modifications induced by experimental manipulation of the thymus are known to alter the neuroendocrine system, age-related changes in the thymic immune system may affect the neuroendocrine axis and vice versa. Studies have been undertaken to verify whether experimental restoration of certain neuroendocrine patterns in old age might return thymic and immune functional activity to levels seen earlier in life (see Figure 8.4). Reacquisition of thymic function may be achieved in several ways: (a) intrathymic transplant of pineal gland or administration of melatonin (Pierpaoli, Dall'Ara, Pedrinis, et al., 1991); (b) implantation of a GH-secreting tumor cell line (Kelley, Brief, Westly, et al., 1986) or treatment with exogenous GH (Davila, Brief, Simon, et al., 1987; Goff, Roth, Arp, et al., 1987); (c) castration (Greenstein, Fitzpatrick, Kendall, et al., 1987) or treatment with exogenous luteinizing hormone–releasing hormone (LH–RH) (Marchetti, Morale, Batticane, et al., 1991); (d) treatment with exogenous thyroxine or triiodothyronine (Fabris & Mocchegiani, 1985; Fabris, Muzziola, & Mocchegiani, 1982); (e) nutritional interventions such as arginine (Mocchegiani, Boemi, Fumelli, et al., 1990b) or zinc supplementation (Fabris et al., 1991).

The recovery of thymulin secretion in old mice is accompanied by an increased number of T lymphocytes in peripheral organs and improved T-cell responses to mitogen stimulation (Fabris et al., 1982; Mocchegiani et al., 1992). Data in humans are still incomplete. Plasma thymulin concentration increases with administration of GH (unpublished data), arginine (Mocchegiani et al., 1990b), and zinc (Chandra, 1989). The potential capacity of thyroid hormones (Fabris et al., 1988) to restore thymic function in old age is indirectly supported by the clinical observation that hyperthyroidism in old humans is associated with thymic enlargement (Simpson, Gray, & Beck, 1975) and with high circulating plasma levels of thymulin

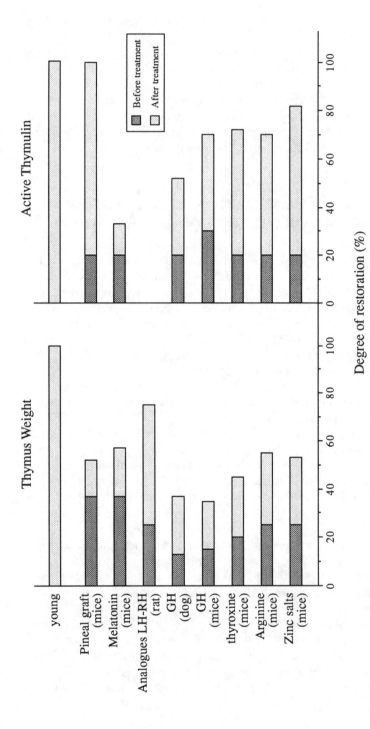

FIGURE 8.4   Restoration of thymic weight and plasma thymulin concentrations in old age by different endocrine and nutritional interventions.

comparable with those recorded in young, normal individuals (Fabris et al., 1986).

The major conclusion from these findings is that the age-related thymic involution is not an irreversible process and that functional recovery can be achieved even in old age. It is, at present, difficult to draw any firm conclusion about the mechanisms involved in such a thymic reconstitution. The effects of GH, thyroid hormones, and LH–RH may be mediated by specific hormone receptors present on thymic epithelial cells (Marchetti et al., 1991). Melatonin or pineal-derived factors may also act through specific receptors, but experimental confirmation is still lacking. Arginine may affect thymic function through an increased release of GH (Isidori, LeMonaco, & Cappa, 1981) and such as action is preserved in old age (Carlson, Gillen, Gorden, et al., 1972). Finally, zinc may act through the reactivation of the pituitary-thyroid axis, as recently demonstrated by its capacity to correct pituitary-thyroid dysfunction in Down's syndrome patients (Licastro, Mocchegiani, Zannotti, et al., 1992).

This interpretation implicates a hormone-mediated reconstitution of thymic activity in old age. Several other interpretations are also possible. In particular, the role played by zinc may not be secondary. In humans, hypersecretion of thyroid hormones and of GH is associated with increased blood levels of zinc (see Figure 8.5). Treatment of animals with triiodothyronine or melatonin augments blood levels of zinc. It is also possible that many hormones including GH, thyroid hormone, and melatonin may increase zinc turnover and thereby influence thymic function. Although speculative at present, this hypothesis cannot be discarded, and it should be considered for future work.

SUMMARY

From the data illustrated in this review, it seems reasonable to deduce the following:

1. The thymus and the neuroendocrine tissues are interrelated in such a way that modifications or manipulations affecting one system are followed by alterations in the other. Such interactions appear to be particularly clear between the thymus and the pituitary.
2. Although these bidirectional interactions operate during the whole life of the organism, they assume greater importance during development and senescence as well as during periods of life characterized by significant and prolonged modifications of the neuroendocrine pathways (e.g., pregnancy [Pepper, 1961]). Furthermore, although the quality and the quantity of signals exchanged between

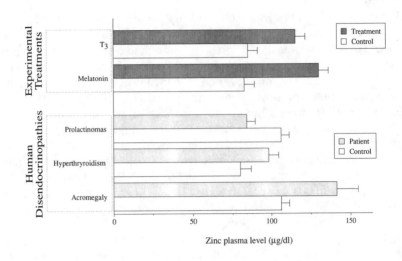

FIGURE 8.5 Increased plasma zinc level in old hyperthyroid and acromegalic humans, and in old triiodothyronine or melatonin-treated mice. Prolactinoma patients show, on the contrary, reduced plasma zinc levels.

the two systems may change in all the preceding reported conditions, the responsivity does not seem to be modified. Provided a given stimulation is of sufficient duration, the target will respond despite age, or other concomitant situations, to reach the predicted efficiency. This fact obliges one to accept the idea that physiologic modifications of the thymus-neuroendocrine interactions are not irreversible. In other words, these interactions possess a high degree of plasticity, which can contribute to functional recovery.

The major remaining question is the understanding of the causes for the progressive involution of the thymus in physiologic aging. In this context one can certainly accept the assumption that the thymus "is the only gland, whose progressive involution with age is a common feature of animals and man" (Korenchevski, 1961). In this context, it is necessary to recall the concept of progressive involution. The involution of the thymus is, in fact, described as an event occurring after puberty, the preceding period being characterized by a steady state if not by a developmental growth stage, and the effect of castration in old age is consequently interpreted as the reverse effect of sexual maturation.

This description does not seem to correspond with reality. If thymus function is measured by the circulating level of thymic peptide, the figure obtained is that of a linear decline, starting at least from birth. No major fluctuations are reported during sexual maturation or menopausal assessment. If modifications occur in these periods, they consist in simply reaching a different size of the organ, which is more evident during development, whereas during menopause a small weight increase is reached followed by the "regular" decline (Simpson et al., 1975). Such a modification is not observed in males. Conversely, there are some exceptions in nature in the age-dependent thymic involution. For example, hens do not show consistent thymic involution (Hammar, 1936), nor do germ-free animals (Moore, 1966). Both situations may encompass different hormonal profiles, though because of different causes, but both are not strictly linked to sexual maturation or involution.

Interpretations of thymic involution as strictly linked to sexual function are somewhat misleading. Recent histologic reexamination of thymic involution seems to be in line with this assumption (Steinman et al., 1985). If so, reasons other than sexual maturation should be found to explain thymus involution. In this context it can be noted that other functions, namely, those described under the concept of linear parameters of aging, show the same linearity as thymic involution. Some of them, such as the response to β-agonist or the polyploidy in the liver, are strictly linked to thymus function and show the same progressive modification with age (Fabris & Piantanelli, 1982).

At present it is difficult to accept a hypothesis based on a single age-related cause for all these phenomena, but their temporal concordance is suggestive. Future work might certainly make understanding such a concordance as well as the plasticity of the systems and tissues involved much clearer (Fabris, 1992b).

REFERENCES

Ban, E., Gagnerault, M. C., Jammes, H., Postel-Vinay, M. C., Haour, F., & Dardenne, M. (1991). Specific binding sites for growth hormone in cultured mouse thymic epithelial cells. *Life Science, 48,* 2141–2148.

Barbul, A., Rettura, G., Levenson, S. M., & Seifter, E. (1983). Wound healing and thymotropic effects of arginine: A pituitary mechanism of action. *American Journal of Clinical Nutrition, 37,* 786–794.

Barbul, A., Wasserkrug, H. L., Seifter, E., Rettura, G., Levenson, S. M., & Efron, G. (1980). Immunostimulatory effects of arginine in normal and injured rats. *Journal of Surgery Research, 29,* 228–235.

Bendrich, A. (1988). Antioxidant, vitamins and immune response. In R. K. Chandra (Ed.), *Nutrition and immunology* (pp. 125–148). New York: Alan R. Liss.

Bernton, E. W., Beach, J. E., Holaday, J. W., Smallridge, R., & Fein, H. G. (1987). Release of multiple hormones by a direct action of interleukin 1 on pituitary cells. *Science, 238*, 519–525.

Besedovsky, H. O., & Sorkin, E. (1984). Thymus involvement in female sexual maturation. *Nature, 249*, 356–358.

Besedovsky, H. O., & Del Rey, A. (1992). Immune-neuroendocrine circuits: Integrative role of cytokines. In *Frontiers in neuroendocrinology* (Vol. 3, pp. 61–94). New York: Raven Press.

Blalock, J. E. (1988). Production of neuroendocrine peptide hormones by the immune system. In J. E. Blalock & K. L. Bost (Eds.), *Neuroimmunendocrinology (progress in allergy)* (Vol. 43, pp. 1–14). Basel: Karger.

Bullock, K. (1987). The innervation of immune system tissues and organs. In C. W. Cotman, R. E. Brinton, A. Galaburda, & B. McEwen (Eds.), *The neuro-immune-endocrine connection* (pp. 33–47). New York: Raven Press.

Carlson, H. E., Gillin, J. C., Gorden, P., & Snyder, F. (1972). Absence of sleep-related growth hormone peaks, in aged normal subjects and in acromegaly. *Journal of Clinical Endocrinology & Metabolism, 34*, 1102.

Chandra, R. K. (1989). Nutritional regulation of immunity and risk of infection in old age. *Immunology, 67*, 141–147.

Daly, J. M., Reynolds, J., Siga, R. K., Shou, J., & Liberman, M. D. (1990). Effect of dietary protein and aminoacids on immune function. *Critical Care Medicine, 18*, 86–93.

Dardenne, M., Itoh, T., & Homo-Delarche, F. (1986). Presence of glucocorticoids receptors in cultured epithelial cells. *Cellular Immunology, 100*, 112–118.

Dardenne, M., Pleau, J., Nabama, B., Lefancier, P., Denien, M., Choay, J., & Bach, J. F. (1982). Contribution of zinc and other metals to the biological activity of the serum thymic factor. *Proceedings of the National Academy of Science, USA, 79*, 5370–5373.

Dardenne, M., Savino, W., Gagnerault, M. C., Itoh, T., & Bach, J. F. (1989). Neuroendocrine control of thymic hormonal production: I. Prolactin stimulates in vivo and in vitro the production of thymulin by human and murine thymic epithelial cells. *Endocrinology, 125*, 3–10.

Davila, D. R., Brief, S., Simon, J., Hammer, R. E., Brinster, R. L., & Kelly, K. W. (1987). Role of growth hormone in regulating T-dependent immune events in aged, nude and transgenic rodents. *Journal of Neuroscience Research, 18*, 108–116.

Fabris, N. (1991). Neuroendocrine-immune interactions: A theoretical approach to aging. *Archives of Gerontology & Geriatrics, 12*, 219–230.

Fabris, N. (1992a). Immune system and aging neuroimmunological implications. *International Journal of Immunopathology & Pharmacology, 5*, 93–102.

Fabris, N. (1992b). Biomarkers of aging in the neuroendocrine-immune domain: Time for a new theory of aging? *Annals of the New York Academy of Science, USA, 663*, 335–348.

Fabris, N. (1993). Neuroendocrine/thymus interactions during development and aging. In C. J. Grossman (Ed.), *Hormones and immunity: Bilateral communications between the endocrine and immune systems*. New York: Springer-Verlag.

Fabris, N., Mocchegiani, E., Amadio, L., Zannotti, M., Licastro, F., & Franceschi, C. (1984). Thymic hormone deficiency in normal aging and Down's syndrome: Is there a primary failure of the thymus? *Lancet, 1,* 983–986.

Fabris, N., Mocchegiani, E., Mariotti, S., Pacini, F., & Pinchera, A. (1986). Thyroid function modulates thymus endocrine activity. *Journal of Clinical Endocrinology & Metabolism, 62,* 474–478.

Fabris, N., Mocchegiani, E., Muzzioli, M., & Imberti, R. (1983). Thymus-neuroendocrine network. In N. Fabris, E. Baraci, J. Hadden, & N. A. Mitchison (Eds.), *Immunoregulation* (p. 341). New York: Plenum Press.

Fabris, N., Mocchegiani, E., Muzzioli, M., & Provinciali, M. (1988). Neuroendocrine-thymus interaction: Perspectives for intervention in aging. In Neuroimmunomodulation: Interventions in aging and cancer. *Annals of the New York Academy of Science, USA, 521,* 72–87.

Fabris, N., Mocchegiani, E., Muzzioli, M., & Provinciali, M. (1991). Role of zinc in neuroendocrine-immune interactions during aging. In Physiological senescence and its postponement: Theoretical approaches and rational interventions. *Annals of the New York Academy of Science, USA, 621,* 314–326.

Fabris, N., Muzzioli, M., & Mocchegiani, E. (1982). Recovery of age-dependent immunological deterioration in BALB/C mice by short-term treatment with L-thyroxine. *Mechanisms of Aging & Development, 18,* 327.

Fabris, N., & Piantanelli, L. (1982). Thymus-neuroendocrine interactions during development and aging. In R. C. Adelman & G. S. Roth (Eds.), *Endocrine and neuroendocrine mechanism of aging* (pp. 186–195). Boca Raton, FL: CRC Press.

Iwara, T., Incefy, G. S., Tanaha, T., Fernandez-Botet, C. J., Pih, K., & Good, R. A. (1979). Circulating thymic hormone levels in zinc deficiency. *Cellular Immunology, 47,* 100–105.

Kelley, K. W., Brief, S., Westly, H. J., Novakofski, J., Bechtel, P. J., Simon, J., & Walker, E. B. (1986). GH3 pituitary adenoma cells can reverse thymic aging in rats. *Proceedings of the National Academy of Science, USA, 83,* 5663–5667.

Kendall, M. D. (1991). Functional anatomy of the thymic microenvironment. *Journal of Anatomy, 177,* 1–29.

Kendall, M. D., Fitzpatrick, F. T. A., Greenstein, B. D., Khóylou, F., Safien, B., & Hamblin, A. (1990). Changes in the thymus of the rat by chemical or surgical castration. *Cell and Tissue Research, 261,* 555–562.

Korenschvski, V. (1961). The aging thymus. In G. H. Bourne (Ed.), *Physiological and pathological aging.* New York: Hafner.

Licastro, F., Mocchegiani, D., Zannotti, M., & Fabris, N. (1992). Normalization of thyroid stimulating hormone and reversal triiodothyronine plasmic levels by dietary zinc supplementation in children with Down's syndrome: Evaluation of clinical impact. *International Journal of Neuroscience, 65,* 259.

Marchetti, B., Morale, M. C., Batticane, N., Gallo, F., Farinelli, Z., & Cioni, M. (1991). Aging of the reproductive-neuroimmune axis. In Physiological senescence and its postponement. *Annals of the New York Academy of Science, USA, 621,* 159–173.

McClain, C. S. (1985). Zinc metabolism in malabsorption syndromes. *Journal of American College of Nutrition, 4,* 49–56.

Meites, J., Goya, R., Takahashi, S. (1986). Why the neuroendocrine system is important in aging processes. *A Review of Experimental Gerontology, 22,* 1.

Meleg-Smith, S. N., & Ossa-Gomex, L. J. (1981). A quantitative histologic comparison of the thymus in 100 healthy and diseased adults. *American Journal of Clinical Pathology, 76,* 657–665.

Mocchegiani, E., Boemi, M., Fumelli, P., & Fabris, N. (1989). Zinc-dependent low thymic hormone level in type I diabetes. *Diabetes, 38,* 932–937.

Mocchegiani, E., Cacciatore, L., Talarico, M., Lingetti, M., & Fabris, N. (1990). Recovery of low thymic hormone levels in cancer patients by lisine-arginine combination. *International Journal of Immunopharmacology, 12,* 365–371.

Mocchegiani, E., Muzzioli, M., Santarelli, L., & Fabris, N. (1992). Restoring effect of oral supplementation of zinc and arginine on thymic endocrine activity and peripheral immune functions in aged mice. *Archives of Gerontology & Geriatrics, 3,* 267–276.

Mocchegiani, E., Paolucci, P., Balsamo, A., Cacciari, E., & Fabris, N. (1990). Influence of growth hormone on thymic endocrine activity in humans. *Hormone Research, 33,* 248–255.

Moore, R. W. (1986). Unpublished observations, cited by Good, R. A. in discussion. In G. E. W. Wolstenholme & R. Porter (Eds.), *The thymus: Experimental and clinical studies* (pp. 179–181). Boston: Little, Brown.

Pepper, F. J. (1961). The effect of age, pregnancy and lactation on the thymus gland and lymphnodes of the mouse. *Journal of Endocrinology, 22,* 335–339.

Pierpaoli, W., Dall'Ara, A., Pedrinis, E., & Regelson, W. (1991). The pineal control of aging. The effects of melatonin and pineal grafting on the survival of older mice. In Physiological senescence and its postponements: Theoretical approaches and rational interventions. *Annals of New York Academy of Science, USA, 621,* 291–313.

Pierpaoli, W., Fabris, N., & Sorkin, E. (1970). Developmental hormones and immunological maturation. In G. E. W. Wolstenholme & J. Knight (Eds.), *Hormones and the immune response* (Vol. 36, pp. 126–143). London: Churchill Ciba Study Group.

Roth, J. A., Laeberle, M. L., Grier, D. L., Hopper, J. G., Spiegel, H. E., & Macallister, H. A. (1984). Improvement in clinical condition and thymic morphological feature associated with growth treatment of immunodeficient dwarf-dogs. *American Journal of Veterinary Research, 45,* 1151–1155.

Roth, J. A., Lamax, L. G., Alszuler, N., Hampshire, J., Laeberle, M. L., Shelton, M., Draper, D. D., & Ledet, A. A. E. (1980). Thymic abnormalities and GH deficient in dogs. *American Journal of Veterinary Research, 41,* 1257–1262.

Savino, W., & Dardenne, M. (1984). Thymic hormone-containing cells: VI. Immunohistologic evidence for the simultaneous presence of thymulin, thymopoietin and thymosin alpha 1 in normal and pathological human thymuses. *European Journal of Immunology, 14,* 987–991.

Seifter, E., Rettura, G., Barbul, A., & Levenson, S. M. (1978). Arginine: An essential aminoacid for injured rats. *Surgery, 84,* 224–230.

Simpson, J. C., Gray, E. S., Michie, W., & Beck, J. S. (1975). The influence of preoperative drug treatment on the extent of hyperplasia of the thymus in primary thyrotoxicosis. *Clinics in Experimental Immunology, 22,* 243–249.

Simpson, J. F., Gray, E. S., & Beck, J. S. (1985). Age involution in the normal human adult thymus. *Clinics in Experimental Immunology, 19*, 261–268.

Spangelo, B. L., Judd, A. M., Ross, P. C., Login, I. S., Jarvis, W. D., Badamchian, M., Goldstein, A. L., & Macleod, R. M. (1987). Thymosin fraction 5 stimulates prolactin and growth hormone release from anterior pituitary cells in vitro. *Endocrinology, 121*, 2035–2040.

Steinmann, G. G., Klaus, B., & Mullerhermelink, H. K. (1985). The involution of aging human thymic epithelium is independent of puberty. *Scandinavian Journal of Immunology, 22*, 536–575.

Travaglini, P., Mocchegiani, E., Togni, E., Muratori, M., Re, T., Bazzoni, S., & Fabris, N. (1990). Thymulin and zinc circulating level in patient with GH and PRL secreting pituitary adenomas. *International Journal of Neuroscience, 51*, 269–271.

Travaglini, P., Micchegiani, E., De Min, C., Re, T., & Fabris, N. (1992). Modifications of thymulin titers in patients affected with prolonged low or high zinc circulating levels are independent of patient's age. *Archives in Gerontology & Geriatrics, 3*, 349–358.

Underwood, E. J. (1977). *Trace elements in human and animal nutrition* (4th ed., pp. 1–302). New York: Academic Press.

Zatz, M., & Goldstein, A. L. (1985). Thymosins, lymphokines and the immunology of ageing. *Gerontology, 31*, 263–272.

Age-Related Alterations in Noradrenergic Sympathetic Innervation of the Immune System

9

Denise L. Bellinger, Kelley S. Madden,
Suzanne Y. Felten, and David L. Felten

Abundant evidence from a variety of fields has accumulated over the last two decades to indicate that bidirectional communication occurs between the major integrative systems of the body, the nervous system, the endocrine system, and the immune system. Further, highly complex interactions between these systems provide biologic signals that are relevant to health and disease in humans. In this chapter, we examine the role of sympathetic neurotransmission in modulation of the immune system, describe the changes that occur in sympathetic innervation of lymphoid organs with age, and discuss the possible implications of age-related changes in sympathetic outflow in immunosenescence.

EPIDEMIOLOGIC AND EXPERIMENTAL EVIDENCE FOR NEURAL-IMMUNE INTERACTIONS

Epidemiologic studies and experimental studies in animals support the hypothesis that various psychological stressors act through the nervous system, and modulate immune response. A large and relatively consistent literature suggests that individuals who experience recent major stressful negative life events are at greater risk for a variety of illnesses including infectious disease, peptic ulcers, essential hypertension, ulcerative colitis, hyperthyroidism, regional enteritis, rheumatoid arthritis, bronchial asthma, and neoplasia (Ader, 1981; Riley, 1981; Weiner, 1977). Many of these studies have focused on classical psychosomatic diseases that involve autoimmune phenomena in their etiology (Geschwind & Behan, 1982; Solomon, 1981), and are associated with acute flare-ups following emotional upheaval (Solomon, 1981). Human studies have shown that a variety of psychosocial factors (i.e., bereavement, depression, marital separation, loneliness, and examination stress in medical students), are associated with altered measures of immune reactivity (reviewed in Kiecolt-Glaser & Gaser, 1991). However, it is difficult to show a causal relationship between these two phenomena. The correlations between these events generally are not large, accounting for only about 10% of the variance (Cohen & Syme, 1985); however, effects are remarkably consistent across populations and different kinds of life events. In particular, life events associated with loneliness and loss of important personal relationships appear to increase risk of illness (Kiecolt-Glaser & Gaser, 1991). Collectively these studies have led investigators to believe that while stressful stimuli alone may not be sufficient to alter immune reactivity with an end point of illness, stressor and psychosocial factors are likely to play a significant role in the health status of individuals already at risk for disease, such as AIDS, autoimmune-linked disorders, and in the elderly whose immunoresponsiveness already may be compromised.

Although exposure to stressful events in humans has been implicated in the development and progression of a variety of disease entities, human studies are complicated by the complexity of human behavior and immunobiology in uncontrolled settings, and limited experimental conditions. Studies in laboratory animals exposed to a variety of stressors have shown a causal relationship between stress and altered immunoresponsiveness. The influence of stressors on in vitro immune parameters, such as mitogen-induced lymphocyte proliferation, antibody responses, and NK cell activity, is generally reported to be suppressive (Gisler et al, 1971; Shavit et al, 1984; Solomon, 1969) with the magnitude of immunosuppression dependent on multiple factors (i.e., stimulus intensity, stimulus duration, age, sex, species, and lymphoid compartment examined). Presentation of stressors to rodents can influence morbidity and mortality from tumors and pathogens (Plaut & Friedman, 1981; Sklar & Anisman, 1979). Studies that examine the effects of stress on in vivo immune responses are more difficult to assess, and clearly emphasize the need to specify the type, intensity, and schedule of stress exposure as well as the specific aspect of immune function assessed. This is borne out in studies demonstrating that stress-induced changes in in vivo immune function are not solely suppressive. Blecha et al. (1982a) showed that immobilization or cold exposure before sensitization decreased delayed-type hypersensitivity (DTH) to sheep red blood cells (SRBC), but enhanced contact sensitivity (CS) to dinitrochlorobenzene. In contrast, exposure to heat potentiated both CS and DTH. Ader and Cohen (1975,1982), as well as others (Gorczynski et al., 1982; Rogers et al., 1976; Wayner et al., 1978) have demonstrated that it is possible to alter immune measures and to alter the progression of an autoimmune disease, using classical Pavlovian conditioning paradigms. These conditioned alterations in immunologic reactivity provide dramatic evidence for signaling between the brain and the immune system.

Localization of brain regions involved in neural modulation of immune reactivity has been examined directly in ablation studies. Discrete lesions in hypothalamus, limbic forebrain structures, brain stem autonomic and reticular regions, and cerebral cortex have been shown to alter immune responses (reviewed by Felten et al., 1991). The magnitude, duration, and direction of the altered immune response are dependent on the site and extensiveness of the lesion. Further, in response to immunization or administration of cytokines, such as IL-1 or interferons, these same brain regions may show altered electrical activity (Korneva, 1987; Saphier et al., 1987a; 1987b) and monoamine metabolism (Besedovsky et al., 1983; Carlson et al., 1987; Kabiersh et al., 1988). Collectively these findings indicate a complex integrated neural circuitry that is involved in modulation of immune function. Although we have not yet elucidated all the neural channels and the mechanisms involved in neural signaling of the immune system, we do know that the central nervous system (CNS) can exert an influence on the immune system via two major outflows, the autonomic nervous system and neuroendocrine system. Conditioning and stress studies examining possible routes for the mediation of altered immunoreactivity indicate that some conditioning effects and stress-induced alterations on the immune response can occur in adrenalectomized, or even hypophysectomized animals (Blecha et al., 1982b; Esterling & Rabin, 1987; Keller et al., 1988). The integrity of the corticotropin-releasing factor (CRF)-ACTH-glucocorticoid

(GC) axis and pituitary appear necessary for stress-induced changes in mitogen-induced proliferation of peripheral blood lymphocytes in one paradigm, whereas noradrenergic (NA) innervation mediates alterations in mitogen-induced proliferation of splenocytes (Cunnick et al., 1988). Irwin et al. (1987) have shown that intracerebroventricular administration of CRF can suppress splenic NK cell responses, and that this response is mediated through sympathetic innervation of the spleen. In addition, brainstem opiate pathways are involved in altered NK cell activity following exposure to stressful stimuli (Shavit et al., 1984).

INNERVATION OF LYMPHOID ORGANS

The autonomic nervous system, through its innervation of lymphoid organs, provides a direct route for communication between the nervous and immune system. NA sympathetic innervation of both primary and secondary lymphoid organs has been well described with fluorescence histochemistry for localization of catecholamines, and with immunocytochemistry for tyrosine hydroxylase (TH), the rate-limiting enzyme in the synthesis of norepinephrine (NE) (Ackerman et al., 1991; Bellinger et al., 1987; Bellinger, Felten, Lorton, & Felten, 1989; Felten & Felten, 1991; Felten & Olschowka, 1987; Felten et al., 1987a, 1987b, 1987c; Livnat et al., 1985; Williams et al., 1981). This innervation is regional and specific, distributing along the vasculature and in the parenchyma among the cells of the immune system. Other studies collectively provide evidence that NE fulfills the criteria for neurotransmission in lymphoid organs with cells of the immune system as targets. In summary these studies demonstrate (a) the presence of NA innervation in lymphoid compartments; (b) the release and availability of NE from nerve terminals on sympathetic nerve stimulation; (c) the presence of adrenoceptors on a variety of cells of the immune system including T and B lymphocytes, thymocytes, macrophages, mast cells, and granulocytes (reviewed by Hall et al., 1985); and (d) predictable immune responses to manipulation of NA innervation, and NE and its receptors (reviewed by Felten et al., 1987c).

Anatomic studies have demonstrated that NA sympathetic nerves innervate both the smooth muscle of blood vessels, and the parenchyma of specific lymphoid compartments within primary and secondary lymphoid organs (Bellinger et al., 1987; Felten & Olschowka, 1987; Felten et al., 1989a, 1987b, 1987c; Williams et al., 1981). Within the parenchyma, NA nerve fibers distribute to zones of T and B lymphocytes and accessory cells including lymphoid compartments where macrophages reside. In the spleen, NA nerves course along the central arteriole and its branches, and extend from these vascular plexuses into the surrounding periarteriolar lymphatic sheath (PALS), a zone where T lymphocytes predominate. NA fibers also course adjacent to arterioles into the marginal zone, and along parafollicular zones where macrophages and B lymphocytes reside. In spleens from adult rodents, few NA nerves are present in the follicles, the B-lymphocyte compartments. In the red pulp, NA nerves reside along the venous sinuses, and in the capsular/trabecular system; few NA fibers course from these compartments into the parenchyma of the red pulp.

Evidence of release and availability of NE for interaction with target cells has been provided from studies showing (a) increased NE content in splenic venous blood following sympathetic nerve stimulation (von Euler, 1946); (b) depletion of NE following intraperitoneal administration of 6-hydroxydopamine (6-OHDA), a neurotoxin that destroys NA nerve terminals, or following removal of sympathetic ganglia that supply NA nerves to lymphoid organs (Bellinger, Felten, Lorton, & Felten, 1989; Wiilliams et al., 1981); and (c) measurement of nanomolar concentrations of NE following in vivo dialysis of the spleen (Felten et al., 1986). These findings suggest that NA nerves are capable of providing high splenic NE concentrations and support a paracrine role for NE in the splenic microenvironment.

The possibility that NA nerves also may interact with cells of the immune system through a mode other than the generally accepted paracrine secretion of NE is indicated from immunocytochemical studies performed at the ultrastructural level. In spleen sections immunocytochemically stained for TH and examined with electron microscopy (EM) (Felten & Olschowka, 1987), we have shown the presence of TH$^+$ nerve terminals adjacent to lymphocytes in the PALS, and adjacent to lymphocytes and to macrophages in the marginal zone. Appositions between TH$^+$ nerve terminals and lymphocytes (macrophages) are characterized by a junction of approximately 6 nm with relatively large regions of membrane apposition and no specialization of either prejunctional or postjunctional membranes. In contrast, NA sympathetic terminals whose targets are presumably smooth muscle cells of the central arteriole show no specialization and have interposed by a basement membrane or cell process within a gap of 250 nm or even greater distances. The presence of TH$^+$ nerve terminals closely apposed to lymphocytes and macrophages suggests direct interaction between TH$^+$ nerve terminals and cells of the immune system; however, the directionality of this interaction is not clear. β-adrenoceptor (βAR) expression on these cells types supports nerve-to-immune cell signaling; conversely it is likely that presumed target cells secrete cytokines that can interact with closely apposed nerve terminals, and regulate the release of NE.

With direct ligand binding assays, βAR expression has been demonstrated on leukocytes (T and B lymphocytes, neutrophils, basophils, macrophages) and on accessory cells of the immune system (mast cells) (reviewed by Hall et al., 1985). βAR on lymphocytes and accessory cells of the immune system are linked with adenylate cyclase and the generation of cAMP. βAR on lymphocytes from young adult rodents appear to be regulated in a similar manner as other tissues innervated by NA sympathetic nerves, with the presence of βAR agonists and antagonists resulting in down-regulation and up-regulation of βAR, respectively. Further, the presence of α-adrenoceptors (αAR) on human lymphocytes (Titinchi & Clark, 1984) and activated murine macrophages (Spengler et al., 1990) has been documented by ligand binding studies. Pharmacologic studies in rodents demonstrating changes in immune parameters mediated via αAR also support the presence of αAR on cells of the immune system (Livnat et al., 1985).

A complex role for NA innervation in modulation of immune function is based on functional studies. Several approaches have been used to evaluate the effect of catecholamines on immunologic reactivity, including the use of relatively selective adrenergic agents in vitro, infusion of adrenergic agents in vivo, and surgical or chemical destruction of sympathetic nerves that distribute to lymphoid organs. Based on these studies several roles have been proposed for NE modulation of immune reactivity including regulation of proliferation and differentiation of lymphocytes (Singh, 1979), lymphocyte trafficking (Ernström & Sandberg, 1974), and immunocompetence (Ackerman et al., 1987a; Felten et al., 1987c; Livnat et al., 1985). T- and B-lymphocyte reactivity in vitro, including mitogen- and cytokine-induced proliferation (Beckner & Farrar, 1988; Johnson et al., 1981); CTL activity (Strom et al., 1973), cytokine production (Didier et al., 1987), and antibody production (Melmon et al., 1974; Watson et al., 1973) were inhibited by βAR stimulation. Sanders and Munson (1985) demonstrated that application of NE (or other β_2-agonists) to unfractionated mouse splenocytes at the start of culture enhanced the plaque-forming cell (PFC) response approximately twofold to fourfold on day 5, the peak of the immune response, in a dose-dependent manner. This effect was blockable in the presence of propranolol within 6 hours of culturing splenocytes. Further, β-blockade also revealed an αAR-mediated enhancement of primary immune response on day 4 and suppression on day 5. Adrenergic agonists also potentiate CTL activity; this effect appears to be mediated via both αAR and βAR. Findings from our laboratory (Felten et al., 1987c; Livnat et al., 1985) demonstrate that the addition of adrenergic agonists in nanomolar to micromolar range to mixed-lymphocyte culture enhanced CTL activity by 25% to 350%.

Macrophages and NK cell functions also can be modified by catecholamines and other adrenergic agents. Catecholamines can suppress the killing of virus-infected cells and tumor cells by IFN-γ–stimulated macrophages (Koff & Dunegan, 1985; 1986), and increase synthesis of complement components in human monocytes (Lappin & Whaley, 1979). Reported effects of catecholamines on NK cell activity in vitro have been variable (enhancement [Hellstrand et al., 1985], and suppression [Katz et al., 1982]). We have not detected significant changes in murine NK cell function using a variety of adrenergic agonists in vitro (S. Livnat, unpublished data); however, chemical sympathectomy in adult mice enhanced NK cell activity in vitro (standard ^{51}Cr-release assay) and in vivo (as measured by clearance of intravenously injected radiolabeled tumor cells from the lung), suggesting that NA innervation supresses NK cell activity in vivo (Livnat et al., 1988).

Epinephrine (EP) hastened the peak and the decline of the PFC response in splenocytes by day 1 when given 6 hours before immunization, but inhibited the primary antibody response at all time points examined when administered 2 to 4 days before immunization (Depelchin & Letesson, 1981). Adoptive transfer of splenocytes that had been either incubated in 10^{-5} M EP for 1 hour or obtained from animals 6 hours after EP administration into syngeneic, irradiated recipients resulted in enhancement of primary antibody response to SRBC challenge compared with recipients of control splenocytes.

Infusion of EP in humans produced a transient increase in the number of circulating lymphocytes and monocytes, and decreased mitogen-induced T-lymphocyte proliferation (Crary et al., 1983a; 1983b). In rodents intracardiac injection of either NE or isoproterenol increased lymphocyte and granulocyte release from the spleen that was blocked by pretreatment with phentolamine and propranolol, respectively. Treatment of sympathectomized (SympX) rodents with NE enhanced leukocyte release from the spleen. In guinea pigs previously immunized with SRBC, release of PFC from the spleen at the peak day of the secondary immune response was enhanced dramatically after intracardiac injection of EP and was sustained beyond the peak day of the response leading to a decrease in spleen PFC number. Findings described above could not be attributed to changes in vascular smooth muscle contractility and altered blood flow, suggesting that catecholamines can modulate lymphocyte migration.

We and others have investigated sympathetic modulation of immune reactivity in vivo using sympathetic denervation strategies. Destruction of NA nerves can be achieved by systemic injection of 6-OHDA, a neurotoxin that is selective for NA nerve fibers, or by surgical removal of sympathetic ganglia that distribute to lymphoid organs. The consequences of NA depletion in spleen can be summarized as follows: (a) denervation with 6-OHDA at birth and surgical SympX in adults results in augmented primary and secondary antibody responses (Williams et al., 1981); (b) chemical SympX in adults results in suppressed primary and variable secondary antibody responses depending on the timing (Felten et al., 1987c; Hall et al., 1982; Livnat et al., 1985). Chemical SympX with 6-OHDA in adult rodents can diminish primary immune responses by 80% in spleens challenged systemically and by 97% in popliteal lymph nodes challenged by foot pad injection (Livnat et al., 1985). Further studies in adult rodents (Felten et al., 1987c; Livnat et al., 1985, 1987, 1988; Madden & Livnat, 1991; Madden et al., 1989), have shown that chemical SympX results in suppression of DTH responses to contact sensitizing agents, reduced CTL responses that are accompanied by lowered IL-2 production, enhanced NK cell activity in vivo and in vitro, augmented B-lymphocyte proliferative responses in lymph nodes, and a complex pattern of mitogen responses in spleen and specific lymph nodes. These responses can be blocked by preventing uptake of the neurotoxin into the nerve terminals with desmethylimipramine (DMI), a tricyclic uptake inhibitor of NE. Moreover, these responses also are not prevented by propranolol, administered concomitantly with the 6-OHDA, indicating that the effect is not mediated through the bolus release of NE from damaged NA terminals, interacting with postsynaptic receptors on lymphocytes. Sympathetic denervation also significantly influences cellular trafficking (Madden & Livnat, 1991). In mice, lymphocytes from nondenervated donors migrate in larger numbers to inguinal and axillary lymph nodes of chemically SympX recipients, whereas lymph node cells taken from SympX donors exhibit decreased migration to lymph nodes in nondenervated recipients. These findings suggest that NA innervation of secondary lymphoid organs in young adult rodents is necessary for competent immune reactivity.

AGE-RELATED DECLINE IN NA INNERVATION OF LYMPHOID ORGANS: FUNCTIONAL IMPLICATIONS

A progressive decline in normal immune functions with the aging process in both humans and in laboratory animals is well documented in the literature. Age-related immunologic dysfunction is associated with an increased occurrence of autoimmune complex diseases, certain types of cancer, and infectious disease. Documented alterations in T-cell–mediated immune function that occur with the normal aging process include decreased T-helper and CTL activity, increased suppressor T-lymphocyte activity, decreased T-lymphocyte proliferation induced by mitogens and antigens, decreased production of a variety of lymphokines, decreased responsiveness of T lymphocytes to thymic hormones, and decline in resistance to tumor cell challenge (Weksler & Siskind, 1984). Although the cause of, and mechanisms involved in, age-associated changes in T-lymphocyte function has not been elucidated, it is clear that both intrinsic (genetic) and extrinsic (environmental) factors play an important role in this process. Studies from our laboratory (Ackerman et al., 1991; Bellinger et al., 1987, 1992a, 199b; Bellinger, Ackerman, Felten, & Felten, 1992; Capocelli et al., 1985; Felten et al., 1987a, 1987b) have demonstrated a decline in NA sympathetic innervation of secondary lymphoid organs in aged rodents that parallel a decline in specific populations of cells of the immune system in secondary lymphoid organs, as well a decline in immune reactivity. Age-related loss of NA innervation of the spleen has been demonstrated by a greater than 50% decline in splenic NE content (Bellinger et al., 1987; Felten et al., 1987), a decrease in the the density of NA nerve fibers in spleen of greater than 80% (assessed with glyoxylic acid induced histofluorescence) (Bellinger et al., 1987), and a loss of TH[+] nerve fibers in spleen with immunocytochemical staining (Bellinger, Ackerman, Felten, & Felten, 1992; Bellinger et al., 1992a, 1992b). Age-associated decline in NA innervation appears to be specific to secondary lymphoid organs, because NA innervation in other organs such as the thymus (Bellinger et al., 1988) and heart (Felten et al., 1982) does not decline with age. Double-label immunocytochemistry for TH and specific markers for cells of the immune system revealed a parallel decline in TH[+] nerves and loss of T lymphocytes and ED3[+] macrophages in spleens from aged rodents (Bellinger, Ackerman, Felten, & Felten, 1992; Bellinger et al., 1992a; 1992b).

The effect of denervation on immunoreactivity in aged rodents has not yet been examined; however, functional studies in neonatal and young adult rodents indicate interaction of the nervous system with the immune system via NA nerves in lymphoid organs that appear to persist throughout the course of life. Altered activity of cells of the immune system with age may contribute to the decline in NA innervation of the spleen. Functional studies in young adult rodents using chemical denervation suggest that altered NE availability from nerves in lymphoid organs contributes to alterations in immune function. Our findings that the direction of change in immune responses following acute chemical SympX with 6-OHDA is often similar to the direction of immune responses measured in aged rodents support the hypothesis that catecholaminergic nerve fiber loss in secondary lymphoid organs causally contributes to altered immunologic reactivity. The presence of NA nerve terminals among T lymphocytes in the PALS, the main cell type showing age-related decline in function, the loss of these nerves in aging spleen, and the decline in T-lymphocyte immunocytochemical staining in spleen reinforce this possibility. The loss of ED3[+] macrophages in the marginal zone of the white pulp of the spleen suggests that other cell populations also are subject to age-related changes. The focus of our studies thus far has been to characterize altered NA innervation of the spleen in aged F344 rats including NE metabolism (synthesis, release, uptake, and turnover) and postsynaptic receptor expression. We also have examined whether nerve fibers are lost as a result of cell loss in sympathetic ganglion that distribute to the spleen degeneration of nerve terminals, or inability to synthesize products to which are chromagen reactions are sensitive (TH and NE).

NA INNERVATION OF THE AGED RAT SPLEEN

Initial studies from our laboratories examined the effect of age on NA innervation using two age groups of male F344 rats, 8- and 27-month-old animals representing young adult and aged populations, respectively (Felten et al., 1987). NA innervation in 8-month-old rats was similar to the innervation described for 3-month-old young adult rats. Spleens from 27-month-old rats showed a loss of NA innervation as assessed by fluorescence histochemistry and neurochemical measures of NE. NE content in the spleen was approximately 50% lower in 27-month-old rats compared with their 3-month-old counterparts. Quantitation of fluorescent varicosities revealed an age-related decrease in NA innervation in all splenic compartments of approximately 70% to 80% (Bellinger et al., 1987). These studies demonstrated a greater loss in NA nerve fibers than is indicated from splenic NE content. This smaller decline in splenic NE content compared with the extent of lost NA nerve fibers results from increased efficiency of NE uptake into, and an increase in NE metabolism in, age-resistant nerve fibers.

Longitudinal studies using fluorescence histochemistry, double-label immunocytochemistry, and neurochemical measurement of NE have been performed to examine the time course and manner in which NA innervation is lost as a function of age, and to examine the relationship of specific populations of lymphoid cells that reside in compartments innervated by NA nerves (Bellinger, Ackerman, Felten, & Felten, 1992). Data from these studies indicate that NA innervation is maintained through 12 months of age and then begins to decline gradually; the density of T lymphocytes in the PALS and ED3+ macrophages in the marginal zone parallel the decline in NA innervation. At 12 months of age, these immune cell compartments (PALS and marginal zone) are reduced as a result of cell loss, and NA innervation of these compartments is still robust. NA nerves appear to retract into smaller lymphoid compartments to maintain their anatomic distribution within these shrinking immune cell zones, giving the appearance of hyperinnervation. By 17 months of age, further loss of T lymphocytes and ED3+ macrophages was apparent; at this time point there was a decline in the density of NA nerve fibers associated with these compartments. This parallel decline in the density of specific populations of cells of the immune system continues through 27 months of age. The pattern of NA nerve loss and decline in T lymphocytes and ED3+ macrophages in these two splenic compartments occur in a regionally specific manner, with nerve fibers first lost in lymphoid compartments that reside most distal from the hilar region. NA innervation continues to decline in a distal to proximal fashion with respect to the hilus, until the only remaining NA nerve fibers in the 27-month-old spleen are distributed near the hilus, the site of entry into the spleen. The density of T lymphocytes in the PALS and ED3+ macrophages in the marginal zone displays a similar regional pattern of loss.

Double-label immunocytochemistry for TH and IgM, a B-lymphocyte marker, indicated little change in the density and distribution of B lymphocytes in the marginal zone or in the follicles of spleens from old rats. A decline in TH+ fibers was apparent in the marginal zone with aging; an occasional TH+ profile was found in the follicle of spleens from 27-month-old rats.

Neurochemical measurement of NE in spleens from rats at 3, 8, 12, 17, 21, and 27 months of age revealed a progressive decline in splenic NE content with age (Bellinger, Ackerman, Felten, & Felten, 1992). This decline was less severe than the corresponding decline in density of NA innervation, similar to our previous findings. We have hypothesized that the time course of splenic NA denervation is dependent on the continued exposure of the adult rat to environmental antigens. Pilot data suggests that splenic NA denervation is accelerated in rats raised under standard vivarium conditions compared with rats raised in a pathogen-free barrier facility. A similar decline in NPY+ nerves and parallel loss of T lymphocytes and ED3+ macrophages occurred with age, supporting colocalization (Felten et al., 1989). Based on immunocytochemical staining and radioimmunoassay measures of splenic content, splenic innervation did not appear to change with the normal aging process (Bellinger, Lorton, Felten, & Felten, 1989).

A loss in NA innervation of the spleen could result from (a) an inability of intact NA nerve terminals to synthesize enough NE to form observable fluorophore (or enough TH for immunostaining since loss of NA nerves in the spleen also is observed with immunocytochemical staining for TH); or (b) an actual loss of NA terminals (Bellinger et al., 1992b; Felten et al., 1987c). In a study to resolve this issue, we administered α-methylnorepinephrine (αMNE) (100 mg/kg body weight, intraperitoneally), a compound that is uptaken by high affinity carriers into NA terminals and persists because it cannot be catabolized by monoamine oxidase (Bellinger et al., 1990, 1992b; Felten et al., 1987c). Preliminary data suggest that αMNE is able to restore fluorescence in only a few nerve profiles in aged rat spleens compared with untreated and vehicle-treated controls, but not even close to the level seen in 3-month-old rats. Increased circulating NE, reported with aging (Ziegler et al., 1976), that would be available for up-take into age-resistant terminals, also would be expected to enhance fluo-rophore-formation in terminals that are intact. These findings support an actual retraction and loss of NA fibers in the aged spleen, presuming that the high affinity uptake system for NE in NA terminals in the aged spleen is not dysfunctional. We have developed a perfused spleen slice model to ex-amine the high affinity uptake, release, and metabolism of [^{3}H]-NE in spleen slices, coupled with fluorescence histochemistry for catechola-mines to quantitate NA innervation in alternate slices (Bellinger et al., 1990). Preliminary studies using spleen slices from 3- and 21-month-old rats indicate that the efficiency of uptake of [^{3}H]-NE per nerve terminal is greatly enhanced in old rats, the result of an increase in the density high-affinity carrier sites on age-resistant nerve terminals acting as a compensa-tory mechanism for declining splenic NE content or the loss of NA nerve terminals.

We measured βAR density on splenocytes of F344 rats as a function of age from the same spleens used for histofluorescence and measurements of splenic NE concentration (Ackerman et al., 1991; Bellinger et al., 1992b). These animals were carefully examined for pathologic abnormalities. These studies revealed an increase in the density of βAR on splenocytes with age, consistent with upregulation of βAR in response to declining NE levels. No differences in receptor affinity were detected.

OTHER LYMPHOID ORGANS AND AGING

Observations in mesenteric and popliteal lymph nodes in aging mice and rats revealed loss of NA nerves similar to that observed in the spleen (Bel-linger, Ackerman, Felten, Lorton, & Felten, 1989a). However, NA nerve loss did not appear to be a general phenomenon for all NA sympathetic in-nervation, because NA sympathetic innervation of other peripheral or-gans in the rat, such as the heart, persists for 2 years or more. In the thymus, a primary lymphoid organ that begins to involute at puberty, we did not find a decrease in NA innervation. Rather, intact innervation with a greatly increased density of varicosities in the cortex, presumably related to the considerable shrinkage of this organ, was observed in 27-month-old rats (Bellinger et al., 1988). It is interesting to note that in preliminary studies examining SP innervation of the spleen and thymus with immunocytoche-mistry for SP and RIA for SP, we found the reverse phenomenon with ag-ing, that is, SP nerves in the spleen appear to be maintained with normal aging, whereas SP innervation of the thymus decline with age (Bellinger et al., 1989c).

PLASTICITY OF NA NERVES IN AGED RODENT SPLEEN FOLLOWING CHEMICAL SYMPX

Using a regimen of 6-OHDA treatment in F344 rats, we have begun a similar study in aged F344 rats. We have demonstrated that NA nerve fibers are still capable of ingrowth back into the spleen following 6-OHDA treatments in aged rodents (27 months of age) compared with 3-month-old rats; however, initial ingrowth of the NA profiles are delayed until day 15 after the last dose, ingrowth occurs over a slower time course, and the density of NA nerve fibers that return to the spleen is reduced at day 56 compared with their young adult counterpart. These findings indicate that the plasticity of NA innervation of the aged spleen is not as robust as it is in young adult animals, but still occurs. Further, while the density of NA nerves that regrow into the spleen appears to be less robust in aged spleens, NE availability reflected in splenic NE concentration appears to compensate for the reduced number of NA nerves in the aged spleen, in a similar fashion as seen in young adult spleens.

NK CELL ACTIVITY AND PRIMARY ANTIBODY RESPONSE IN YOUNG AND OLD F344 RATS

In pilot studies, NK cell activity in 21-month-old F344 rats is suppressed by greater than 50% compared with 3-month-old controls ($n=6$ for each age group). Administration of keyhole limpet hemocyanin (50, 150, and 450 µg intraperitoneally) to 3-month-old F344 rats demonstrates a robust primary antibody response on day 7 after immunization ($n=4$). IgG and IgM production by splenocytes ($n=4$) rise by day 3 and peaks at day 7. Furthermore, both IgG and IgM production by splenocytes from 21-month-old rats are enhanced compared with 3-month-old control splenocytes.

SUMMARY

We have described the presence of NA innervation of both primary and secondary lymphoid organs. Further we have demonstrated the dynamic changes that occur in sympathetic innervation of lymphoid organs throughout the life-span of the animal, and the plasticity of NA nerves in the spleen following insult. An abundance of evidence has accumulated to indicate a role for sympathetic innervation, and neuroendocrine outflow, in modulation of the immune system across the life-span of the individual. There is evidence supporting involvement of NA sympathetic innervation during development of the immune system, in age-associated changes in immune function, and in disease processes, such as autoimmune disorders. Collectively, these findings indicate that the development of disease states, including autoimmune disorders that increase in frequency with normal aging, depends on highly complex interactions between the nervous and immune systems at multiple sites of information processing. The mechanisms of action, routes of communication between these sites, and the neural and immune mediators that determine the overall health status of an individual awaits further investigation. Studies described in this chapter demonstrate that innervation of lymphoid organs can play an important role in health and illness, and under conditions of marginal functioning of the immune system, the outflow of neural signals may be a critical factor. Future research to elucidate pathways for neural-immune interactions, the identity of neural and immune signal molecules and their mechanism of action in models of aging, disease, and autoimmunity may ultimately lead to unique pharmacologic approaches in the maintenance of immune system homeostasis and host defense mechanisms throughout the life of an individual, and for the intervention of disease.

REFERENCES

Ackerman, K. D., Bellinger, D. L., Felten, S. Y., & Felten, D. L. (1991). Ontogeny and senescence of noradrenergic innervation of the rodent thymus and spleen. In R. Ader, D. L. Felten, & N. Cohen (Eds.), *Psychoneuroimmunology* (2nd ed., Vol. 2, pp. 72–125). New York: Academic Press.

Ader, R., & Cohen, N. (1975). Behaviorally conditioned immunosuppression. *Psychosomatic Medicine, 37,* 333–340.

Ader, R. (1981). *Psychoneuroimmunology.* New York: Academic Press.

Ader, R., & Cohen, N. (1982). Behaviorally conditioned immunosuppression and murine systemic lupus erythematosus. *Science, 215,* 1534–1536.

Beckner, S. K., & Farrar, W. L. (1988). Potentiation of lymphokine-activated killer cells differentiation and lymphocyte proliferation by stimulation of protein kinase C or inhibition of adenylate cyclase. *Journal of Immunology, 140,* 208–214.

Bellinger, D. L., Ackerman, K. D., Felten, S. Y., & Felten, D. L. (1992). A longitudinal study of age-related loss of noradrenergic nerves and lymphoid cells in the aged rat spleen. *Experimental Neurology, 116,* 295–311.

Bellinger, D. L., Felten, S. Y., & Felten, D. L. (1992a). Neural-immune interactions: Neurotransmitter signaling of cells of the immune system. *Annual Review of Psychiatry, 11,* 127–144.

Bellinger, D. L., Felten, S. Y., & Felten, D. L. (1992b). Noradrenergic sympathetic innervation of lymphoid orans during development, aging, and autoimmunity. In F. Amenta (Ed.), *Aging of the autonomic nervous system.*

Bellinger, D. L., Ackerman, K. D., Felten, S. Y., Lorton, D., & Felten, D. L. (1989). Noradrenergic sympathetic innervation of thymus, spleen, and lymph nodes:

Aspects of development, aging and plasticity in neural immune interaction. In *Proceedings of a symposium on interactions between the neuroendocrine and immune systems* (pp. 35–66). Roma, Milano: Pythagora Press.

Bellinger, D. L., Felten, S. Y., Collier, T. J., & Felten, D. L. (1987). Noradrenergic sympathetic innervation of the spleen: IV. Morphometric analysis in adult and aged F344 rats. *Journal of Neuroscience Research, 18,* 55–63.

Bellinger, D. L., Felten, S. Y., & Felten, D. L. (1988). Maintenance of noradrenergic sympathetic innervation in the involuted thymus of the aged Fischer 344 rat. *Brain Behavior & Immunity, 2,* 133–150.

Bellinger, D. L., Felten, S. Y., Lorton, D., & Felten, D. L. (1989). Origin of noradrenergic innervation of the spleen in rats. *Brain Behavior & Immunity, 3,* 291–311.

Bellinger, D. L., Lorton, D., Felten, S. Y., & Felten D. L. (1989). Effects of age on substance P (SP)+ nerve fibers in the spleen of Fischer 344 rats. *Society of Neurosciences Abstract, 15,* 714.

Bellinger, D. L., Lorton, D., Felten, S. Y., & Felten, D. L. (1990). Age-related alterations in norepinephrine uptake in the rat spleen [Abstract]. *Society of Neurosciences Abstract, 16,* 1210.

Besedovsky, H. O., Rey, A. del, Sorkin, E., Da Prada, M., Burri, R., & Honegger, C. (1983). The immune response evokes changes in brain noradrenergic neurons. *Science, 221,* 564–565.

Blecha, F., Barry, R. A., & Kelley, K. W. (1982a). Stress-induced alterations in delayed-type hypersensitivity to SRBC and contact sensitivity to DNFB in mice. *Proceedings of the Society for Experimental Biology and Medicine, 169,* 239–246.

Blecha, F., Barry, R. A., Kelley, K. W., & Satterlee, D. G. (1982b). Adrenal involvement in the expression of delayed-type hypersensitivity to SRBC and contact sensitivity to DNFB in stressed mice. *Proceedings of the Society of Experimental Biology and Medicine, 169,* 247–252.

Capocelli, A., Bellinger, D. L., Felten, D. L., & Coleman, P. D. (1985). Age-related decrease in the catecholaminergic innervation of the mouse spleen [Abstract]. *Society of Neuroscience, 11,* 662.

Carlson, S. L., Felten, D. L., Livnat, S., & Felten, S. Y. (1987). Alterations of monoamines in specific central autonomic nuclei following immunization in mice. *Brain Behavior & Immunity, 1,* 52–63.

Cohen, S., & Syme, S. L. (1985). *Social support and health.* New York: Academic Press.

Crary, B., Borysenko, M., Sutherland, D. C., Kutz, I., Borysenko, J. Z., & Benson, H. (1983a). Decreased in mitogen responsiveness of mononuclear cells from peripheral blood after epinephrine administration in humans. *Journal of Immunology, 130,* 694–697.

Crary, B., Hauser, S. L., Borysenko, M., Kutz, I., Hoban, C., Ault, K. A., Weiner, H. L., & Benson, H. (1983b). Epinephrine-induced changes in the distribution of lymphocyte subsets in peripheral blood of humans. *Journal of Immunology, 131,* 1178–1181.

Cunnick, J. E., Lysle, D. T., Armfield, A., & Rabin, B. S. (1988). Shock-induced modulation of lymphocyte responsiveness and natural killer activity: Differential mechanisms of induction. *Brain Behavior & Immunity, 2,* 102–113.

Depelchin, A., & Letesson, J. J. (1981). Adrenaline influence on the immune response: I. Accelerating or suppressor effects according to the time of application [Letter]. *Immunology Letters, 3,* 199–205.

Didier, M., Aussel, C., B, Ferrua, & Fehlmann, M. (1987). Regulation of interleukin 2 synthesis by cAMP in human T cells. *Journal of Immunology, 39,* 1179–1184.

Ernström, U., & Sandberg, G. (1974). Stimulation of lymphocyte release from the spleen by theophylline and isoproternol. *Acta Physiolojica Scandinavia, 90,* 202–209.

Esterling, B., & Rabin, B. S. (1987). Stress-induced alteration of T-lymphocyte subsets and humoral immunity in mice. *Behavioral Neuroscience, 101,* 115–119.

Felten, D. L., Ackerman, K. D., Bellinger, D. L., & Felten, S. Y. (1987a). Time course of depletion of noradrenergic innervation of the splenic white pulp in aged Fischer 344 rats and its relationship to declining populations of specific immune cells [Abstract]. *Society of Neuroscience, 13,* 1380.

Felten, D. L., Ackerman, K. D., Wiegand, S. J., & Felten, S. Y. (1987b). Noradrenergic sympathetic innervation of the spleen: I. Nerve fibers associate with lymphocytes and macrophages in specific compartments of the splenic white pulp. *Journal of Neurosciences Research, 18,* 28–36.

Felten, D. L., Felten, S. Y., Bellinger, D. L., Carlson, S. L., Ackerman, K. D., Madden, K. S., Olschowka, J. A., & Livnat, S. (1987c). Noradrenergic sympathetic neural interactions with the immune system: Structure and function. *Immunology Reviews, 100,* 225–260.

Felten, D. J., Bellinger, D. L., & Felten, S. Y. (1989). Age-related alterations in the distribution of neuropeptide Y (NPY)-positive nerve fibers in the rat spleen. [Abstract]. *Society for Neuroscience, 15,* 714.

Felten, D. L., Cohen, N., Ader, R., Felten, S. Y., Carlson, S. L., & Roszman, T. L. (1991). Central neural circuits involved in neural-immune interactions. In R. Ader, D. L. Felten, & N. Cohen (Eds.) *Psychoneuroimmunology* (2nd ed., Vol. 2, pp. 1–26). New York: Academic Press.

Felten, S. Y., Peterson, R. G., Shea, P. A., Besch, H. R. Jr., & Felten, D. L. (1982). Effects of streptozotocin diabetes on the noradrenergic innervation of the rat heart: A longitudinal histofluorescence and neurochemical study. *Brain Research Bulletin, 8,* 593–607.

Felten, S. Y., Housel, J., & Felten, D. L. (1986). Use of in vivo dialysis for evaluation of splenic norepinephrine and serotonin [Abstract]. *Society of Neuroscience, 12,* 1065.

Felten, S. Y., Bellinger, D. L., Collier, T. J., Coleman, P. D., & Felten, D. L. (1987). Decreased sympathetic innervation of spleen in aged Fischer 344 rats. *Neurobiology of Aging, 8,* 159–165.

Felten, S. Y., & Olschowka, J. A. (1987). Noradrenergic sympathetic innervation of the spleen: II. Tyrosine hydroxylase (TH)-positive nerve terminals form synaptic-like contacts on lymphocytes in the splenic white pulp. *Journal of Neurosciences Research, 18,* 37–48.

Felten, S. Y., & Felten, D. L. (1991). The innervation of lymphoid organs. In R. Ader, D. L. Felten, & N. Cohen (Eds.), *Psychoneuroimmunology* (2nd ed., Vol. 2, pp. 27–69). New York: Academic Press.

Geschwind, N., & Behan, P. (1982). Left-handedness: Association with immune disease, migraine, and developmental learning disorder. *Proceedings of the National Academy of Science, USA, 79,* 5097–5100.

Gisler, R. H., Bussard, A. E., Mazié, J. C., & Hess, R. (1971). Hormonal regulation of the immune response: I. Induction of an immune response in vitro with lymphoid cells from mice exposed to acute systemic stress. *Cellular Immunology, 2,* 634–645.

Gorczynski, R. M., Macrae, S., & Kennedy, M. (1982). Conditioned immune response associated with allogeneic skin grafts in mice. *Journal of Immunology, 129,* 704–709.

Hall, N. R., McGillis, J. P., Spangelo, B. L., Henly, D. L., Chrousos, G. P., Schulte, H. M., & Goldstein, A. L. (1985. Thymic hormone effects on the brain and neuroendocrine circuits. In R. Guillemin, M. Cohn, & T. Melnechuk (Eds.), *Neural modulation of immunity* (pp. 179–196). New York: Raven Press.

Hellstrand, K., Hermodsson, S., & Strannegård, Ö. (1985). Evidence for a β-adrenoceptor-mediated regulation of human natural killer cells. *Journal of Immunology, 134,* 4095-4099.

Irwin, M., Vale, W., & Britton, K. T. (1987). Central corticotropin-releasing factor suppresses natural killer cytotoxicity. *Brain Behavior & Immunity, 1,* 81–87.

Johnson, D. L., Ashmore, R. C., & Gordon, M. A. (1981). Effects of beta-adrenergic agents on the murine lymphocyte response to mitogen stimulation. *Journal of Immunopharmacology, 3,* 205–219.

Kabiersh, A., del Rey, A., Honegger, C. G., & Besedovsky, H. D. (1988). Interleukin-1 induces changes in norepinephrine metabolism in the rat brain. *Brain Behavior & Immunity, 2,* 267–274.

Katz, P., Zaytoun, A. M., & Fauci, A. S. (1982). Mechanisms of human cell-mediated cytotoxicity: I. Modulation of natural killer cell activity by cyclic nucleotides. *Journal of Immunology, 129,* 287–296.

Keller, S. E., Schleifer, S. J., Liotta, A. S., Bond, R. N., Farhoody, N., & Stein, M. (1988). Stress-induced alterations of immunity in hypophysectomized rats. *Proceedings of the National Academy of Sciences, 85,* 9297–9301.

Kiecolt-Glaser, J. K., & Gaser, R. (1991). Stress and immune function in human. In R. Ader, D. L. Felten, & N. Cohen (Eds), *Psychoneuroimmunology* (2nd ed., pp. 849–867). New York: Academic Press.

Koff, W. C., & Dunegan, M. A. (1985). Modulation of macrophage-mediated tumoricidal activity by neuropeptides and neurohormones. *Journal of Immunology, 135,* 350–354.

Koff, W. C., & Dunegan, M. A. (1986). Neuroendocrine hormones suppress macrophage-mediated lysis of herpes simplex virus-infected cells. *Journal of Immunology, 136,* 705–709.

Korneva, E. A. (1987). Neuroimmune interactions. *Annals of the New York Academy of Science, 496,* 318–337.

Krall, J. F., Connelly, M., Weisbart, R., & Tuck, M. L. (1981). Age-related elevation of plasma catecholamine concentration and reduced responsiveness of lymphocyte adenylate cyclase. *Journal of Clinical Endocrinology of Metabolism, 52,* 863–867.

Lappin, D., & Whaley, K. (1979). Adrenergic receptors on monocytes modulate complement component synthesis. *Journal of Histochemistry, Cytochemistry, 27*, 936.

Livnat, S., Eisen, J., Felten, D. L., Felten, S. Y., Irwin, J., Madden, K. S., & Sundaresan, P. J. (1988). Behavioral and sympathetic neural modulation of immune function. In A. Dahlstrom, R. M. Belmaker & M. Sandler (Eds.), *Progress in catecholamine research, Part A: Basic aspects and peripheral mechanisms* pp. 539–546. New York: Alan R. Liss.

Livnat, S., Felten, S. Y., Carlson, S. L., Bellinger, D. L., & Felten, D. L. (1985). Involvement of peripheral and central catecholamine systems in neural-immune interactions. *Journal Neuroimmunology, 10*, 5–30.

Livnat, D., Madden, K. S., Felten, D. L., & Felten, S. Y. (1987). Regulation of the immune system by sympathetic neural mechanisms. *Progress Neuro-psychopharmacologic & Biologic Psychiatry, 11*, 145–152.

Madden, K. S., Felten, S. Y., Felten, D. L., & Livnat, S. (1989). Sympathetic neural modulation of the immune system: I. Depression of T cell immunity in vivo and in vitro following chemical sympathectomy. *Brain Behavior & Immunity, 3*, 72–89.

Madden, K. S., & Livnat, S. (1991). Catecholaminergic influences on immune reactivity. In R. Ader, D. L. Felten, & N. Cohen (Eds), *Psychoneuroimmunology* (2nd ed., vol. 2, pp. 283–310). New York: Academic Press.

Melmon, K. L., Bourne, H. R., Weinstein, Y., Shearer, G. M., Kram, J., & Bauminger, S. (1974). Hemolytic plaque formation by leukocytes in vitro: Control by vasoactive hormones. *Journal of Clinical Investigation, 53*, 13–21.

Plaut, S. M., & Friedman, S. B. (1981). Psychosocial factors in infections disease. In R. Ader (Ed.), *Psychoneuroimmunology* (pp. 3–30). New York: Academic Press.

Riley, V. (1981). Psychoneuroendocrine influences on immunocompetence and neoplasia. *Science, 212*, 1100–1109.

Riley, V., Fitzmaurice, M. A., & Spackman, D. H. (1981). Psychoneuroimmunologic factors in neoplasia. In R. Ader (Ed.), *Psychoneuroimmunology*, New York: Academic Press.

Rogers, M. P., Reich, P., Strom, T. B., & Carpenter, C. B. (1976). Behaviorally conditioned immunosuppression: Replication of a recent study. *Psychosomatic Medicine, 38*, 447–451.

Sanders, V. M. & Munson, A. E. (1985). Norepinephrine and the antibody response. *Pharmacology Review, 37*, 229–248.

Saphier, D., Abramsky, O., Mor, G., & Ovadia, H. (1987a). A neurophysiological correlate of an immune response. *Annals of the New York Academy of Science, 496*, 354–359.

Saphier, D., Abramsky, O., Mor, G., & Ovadia, H. (1987b) Multiunit electrical activity in conscious rats during an immune response. *Brain Behavior & Immunity, 1*, 40–51.

Shavit, Y., Lewis, J. W., Terman, G. W., Gale, R. P., & Liebeskind, J. C. (1984). Opioid peptides mediate the suppressive effect of stress on natural killer cell cytotoxicity. *Science, 223*, 188–190.

Singh, U. (1979). Effect of catecholamines on lymphopoiesis in fetal mouse thymic explants. *European Journal of Immunology, 14*, 757–759.

Sklar, L. S. & Anisman, H. (1979). Stress and coping factors influence tumor growth. *Science, 205*, 513–515.

Solomon, G. F. (1969). Stress and antibody response in rats. *International Archives of Allergy & Applied Immunology, 35*, 97–104.

Solomon, G. F. (1981). Emotional and personality factors in the onset and course of autoimmune disease, particularly rheumatoid arthritis. In R. Ader (Ed.) *Psychoneuroimmunology,* New York: Academic Press.

Spengler, R. N., Allen, R. M., Remick, D. G., Strieter, R. M., & Kunkel, S. L. (1990). Stimulation of alpha-adrenergic receptor augments the production of macrophage-derived tumor necrosis factor. *Journal of Immunology, 145*, 1430–1434.

Strom, T. B., Carpenter, C. B., Garovoy, M. R., Austen, K. F., Merrill, J. P., & Kaliner, M. (1973). The modulating influence of cyclic nucleotides upon lymphocyte-mediated cytotoxicity. *Journal of Experimental Medicine, 138*, 381–393.

Titinchi, S., & Clark, B. (1984). Alpha2-adrenoceptors in human lymphocytes: Direct characterisation by [3H]yohimbine binding. *Biochemistry Biophysics Research Community, 121*, 1-7.

Watson, J., Epstein, R., & Cohn, M. (1973). Cyclic nucleotides as intracellular mediators of the expression of antigen-sensitive cells. *Nature, 246*, 405–409.

Wayner, E. A., Flannery, G. R., & Singer, G. (1978). Effect of taste aversion conditioning on the primary antibody response to sheep red blood cells and Brucella abortus in the albino rat. *Physiology & Behavior, 21*, 995–1000.

Weiner, H. (1977). *Psychobiology and human disease.* New York: Elsevier.

Weksler, M. E. & Siskind, G. W. (1984). The cellular basis of immune senescence. *Monographs in Developmental Biology, 17*, 110–121.

Williams, J. M., Peterson, R. G., Shea, P. A., Schmedtje, J. F., Bauer, D. C., & Felten, D. L. (1981). Sympathetic innervation of murine thymus and spleen: Evidence for a functional link between the nervous and immune systems. *Brain Research Bulletin, 6*, 83–94.

Ziegler, M. G., Lake, C. R., & Kopin, I. J. (1976). Plasma noradrenaline increases with age. *Nature* (London), *261*, 333–335.

Endogenous Opioids, Immune Function, and Aging

10

John E. Morley

The last decade has seen an explosion in studies on mind-body interactions. The concept that complete healing involves both physical and mental components is slowly becoming firmly established among physicians. The pioneering observations by Galen that breast cancer does better in sanguine than in melancholy women finds its modern counterpart in support groups for women with breast cancer. Before the development of antituberculous drugs, William Osler suggested that the cure of tuberculosis depended far more on factors in the mind than in the chest. Today we know that stressed caregivers and bereaved persons develop abnormalities in immune function that make them at greater risk to develop infection. Older persons who have aged successfully have greater NK cell activity than do younger persons, suggesting that these cells confer a survival advantage. NK cell activity can be increased by exercise and mental activity.

The ways in which the mind can modulate immune function and in which immune function can modulate mental activity have only been illuminated in the last decade. For example, Bellinger and colleagues (1992) have shown that sympathetic nerve fibers to the spleen impinge not only on blood vessels in this organ but also on the lymphocytes. Chemical sympathectomy produces immune system changes in young rodents that closely parallel the immune system changes in older rodents. Older rodents show immunohistochemical evidence of sympathetic nervous system degeneration. Other studies have shown that cytokines can modulate acetylcholine synthesis in the hippocampus and thus play a role in memory function and the pathogenesis of delirium. Activated human T cells cause rat brain astrocytes and oligodendrocytes to proliferate, and this has been demonstrated to be due to the release of IL-1 and IL-2 (Kemeny, Solomon, Morley, et al., 1992).

β-Endorphin (the body's own morphine) not only plays a role centrally and at the level of the spinal cord in producing analgesia, but is also released from the pituitary gland, together with ACTH, into the circulation where it can act as a hormone. There is increasing evidence that the major target tissue of circulating β-endorphin is the immune system. Further endogenous opioid modulation of immune function may be mediated by the release of methionine- and leucine-enkephalin–related peptides from the adrenal medulla at times of stress.

Endogenous opioid secretion and receptor activity tends to decline with age (Morley, Flood, & Silver, 1990). Both the circadian rhythm of β-endorphin secretion and cerebrospinal fluid levels decline with age. These changes in opioid activity with aging have been shown to be associated with some of the common physiologic changes of aging (see Table 10.1). This chapter briefly explores the potential role of endogenous opioids as a link in the ability of the brain to modulate immune function and its relationship to aging.

β-ENDORPHIN AND IMMUNE FUNCTION

Endogenous opioids have been shown to have a variety of effects on the immune system (Morley, Solomon, & Benton, 1991) (see Table 10.2). β-Endorphin has been demonstrated, in particular, to increase NK activity (Kay, Allen, & Morley 1984; Kay, Morley, & VonRee, 1987). This effect is reversed by naloxone administration and is therefore dependent on activation of an opioid receptor. Nonopioid fragments of β-endorphin (amino acids 2–7, 2–9, 12–16, 6–17) also enhance NK activity, and this effect is naloxone reversible. The 10–13 and 10–16 fragments are inactive. This demonstrates an important role for the α-helical portion (amino acids 6–9) of the molecule in modulation of NK-cell activity. Overall, these findings suggest that the β-endorphin-lymphocyte receptor is of the "address-message" type with the α-helical portion representing the address portion and the opioid moiety representing the message portion (Morley & Kay, 1986).

TABLE 10.1 Physiological Changes with Aging That Are Associated with Decline in the Opioid System

1. **Decreased food intake (kappa opioids)**

2. **Decreased fluid intake (mu opioids)**

3. **Age-related memory dysfunction (continued amnestic effect of beta-endorphin in presence of a decline in acetylcholine function)**

4. **Secondary hypogonadism (beta-endorphin inhibits luteinizing hormone secretion)**

5. **Increased free radical (superoxide) production leading to age-related tissue destruction.**

6. **Immune dysfunction**

TABLE 10.2   Effects of β-Endorphin on the Immune System

1. **Enhancement of chemotaxis for neutrophils and monocytes**

2. **Enhancement of lymphocyte proliferative response to mitogens**

3. **Enhancement of primary antibody response**

4. **Enhancement of natural killer cell activity**

5. **Enhancement of gamma-interferon production**

6. **Stimulation of superoxide production**

Several lines of evidence suggest that receptors for IL-2 and opioids on lymphocytes appear are able to directly modulate one another. Interferon and IL-2 both produce naloxone-reversible increases in NK activity (Kay, Morley, & Allen, 1990). Naloxone and β-endorphin both displace radiolabeled IL-2 receptors. Radiolabeled naloxone binding to phytohemagglutinin-stimulated lymphocytes is inhibited by IL-2. Norman, Morley, and Chang (1988) have demonstrated that the spleen cell mitogenic response to Con A is stimulated by β-endorphin in young mice but not in old mice. This suggests a decline in opioid ability to stimulate immune function with aging.

Physiologic Effects

Physical exercise causes an increase in both NK cell numbers and activity (Fiatarone, Morley, Bloom, et al., 1988). The increase in NK activity is partially blocked by the opioid antagonist naloxone which also inhibits the ability of β-endorphin to stimulate NK cells in vitro. In other studies, stressful mental activity was demonstrated to enhance NK cell activity (Naliboff, Benton, Solomon, et al., 1991).

Exercise is equally effective in enhancing NK activity in both young and old individuals (Solomon, Fiatarone, Morley, Bloom, et al., 1989). However, stressful mental activity does not enhance NK activity in old persons (Naliboff et al., 1991). These studies suggest that NK cells from older persons are capable of responding to severe but not minor stressors.

There are several studies suggesting that cancer prevalence is decreased in persons who perform moderate exercise over their lifetime. There is an inverse correlation between moderate exercise and colon cancer in males (Vera, Graham, & Zielezny, 1984). Breast and reproductive malignancies are reduced in women who regularly exercise (Frisch, Wyshak, & Albright, 1985). Overall, these studies suggest that exercise may inhibit tumor growth through β-endorphin stimulated NK cell activity.

STRESS, β-ENDORPHIN, AND THE AGING PROCESS

Hans Selye originally suggested that there were two types of stress: good, or eustress, and bad, or distress. We have found that older persons who have good psychologic coping mechanisms often have better NK cell activity than those who cope less well with stress (Fiatarone et al., 1988). The data presented above has led us to develop an aging theory based on the effects of β-endorphin release on the immune system, in response to stress and the organism's response to stress (Figure 10.1). Stress, either physical

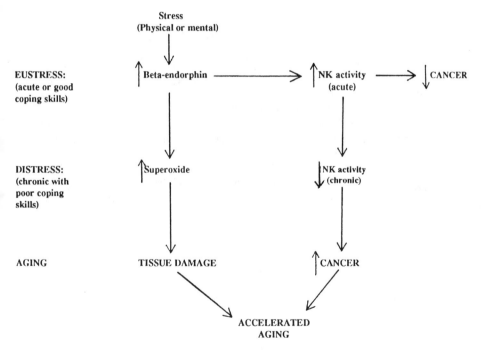

FIGURE 10.1 Stress, β-Endorphin, Immune Dysfunction and the Aging Process (↑ = increase and ↓ = decrease)

or mental, leads to the release of β-endorphin from the pituitary and the acute increase in NK cell activity, decreasing the propensity to develop cancer (eustress). However, if the stress is prolonged or overwhelms individuals' ability to cope with the stress, there is eventually a tolerance to the β-endorphin response and an increase in tumorigenesis. In addition, prolonged β-endorphin release also increases superoxide free radical formation, which would result in tissue destruction(distress).

These formulations clearly suggest that mind-body interactions play a major role in the modulation of the immune system and possibly in the aging process itself. β-Endorphin represents one of the putative mediators through which these complex interactions may occur. However, it should be recognized that it is likely that there are multiple mediators and that it is the interplay between these numerous actors that eventually is responsible for these mind-body interactions. As succinctly stated by the English philosopher, Emerson Pugh: "If the human brain were so simple that we could understand it, we would be so simple that we couldn't."

REFERENCES

Bellinger, D. L., Ackerman, K. D., Felten, S. Y., & Felten, D. L. (1992). A longitudinal study of age-related loss of noradrenergic nerves and lymphoid cells in the rat spleen. *Experimental Neurology, 116,* 295–311.

Fiatarone, M. A., Morley, J. E., Bloom, E. T., Benton, D., Makinodan, T., & Solomon, G. F. (1988). Endogenous opioids and the exercise-induced augmentation of natural killer cell activity. *Journal of Laboratory and Clinical Medicine, 112,* 544–552.

Fiatarone, M. A., Morley, J. E., & Bloom, E. T., Benton, D., Makinodan, T., & Solomon, G. F. (1989). The effect of exercise on natural killer cell activity in young and old subjects. *Journal of Gerontology: Medical Science, 44,* M37–45.

Frisch, R. E., Wyshak, G., & Albright, N. L. (1985). Lower prevalence of breast cancer and careers of the reproductive system among former college athletes compared to non-athletes. *British Journal of Cancer, 52, 885–891.*

Kay, N., Allen, J., & Morley, J. E. (1984). Endorphins stimulate normal human peripheral blood lymphocyte natural killer activity. *Life Sciences, 35,* 53–59.

Kay, N. E., Morley, J. E., & Allen, J. I. (1990). Interaction between endogenous opioids and IL-2 on PHA-stimulated human lymphocytes. *Immunology, 70,* 485–491.

Kay, N., Morley, J. E., & Von Ree, J. M. (1987). Enhancement of human lymphocyte natural killing function by non-opioid fragments of beta-endorphin. *Life Sciences, 40,* 1083–1087.

Kemeny, M. E., Solomon, G. F., Morley, J. E., & Herbert, T. L. (1992). Psychoneuroimmunology. In C. B. Nemeroff (Ed.), *Neuroendocrinology* (pp. 563–591). Boca Raton: CRC Press.

Morley, J. E., Flood, J. F., & Silver, A. J. (1990). Opioid peptides and aging. *Annals of the New York Academy of Sciences USA, 579,* 123–132.

Morley, J. E., Kay, N. (1986). Neuropeptides as modulators of immune function. *Psychopharmacological Bulletin, 22,* 1089–1092.

Morley, J. E., Solomon, G. F., & Benton, D. (1991). Opioids and physiological regulation of natural killer cell activity and flushing. In N. Plotnikoff, A. Murgo, R. Faith, & J. Wybran (Eds.), *Stress and immunity* (pp. 409–415). Boca Raton: CRC Press.

Naliboff, B. D., Benton, D., Solomon, G. F., Morley, J. E., Fahey, J. L., Bloom, E. T., Makinodan, T., & Gilmore, S. L. (1991). Immunological changes in young and old adults during brief laboratory stress. *Psychosomatic Medicine, 53,* 121–132.

Norman, D. C., Morley, J. E., & Chang, M. -P. (1988). Aging decreases beta-endorphin enhancement of T-cell mitogenesis in mice. *Mechanisms of Aging and Development, 44,* 185–191.

Solomon, G. F., Fiatarone, M. A., Benton, D., & Morley, J. E. (1988). Psychoimmunologic and endorphin function in the aged. *Annals of the New York Academy of Sciences, 321,* 43–58.

Vera, J. E., Graham, S., & Zielezny, M. (1984). Lifetime occupational exercise and colon cancer. *American Journal of Epidemiology, 119,* 1005–1014.

Aging, Stress, and Immune Function:

Neural Regulation of Natural Killer Cell Activity

Michael Irwin

Aging is associated with an elevation of sympathetic tone, impairment of immune function, and an increased susceptibility to stress-induced immune suppression. Our recent clinical studies show that sympathetic activation has a role in the reduction of cellular immunity in persons who are aged and undergoing life stress or depression. This suggests that abnormal regulation of sympathetic outflow by the central nervous system might contribute to stress-induced changes of immune function in aging (Irwin, Brown, Patterson, et al., 1991). In support of this hypothesis, this chapter reviews the role of central corticotropin releasing hormone (CRH) in the regulation of autonomic outflow and immunity. Release of this neuropeptide following stress has been found to elevate sympathetic activity and reduce cellular immune function. Furthermore, aged rats show an increased responsivity to central CRH with exaggerated activation of the sympathetic nervous system and reduction of NK cell activity. The implications of these data, i.e., that central CRH systems modulate sympathetic activity and reduce immune function in aged organisms, are discussed.

AGED-RELATED CHANGES IN NK ACTIVITY:
RELEVANCE TO HEALTH

Aging is associated with an "impaired adaptive response" (Ackerman, Bellinger, & Felten, 1991) that is characterized by a decline of immune responses to exogenous stimuli (mainly involving T-cell dependent functions), dysregulation, and a loss of self-tolerance (Hallgren, Buckley, Gilbertson, et al., 1973; Makinodan & McKay, 1980; O'Leary & Hallgren, 1991), which are likely to contribute to the increased morbidity in the elderly (Makinodan & Kay, 1980).

In animal models of aging, there is general agreement that NK activity is diminished with age, despite no change or even an increase in the numbers of circulating NK cells (Bash & Vogel, 1984; Blair, Staskawicz, & Sam, et al., 1987; Shigemoto, Kishimoto, & Yamamura, 1975; Weindruch, Devens, Raff, et al., 1983). In humans, some studies (Irwin, Brown, Patterson, et al., 1991; Facchini, Mariani, Mariani, et al., 1987; Sato, Fuse, & Kuwata, 1979) but not all (Krishnaraj & Blandford, 1987) have demonstrated an age-related reduction of NK activity. However, variation in the distribution of NK activity is greater in an elderly population. More than 10% of persons in the 50- to 80-year span have a marked reduction of NK activity with lytic values one-third to one-fourth of the level found in other age groups (Adler & Nagel, 1977).

A series of recent observations collectively argues that NK cells play a salient role in host defense against viral illness. In animals, an enhanced susceptibility to herpes simplex virus type 1 and cytomegalovirus has been found to occur in the absence of NK cells (Bancroft, Shellam, & Chalmer, 1981; Bukowski, Warner, Dennert, et al., 1985; Habu, Akamatsu, Tamaoki, et al., 1984). In humans, positive correlations have been made between sensitivity to viral infection and depressed NK cell function (Padgett, Reiquam, Henson, et al., 1968; Sullivan, Byron, Brewster, et al., 1980). Futhermore, Biron, Byron, and Sullivan (1989) described a case with an extreme susceptibility to herpes virus infections and a complete and specific loss of NK cells, NK-cell function, and inducible NK cell activity.

AGING AND ELEVATED SYMPATHETIC ACTIVITY:
ROLE OF STRESS AND CRH

Clinical studies have shown that blood pressure (Pfeifer, Weinberg, Cook, et al., 1983), sympathetic nerve activity (Iwase, Mano, Watanabe, et al., 1991), and plasma concentrations of norepinephrine and neuropeptide Y are increased with age (Irwin et al., 1991; Pfeifer et al., 1983; Ziegler, Lake, & Kopin, 1976). The latter changes are secondary to increased hormone production rather than a decrease in their clearance (Supiano, Linares, Smith, et al., 1990; Veith, Featherstone, et al., 1986). In addition to an age-related increase of basal levels of sympathetic activity, an enhanced responsivity of the sympathetic nervous system has also been found. Aged humans and animals show an exaggerated release of catecholamines following physical stressors such as exercise or postural change (Sowers, Rubenstein, & Stern, 1983; Supiano et al., 1990).

To test whether increases of sympathetic outflow contribute to the decrease of NK activity in aging, we evaluated the presence of severe life stress and depression, and measured levels of circulating catecholamines and neuropeptide Y as well as NK activity in stressed Alzheimer's caregivers, depressed patients, normal aged individuals (controls 2) and normal middle-aged subjects (controls 1) (Irwin et al., 1991). The effect of age, chronic stress of Alzheimer's caregiving, and depression on sympathetic activity was evaluated by the measurement of basal and dynamic levels of epinephrine, norepinephrine, and neuropeptide Y following orthostatic challenge.

The findings of this study suggested that activation of the sympathetic nervous system and release of neuropeptide Y is associated with a reduction of values of NK cytotoxicity in aging, life stress, and depression (Irwin et al., 1991). First, sympathetic activity as measured by plasma levels of neuropeptide Y was elevated both in depressed patients and in Alzheimer's caregivers compared with respective age-matched controls. In addition, old controls 2 had higher levels of neuropeptide Y compared with the middle-aged controls 1. Second, a reduction of NK activity was found in the depressed patients and in the old controls 2 compared with controls 1. However, NK lytic activity was similar in the Alzheimer's caregivers and controls 2. Third, the circulating concentration of the sympathetic neurotransmitter neuropeptide Y was inversely correlated with NK activity in the total sample. Finally, regression analyses demonstrated that plasma levels of neuropeptide Y appear to be a distinct correlate of NK cell activity, independent of the contribution of age and circulating levels of catecholamines.

Neuropeptide Y has been previously implicated as a potential immunomodulatory transmitter (Ackerman et al., 1991). However, the mechanisms of action of neuropeptide Y on lymphocytes such as the NK cell are not yet known, even though neuroanatomic observations have demonstrated that neuropeptide Y–containing nerve fibers innervate immune compartments of the secondary lymphoid tissue such as the spleen (Ackerman et al., 1991). Neuropeptide Y might bind to the NK cell and alter cytotoxicity, or this sympathetic cotransmitter might produce changes in immune activity by potenting the action of norepinephrine at β_2-adrenergic receptors on lymphocytes.

In summary, elevated plasma levels of neuropeptide Y were found in aged individuals, stressed persons caregiving for a spouse with Alzheimer's disease, and patients with major depressive disorder compared with middle-aged controls. Importantly, aged and stressed Alzheimer's caregivers were likely to show an elevation of plasma levels of neuropeptide Y that was even greater than that found in aged persons who were not stressed. Finally, circulating levels of neuropeptide Y were inversely correlated with NK activity distinct from any immunomodulatory effects of epinephrine and norepinephrine. These data suggested that chronic activation of the sympathetic nervous system and release of neuropeptide Y is associated with a reduction of NK activity in aged persons and subjects undergoing severe life stress or depression.

Animal Studies

Consistent with these clinical findings, animal studies have found an interaction between age and stress in the increase of sympathetic tone. Adrenal medullary stores of norepinephrine are elevated in aged rats (Kingsley, Nekvasil, & Snyder, 1991). McCarty (1985) described a hypersecretory profile of catecholamines following acute cold stress in aged animals. To evaluate further the effects of aging on the regulation of sympathetic activity as well as immune function following stress, responses of the autonomic and immune systems have been examined using exogenous CRH.

CRH has been implicated as a neurotransmitter in the central nervous system that coordinates neuroendocrine (Rivier, Rivier & Vale, 1982) and autonomic outflow (Brown, 1986; Brown, Fisher, Webb, et al., 1985; (Brown, Fisher, Spiess, et al., 1982), and thereby modulates immune responses (Irwin, Hauger, Jones, et al., 1990; Irwin, Vale, & Britton, 1987; Stausbaugh & Irwin, 1992). Indeed, the release of endogenous CRH following stress has been demonstrated to induce elevations in plasma levels of norepinephrine and epinephrine (Brown et al., 1982), which mediate the suppression of NK activity independent of the activation of the pituitary adrenal axis (Irwin et al., 1990; Irwin, Vale, & Rivier, 1990).

An age-related dysregulation of CRH and other physiologic systems has been proposed (Sapolsky, Krey, & McEwen, 1986), and hypothalamic CRH might be hypersecreted in aged animals. For example, release of CRH from hypothalamic fragments of aged rates is increased at rest and following acetylcholine stimulation in vitro (Scaccianoce, DeSciullo, & Angelucci, 1990), anterior pituitary response to CRH in vivo is dampened in aged animals (Hylka, Sonntag, & Meites, 1984), and an age-related decrease in hypothalamic- and anterior pituitary CRH receptors has been found (Heroux, Grigoriadis, & DeSouza, 1991).

Based on the key role of CRH in the regulation of both the autonomic nervous system and NK cells and the possibility of age-related changes CRH systems, we have examined CRH-induced activation of the sympathetic nervous system and suppression of immunity. Because responses of plasma levels of catecholamines following stress are increased in aged rats (McCarthy, 1985), we hypothesized that CRH will also induce an exaggerated release of epinephrine, norepinephrine, and neuropeptide Y in the aged animals. Furthermore, this increased sympathetic response following CRH was proposed to be associated with a further decrement of NK activity in aged rats compared with young animals independent of adrenocortical responses. To test these predictions, splenic NK activity was assayed, and basal levels and responses of epinephrine, norepinephrine, neuropeptide Y, and corticosterone were determined following the central administration of CRH in aged and young rats (Irwin, Hauger, & Brown, 1992).

For epinephrine, basal levels were similar in the aged and young animals. However, CRH induced an elevation of epinephrine in the aged rats that occurred more rapidly, reached a higher peak value, and was sustained throughout the blood sampling period compared with responses in the young rats.

In contrast with similar basal levels of epinephrine in the aged and young rats, basal levels of norepinephrine were significantly higher in the aged rats than those in the young animals. Responses of plasma norepinephrine in the aged animals following CRH infusion again occurred more rapidly, reached higher peak values, and were sustained throughout the experimental sampling period, whereas the young Fischer rats showed only a modest increase in norepinephrine 15 minutes following CRH, which returned to baseline at 60 minutes. Basal plasma levels of neuropeptide Y were also elevated in the aged animals compared with the young rats, similar to the aged-related increase in plasma norepinephrine. In addition, CRH induced a transient increase in circulating concentrations of neuropeptide Y in the aged animals but not in the young rats. Neither basal levels nor responses of corticosterone to CRH infusion differed between the aged and young rats. CRH induced a similar increase in plasma corticosterone, which was sustained in both age groups of animals throughout the testing interval.

NK activity was significantly different between the four groups 1 hour following intracerebroventricular (ICV) infusion. The aged rats had lower values of NK activity than those found in the young animals. In addition, ICV CRH produced a further reduction of splenic NK cytotoxicity in the aged animals, but did not alter lytic activity in the young animals.

The present study investigated differences in the responses of the autonomic nervous system and NK cell activity following central administration of CRH in aged rats compared with young animals. First, an increase in resting sympathetic tone as measured by elevated basal levels of plasma norepinephrine and neuropeptide Y was found in the aged rats. Although an increased concentration of plasma norepinephrine had been previously reported in some (Chiueh, Nespor, & Rapoport, 1980) but not all studies (McCarty, 1985) of aged rats, measurement of plasma norepinephrine levels alone could reflect a diminished clearance of norepinephrine from the plasma rather than an increase in sympathetic nervous activity. However, in aged humans the increase of plasma norepinephrine has been found to be due to increased rate of plasma norepinephrine appearance rather than a decreased norepinephrine clearance (Veith et al., 1986). The present findings that both norepinephrine and neuropeptide Y are increased in the aged rat has provided firm support for an increased level of sympathetic nervous system activity in aging, because norepinephrine and neuropeptide Y are colocalized and are coreleased during sustained sympathetic nervous stimulation (Castagne, Corder, Gaillard, et al., 1987; Lundberg, Martinsson, Hemson, et al., 1985; Pernow, Lundberg, Kaijsen, et al., 1986; Waeber, 1990).

In addition to the age-related difference in basal levels of sympathetic activity, the present data also demonstrated an increase in the response of the sympathetic-adrenal medullary system to central CRH in the aged rats. Peak responses of plasma epinephrine were greater in the aged rats than in the young animals, even though basal concentrations were similar. Likewise in the aged rats, CRH-induced elevations of plasma concentrations of norepinephrine and neuropeptide Y were greater than responses in the young animals. Finally, the duration of the responses of epinephrine and norepinephrine was prolonged in the aged animals. Age differences in the duration of activation of the sympathetic nervous system are not likely to be due to age-related differences in the central metabolism of CRH, because the magnitude and duration of corticosterone responses were similar in the aged and young animals. Rather, this hypersecretory profile of catecholamines following central CRH in the aged rat is consistent with the findings of McCarty (1985) in which acute cold stress induced a greater elevation of plasma levels of epinephrine and norepinephrine in aged animals, suggesting an age-related alteration in the regulation of the sympathetic nervous system.

Of unique and considerable interest in the present study was the age-related association between NK cytotoxicity and sympathetic activity as measured by plasma levels of catecholamines and neuropeptide Y both at rest and following central administration of CRH. For example, at rest the aged rats showed increased basal levels or norepinephrine and neuropeptide Y and a reduction of NK activity. Anatomic studies have revealed an extensive presence of noradrenergic fibers in both primary and secondary lymphoid organs (Felten, Felten, Bellinger, et al., 1988; Livnat, Felten,

Carlson, et al., 1985), in which noradrenergic neurons innervate both the vasculature and the parenchyma of the spleen and end in synaptic-like contacts with lymphocytes (Felten et al., 1988). Norepinephrine acts as a neurotransmitter that binds to lymphocyte β-adrenergic receptors and reduces cellular function in vitro as measured by NK activity (Hellstrand, Hermodsson, & Strannegård, 1985). Likewise, in vivo studies involving young animals have demonstrated that either autonomic blockade, chemical sympathectomy, or β-receptor antagonism abolished the suppression of cellular immunity following administration of central CRH (Irwin, Hauger, Brown, et al., 1988; Irwin, Vale, & Rivier, 1990), IL-1 (Sundar, Cierpial, Kilts, et al., 1990) or footshock stress (Cunnick, Lysle, Kucinski, et al., 1990). In humans, we have also demonstrated that acute release of catecholamines during physical exercise mediates suppression of lymphocyte proliferation via β_2-adrenergic mechanisms (Murray, Irwin, Reardon, et al., 1992). Finally, our data described earlier have demonstrated that *chronic*, sustained elevation of sympathetic tone and release of neuropeptide Y were negatively correlated with NK activity in aged individuals, as well as in depressed patients and persons undergoing severe life stress (Irwin et al., 1991).

CRH induced a further decrement of NK activity in aged but not in adult rats, which might be due to the greater activation of the sympathetic adrenal medullary system, exaggerated release of epinephrine, norepinephrine, and neuropeptide Y, and dose-dependent suppression of cytotoxicity by these neurotransmitters (Hellstrand & Hermodsson, 1989). Alternatively, the lymphocytes of aged rats may have an increased sensitivity to the inhibitory effects of catecholamines, particularly epinephrine. Recently, Ackerman and colleagues (1991) and Bellinger, Felten, Collier, et al. (1987) have found an age-related denervation of splenic lymphoid tissue with an associated up-regulation of splenocyte β_2-adrenergic receptors (Ackerman et al., 1991). Because epinephrine preferentially binds at β_2-adrenergic receptors and produces a suppression of NK activity at physiologic concentrations (10^{-9}M) (Hellstrand & Hermodsson, 1989), CRH-induced elevations in the circulating concentration of epinephrine are likely to produce a greater inhibitory effect on the lytic activity of lymphocytes from aged versus young animals. These data are consistent with those of Zalcman, Henderson, Richter, et al. (1991), who found that immune responses of aged mice are more susceptible to increased sympathetic activity following stress. Finally, regulation of β-receptors may be impaired in the aged rat, exacerbating the immunosuppressive effects that follow acute elevations of circulating plasma epinephrine. For example, DeBlasi, Lipartiti, Algeri, et al. (1986) have reported that down-regulation of β-receptors following restraint stress is slowed and diminish in aged rats compared with young animals, suggesting that aged rats lose the ability to regulate β-receptor number in response to agonist availability.

These findings of increased sympathetic activity as measured by circulating concentrations of the sympathetic neurotransmitters norepinephrine and neuropeptide Y contrast with anatomic and biochemical data, which show sympathetic denervation of the splenic tissue during senescence (Ackerman et al., 1991) and a decrease of norepinephrine content in the spleens of aged rats (Ackerman et al., 1991; Bellinger et al., 1987). Because inhibition of NK cells in vitro requires micromolar concentrations of norepinephrine (Hellstrand et al., 1985; Hellstrand & Hermodsson, 1989), further studies using such techniques as in vivo microdialysis are necessary to quantitate the amount of norepinephrine released within the spleen by CRH and to define further the role of increase of sympathetic tone within splenic tissue in the suppression of immune function in aged rats.

The central mechanisms that mediate the differential effects of age on CRH-induced elevations in catecholamines and NK activity remain to be elucidated including an age-associated increase in release of CRH in vivo (Sapolsky et al., 1986) and augmentation of an ultrashort positive feedback loop of CRH on its own release (Ono, DeCastro, & McCann, 1985). In addition, the persistent elevation of plasma catecholamines following central CRH in the aged rats suggests a decreased sensitivity with age to the inhibitory feedback signal of increased of sympathetic activity.

In summary, CRH acts within the brain to stimulate the activity of the sympathetic nervous system and to reduce splenic NK activity. These findings show an age-related increase of autonomic outflow following CRH. Furthermore, these data are consistent with the hypothesis that age-related changes in central nervous system regulation of sympathetic activity may influence in vivo modulation and suppression of natural cytotoxicity in aging.

SUMMARY

This chapter has provided a review of recent data from clinical and animal studies showing the role of the sympathetic nervous system in the modulation of immune function. Because aging is associated with an activation of the sympathetic nervous system as reflected in elevated basal levels as well as increased release of catecholamines and neuropeptide Y following stress or central administration of CRH, dysregulation of sympathetic activity may contribute to the increased susceptibility of aged humans and animals to stress-induced decrement of cell-mediated immune responses.

REFERENCES

Ackerman, K. D., Bellinger, D. L., Felten, D. L. (1991). Ontogeny and senescence of noradrenergic innervation of the rodent thymus and spleen. In R. Ader, D. L. Felten, & N. Cohen (Eds.), *Psychoneuroimmunology* (2nd. ed., pp. 71–125). San Diego: Academic Press.

Adler, W. H., & Nagel, J. E. (1977). Studies of immune function in a human population. In D. Segre & L. Smith (Eds.), *Immunological aspects of aging* (pp. 295–310). New York: Dekker.

Bancroft, G. J., Shellam, G. R., & Chalmer, J. E. (1981). Genetic influences on the augmentation of natural killer cells (NK) during murine cytomegalovirus infection: Correlation with patterns of resistance. *Journal of Immunology, 124,* 988–994.

Bash, J. A., & Vogel, D. (1984). Cellular immunosenescence in F344 rats: Decreased natural killer (NK) cell activity involves changes in regulatory interactions between NK cells, interferon, prostaglandin and macrophages. *Mechanisms of Aging and Development, 24,* 49–65.

Bellinger, D. L., Felten, S. Y., Collier, T. J., & Felten, D. L. (1987). Noradrenergic sympathetic innervation of the spleen: IV. Morphometric analysis in adult and aged F344 rats. *Journal of Neurosciences Research, 18,* 55–63.

Biron, C. A., Byron, K. S., & Sullivan, J. L. (1989). Severe herpes virus infections in an adolescent without natural killer cells. *New England Journal of Medicine, 320,* 1731–1735.

Blair, P. B., Staskawicz, M. O. & Sam, J. S. (1987). Suppression of natural killer cell activity in young and old mice. *Mechanisms of Aging and Development, 40,* 57–70.

Brown, M. R. (1986). Corticotropin releasing factor: Central nervous system sites of action. *Brain Research, 399,* 10–14.

Brown, M. R., Fisher, L. A., Spiess, J., Rivier, C., Rivier, J., & Vale, W. (1982). Corticotropin releasing factor: Actions on the sympathetic nervous system and metabolism. *Endocrinology, 111,* 928–931.

Brown, M. R., Fisher, L. A., Webb, V., Vale, W., W., & Rivier, J. E. (1985). Corticotropin-releasing factor: A physiologic regulator of adrenal epinephrine secretion. *Psychiatry Research, 328,* 355–357.

Bukowski, J. F., Warner, J. F., Dennert, G., & Welsh, R. M. (1985). Adoptive transfer studies demonstrating the antiviral affect of natural killer cells in vivo. *Journal of Experimental Medicine, 131,* 1531–1538.

Castagne, V., Corder, R., Gaillard, R., & Mormede, P. (1987). Stress-induced changes of circulating neuropeptide Y in the rat: Comparison with catecholamines. *Regulators Peptides, 19,* 55–63.

Chiueh, C. C., Nespor, S. M., & Rapoport, S. I. (1980). Cardiovascular, sympathetic and adrenal cortical responsiveness of aged fischer-344 rats to stress. *Neurobiology and Aging, 1,* 157–163.

Cunnick, J. E., Lysle, D. T., Kucinski, B. J., & Rabin, B. S. (1990). Evidence that shock-induced immune suppression is mediated by adrenal hormones and peripheral β-adrenergic receptors. *Pharmacology and Biochemistry of Behavior, 36,* 645–651.

De Blasi, A., Lipartiti, M., Algeri, S., et al. (1986). Stress induced desensitization of lymphocyte β-adrenoceptors in young and aged rats. *Pharmacology and Biochemistry of Behavior, 24,* 991–998.

Facchini, A., Mariani, E., Mariani, A. R., Papa, S., Vitale, M., & Manzoli, F. A. (1987). Increased number of circulating Leu 11+ (CD16) large granular lymphocytes and decreased NK activity during human aging. *Clinics in Experimental Immunology, 68,* 340–347.

Felten, S. Y., Felten, D. L., Bellinger, D. L., et al. (1988). Noradrenergic sympathetic innervation of lymphoid organs. *Progress in Allergy, 43,* 14–36.

Habu, S., Akamatsu, K., Tamaoki, N., & Okumura, K. (1984). In vivo significance of NK cell in resistance against (HSV-1) infections in mice. *Journal of Immunology, 133,* 2743–2747.

Hallgren, H. M., Buckley, C. E., Gilbertson, V. A., & Yunis, E. J. (1973). Lymphocyte phytohemagglutinin responsiveness, immunoglobulins and autoantibodies in aging humans. *Journal of Immunology, 111,* 1101–1107.

Hellstrand, K., & Hermodsson, S. (1989). An immunopharmacological analysis of adrenaline-induced suppression of human natural killer cell cytotoxicity. *International Archives of Allergy and Applied Immunology, 89,* 334–341.

Hellstrand, K., Hermodsson, S. & Strannegård, Ö. (1985). Evidence for a β-adrenoceptor-mediated regulation of human natural killer cells. *Journal of Immunology, 134:* 4095–4099.

Heroux, J. A., Grigoriadis, D. E., & DeSouza, E. B. (1991). Age-related decreases in corticotropin-releasing factor (CRF) receptors in rat brain and anterior pituitary gland. *Brain Research, 542,* 155–158.

Hylka, V., Sonntag, W., & Meites, J. (1984). Reduced ability of old male rats to release ACTH and corticosterone in response to CRF administration. *Proceedings of the Society of Experimental Biology and Medicine, 175,* 1.

Irwin, M., Brown, M., Patterson, T., Hauger, R., & Mascovich, A., & Grant, I. (1991). Neuropeptide Y and natural killer cell activity: Findings in depression and Alzheimer caregiver stress. *Federation of the American Society for Experimental Biology Journal, 5,* 3100–3107.

Irwin, M. R., Hauger, R., & Brown, M. (1992). Central corticotropin-releasing hormone activates the sympathetic nervous system and reduces immune function: Increased responsivity of the aged rat. *Endocrinology, 131,* 1047–1053.

Irwin, M., Hauger, R. L., Brown, M., & Britton, K. T. (1988). CRF activates autonomic nervous system and reduces natural killer cytotoxicity. *American Journal of Physiology, 255,* R744–747.

Irwin, M., Hauger, R. L., Jones, L., Provencio, M., & Britton, K. T. (1990). Sympathetic nervous system mediates central corticotropin-releasing factor induced suppression of natural killer cytotoxicity. *Journal of Pharmacology and Experimental Therapy, 255,* 101–107.

Irwin, M. R., Vale, W., & Rivier, C. (1990). Central corticotropin-releasing factor mediates the suppressive effect of stress on natural killer cytotoxicity. *Endocrinology, 126,* 2837–2844.

Irwin, M. R., Vale, W., & Britton, K. T. (1987). Central corticotropin-releasing factor suppresses natural killer cytotoxicity. *Brain Behavior and Immunity, 1*, 81–87.

Iwase, S., Mano, T., Watanabe, T., Saito, M., & Kobayashi, F. (1991). Age-related changes of sympathetic outflow to muscles in humans. *Journal of Gerontology, 46*, M1–M5.

Kingsley, T. R., Nekvasil, N. P., & Snyder, D. L. (1991). The influence of dietary restriction, germ free status, and aging on adrenal catecholamines in Lobund-Wistar rats. *Journal of Gerontology, 46*, B135–141.

Krishnaraj, R., & Blandford, G. (1987). Age-associated alterations in human natural killer cells: increased activity as per conventional and kinetic analysis. *Clinical Immunology and Immunopathology, 45*, 268–285.

Livnat, S., Felten, S. Y., Carlson, S. L., Bellinger, D. L., & Felten, D. L. (1985). Involvement of peripheral and central catecholamine systems in neural-immune interactions. *Journal of Neuroimmunology, 10*, 5–30.

Lundberg, J. M., Martinsson, A., & Hemson, A., et al. (1985). Co-release of neuropeptide Y and catecholamines during physical exercise in man. *Biochemistry and Biophysics Research Communication, 133*, 30–36.

Makinodan, T., & Kay, M. M. (1980). Age influence on the immune system. *Advances in Immunology, 29*, 287–330.

McCarty, R. (1985). Sympathetic-adrenal medullary and cardiovascular responses to acute cold stress in adult and aged rats. *Journal of the Autonomic Nervous System, 12*, 15–22.

Murray, D. R., Irwin, M., Rearden, C. A., Ziegler, M., Motulsky, H., & Maisel, A. S. (1992). Sympathetic and immune interactions during dynamic exercise: Mediation via a β2-adrenergic dependent mechanism. *Circulation, 86*, 203–213.

O'Leary, J. J., & Hallgren, H. M. (1991). Aging and lymphocyte function: A model for testing gerontologic hypotheses of aging in man. *Archives of Gerontology and Geriatrics, 12*, 199–218.

Ono, N., De Castro, J. C. B., McCann, S. M. (1985). Ultrashort-loop positive feedback of corticotropin (ACTH)-releasing factor to enhance ACTH in stress. *Proceedings of the National Academy of Sciences, USA, 82*, 3528–3531.

Padgett, G. A., Reiquam, C. W., Henson, J. B., & Gorham, J. R. (1968). Comparative studies of susceptibility to infection in the Chediak-Higashi syndrome. *Journal of Pathology and Bacteriology, 95*, 509–522.

Pernow, J., Lundberg, J. M., Kaijser, L., et al. (1986). Plasma neuropeptide Y-like immunoreactivity and catecholamines during various degrees of sympathetic activation in man. *Clinical Physiology, 45*, 355–365.

Pfeifer, M. A., Weinberg, C. R., Cook, D., Best, J. D., Reenan, A., & Halter, J. B. (1983). Differential changes of autonomic nervous system function with age in man. *American Journal of Medicine, 75*, 249–258.

Rivier, C., Rivier, J. & Vale, W. (1982). Inhibition of adrenocorticotropic hormone secretion in the rat by immunoneutralization of corticotropin-releasing factor. *Science, 218*, 377–379.

Sapolsky, R. M. Krey, L. C., McEwen, B. S. (1986). The neuroendocrinology of stress and aging: The glucocorticoid cascade hypothesis. *Endocrinology Review, 7*, 284–300.

Sato, T., Fuse, A., & Kuwata, T. (1979). Enhancement by interferon of natural cytotoxic activities of lymphocytes from human cord blood and peripheral blood of aged persons. *Cellular Immunology, 45*, 458–463.

Scaccianoce, S., DeSciullo, A., & Angelucci, L. (1990). Age-related changes in hypothalamo-pituitary-adrenocortical axis activity in the rat. *Neuroendocrinology, 52*, 150–155.

Shigemoto, S., Kishimoto, S., & Yamamura, Y. (1975). Change of cell-mediated cytotoxicity with aging. *Journal of Immunology, 115*, 307–309.

Sowers, J. R., Rubenstein, L. Z., & Stern, N. (1983). Plasma norepinephrine responses to posture and isometric exercise increase with age in the absence of obesity. *Journal of Gerontology, 38*, 315.

Stausbaugh, H., & Irwin, M. (1992). Central corticotropin releasing hormone reduces cellular immunity. *Brain Behavior and Immunity, 6*, 11–17.

Sullivan, J. L., Byron, K. S., Brewster, F. E., & Purtilo, D. T. (1980). Deficient natural killer activity in X-linked lymphoproliferative syndrome. *Science, 210*, 535.

Sundar, S. K., Cierpial, M. A., Kilts, C., Ritchie, J. C., & Weiss, J. M. (1990). Brain IL-1-induced immunosuppression occurs through activation of both pituitary-adrenal axis and sympathetic nervous system by corticotropin-releasing factor. *Journal of Neurosciences, 10*: 3701–3706.

Supiano, M. A., Linares, O. A., Smith, M. J., & Halter, J. B. (1990). Age-related differences in norepinephrine kinetics: Effect of posture and sodium-restricted diet. *American Journal of Physiology, 259*, E422–E431.

Veith, R. C., Featherstone, J. A., Linares, O. A., Halter, J. B. (1986). Age differences in plasma norepinephrine kinetics in humans. *Journal of Gerontology, 41*, 319–324.

Waeber, B. (1990). Neuropeptide Y: A missing link? *Hospital Practice, 25*, 101–120.

Weindruch, R., Devens, B. H., Raff, H. V., Walford, R. L. (1983). Influence of dietary restriction and aging on natural killer cell activity in mice. *Journal of Immunology, 130*, 993–996.

Zalcman, S., Henderson, N., Richter, M., & Anisman, H. (1991). Age-related enhancement and suppression of a T-cell-dependent antibody response following stressor exposure. *Behavioral Neurosciences, 105*, 669–676.

Ziegler, M. G., Lake, C. R., & Kopin, J. J. (1976). Plasma noradrenaline increases with age. *Nature, 261*, 333–335.

Immunologic and Psychological Correlates in Older Females

12

Donna Benton and George F. Solomon

A discussion of gender differences in immune responsivity as it relates to psychological function is made difficult by the complexities involved in unraveling the links among various aspects of mood, coping skills, stress appraisal, health and a variety of other biopsychosocial factors. The complexity is further compounded by the process of aging, which affects both immunologic and psychological processes. However, this type of challenge is not new to those involved in the fields of psychoneuroimmunology (PNI) or gerontology. PNI primarily focuses on bidirectional communication of the CNS and the immune system, and their clinical and bioregulatory implications. Many studies have provided evidence of reciprocal interactions between the CNS and the immune system in humans (Kemeny, Solomon, Morley, & Herbert, 1992; Kiecolt-Glaser & Glaser, 1991). The interaction of these systems is neither straightforward or simple (Fabris, 1991).

Immunosenescence may be defined as those alterations in immune function that occur to some degree in all older individuals, and that are distinguishable from immunodeficiency secondary to underlying disease, malnutrition, toxic exposure, or genetic disorder. Immunosenescence is characterized by its high prevalence, interindividual variability, and complexity. The immune system is not uniformly affected by the aging process. An already compromised immune system may be more vulnerable to or be influenced differently by psychosocial factors. Coversely, an argument could be made that an impaired immune system is less able to be influenced by neuroendocrine regulators that are impacted by experiential factors. Aging is associated with decrements in cellular immune function, and with increased susceptibility to infectious and neoplastic disease. Although many studies have looked at stress, immunity, and aging, few studies have integrated these factors or looked for gender differences. A better understanding of how these factors relate may have predictive health significance. The fact that immune-related (not immune-resisted) diseases are more prevalent in women emphasizes the importance of understanding psychoneuroimmunologic factors that can affect health in older women.

To attempt this integration, we briefly review several issues using psychological stress and distress as a framework for this discussion. It is beyond the scope of this chapter to review all the human and animal studies of PNI and stress. Therefore, we review human studies in aging, which present information on the following: (a) gender, health, and aging; (b) gender, hormones, immunity, and aging; (c) gender, depression, immunity, and aging; and (d) gender, immunity, stress, and psychological distress.

GENDER, HEALTH, AND AGING

Epidemiologic health research has shown that men and women differ in the types of illnesses that they develop and in causes of death. For primary illnesses, the differences are not apparent; both men and women exhibit highest death rates from cardiovascular diseases, cancers, and cerebrovascular diseases (Brock, Guralnik, & Brody, 1990). However, incidence of chronic obstructive pulmonary diseases and death from accidents are among the top five causes of death for men; whereas pneumonia and influenza complete the list for women (Verbrugge, 1985). Although life expectancy for women is about 7 years longer than for men, the difference is reduced once women are older than 60 years old (Cleary, 1987; Rodin, 1986; U.S. Bureau of the Census, 1991). The longevity gap between men and women appears to be diminishing. Possible reasons include changes in disease patterns for women, changes in health behaviors in women, and changes in the participation of women in the workplace. Although employment appears to have a positive effect on women's health (Repetti, Matthews, & Waldron 1989), some behavior changes, such as increased smoking, alcohol consumption, and illicit drugs use have had a detrimental effect on women's health.

The advantage women hold in mortality compared with men is not maintained when looking at morbidity. Morbidity can be defined as generalized poor health, a specific illness, or the sum of a number of illnesses (Rodin, 1986). Women tend to live longer with disability. Much of the disability is related to arthritis and dementia (Manton, 1989). Moreover, women are more likely to develop autoimmune diseases and are at greater relative risk for pneumonia and influenza than are men (Strickland, 1988). It has been asserted that the differences in morbidity can be attributed to a variety of factors including gender differences in stress, distress, and age. A great many differences in health associated with gender are stress related. Research suggests that men and women differ in bodily reactions to stress or challenge and that these differences appear to be more than reflections of intensity of experience or of perceived threat. Autoimmune disease, such as rheumatoid arthritis and systemic lupus erythematosus, are 3 to 10 times more common in women than men (Inman, 1978; Lahita, 1984).

Knowledge about what factors assist in the initiation and maintenance of the autoimmune process in these diseases is complex and not fully understood. Tolerance to self-antigens is related to multiple distinct safety valves that are connected in series and intervene at defined points of the life cycle of the developing lymphocyte to guarantee the physical elimination, functional inactivation, or regulated inhibition of self-reactive, potentially autoaggressive B and T cells (Kroemer & Marinez, 1992). Regarding the latter, suppressor T cells, which can be stress influenced, are important.

Although overt autoimmune diseases generally have their onset in younger life, they can have their onset in later years. Psychosocial factors appear to be related to the onset and course in the elderly as they are in the young (Solomon, 1981a). For example, Solomon (1981b) reported the onset of rheumatoid arthritis in a previously healthy 84-year-old man (who achieved a black belt in judo at age 60) when he was persuaded to give up the independence he cherished and move in with his son. In a series of studies by Moos and Solomon (1964, 1965), psychological distress was found to be negatively related to rate of progression of, degree of incapacition by, and response to treatment in rheumatoid arthritics.

Some studies of AIDS have suggested that compared with men, women with HIV infection die sooner of AIDs when factors of intravenous drug abuse and socioeconomic status are controlled, possibly as a result of autoimmune components of that disease (Solomon, 1989). In contrast, an epidemiologic study of more than 1,000 HIV-infected men and women (mostly men) found no significant association with progression of disease and gender. However, older age was associated with disease progression in both late- and early-stage HIV groups (Gardner, Grundage, McNeil et al., 1992).

Moreover, being older than 50 years of age was found to have negative prognostic implications in men with AIDS (Ferro & Salit, 1992).

Another risk factor related to health impairments in women is the role of caregiver. Although both men and women provide informal care to older adults, estimates indicate that from two-thirds to three quarters of caregivers are women (Barr, Johnson, & Warshaw, 1992). Studies of caregivers found that caregiving responsibilities have been associated with self-reported health impairments (Brocklehurst, Morris, Andrews, et al., 1981; Sainsbury & Grad de Alarcon 1970). Moreover, many caregivers are often older than 60 years of age (Cohen, Luchins, Eisdorfer, et al., 1990). The range of psychosocial responses associated with the stress of caregiving includes depression, depressed mood, and anxiety. Caregivers to Alzheimer's disease patients and those with dementias have been found to be at increased risk for clinical depression and anxiety (e.g., Cohen et al., 1990), and older caregivers use psychotropic drugs more frequently than age-matched controls (Clipp & George, 1990).

GENDER, HORMONES, IMMUNITY, AND AGING

Women have higher immunoglobulin levels than do men and mount larger antibody responses to a variety of pathogens, although cell-mediated immune responses appear to be weaker than those seen in men (Baum & Grunberg, 1991). It has been well established that the aging immune system is characterized by a decline in most measures of T-cell function, although helper T-cell numbers may be normal or reduced with age. Function is usually found to be diminished secondary to both impaired IL-2 production and responsiveness (Ershler, Moore, Roessner, et al., 1985; Thomas, 1985). For a long time it has been known that autoantibodies (which are not necessarily correlated with overt clinical autoimmune disease) are more common in older people and those suffering from schizophrenia, probably reflective of disordered immune dysregulation in both aging and mental illness (Goodman, Rosenblatt, Gottlieb, et al., 1963; Solomon, 1981a).

The T-cell proliferative response to mitogenic lectins in older humans is usually diminished, but gender differences have not been noted (Hashimoto & Wakabayashi 1990; Matour, Melnicoff, Kaye, et al., 1989; Pieri, Recchioni, Moroni, et al., 1992; Thompson, Wekstein, Rhoades, et al., 1984;). Suppressor T cells have been reported to increase (Gupta & Good 1979), decrease (Hallgren & Yunis, 1977), or not change (Chopra, 1990) with age. Natural killer (NK) cells are a heterogeneous subpopulation of lymphocytes contained within the null (non-B, non-T) cell population and comprise approximately 5% to 15% of peripheral blood lymphocytes

(Herberman, Ortaldo, & Bonnard, 1979). Data regarding NK cell activity in the aged are controversial, as NK cell activity has been reported to be maintained, increased, or decreased in the elderly (Fiatarone, 1989). NK cells in healthy elders, have been found to remain stable across the life-span (Miller, 1990). Moreover, in healthy centenarians, NK cell activity is normal, whereas phenotypes of NK cells are increased (Thompson et al., 1984). In a study by Solomon (1989), we found that in 45 healthy elderly women, NK activity was significantly higher in older healthy women compared with young healthy women. Moreover, lymphocyte phenotypes associated with NK activity were also significantly higher in the older female sample. T-cell function of these healthy elderly women was equivalent to that of young women. The preceding studies strongly suggest that immune functions in older healthy adults not only may not be significantly diminished with age, but that a cohort effect may operate allowing only individuals with superior immune functions to survive to a healthy old age.

Receptors for both GH (Kiess & Butenandt, 1985) and prolactin (Haddock, Russell, Kibler, 1985) are found on lymphocytes. GH appears to peak during early adulthood and decline with age (Weksler, 1981). The level of GH may be sex linked with more decline of basal GH level with age in women (Prinz, Weithzman, Cunningham, et al. 1983; Vidalon, Khurana, Chae, et al., 1973). GH is also affected by obesity and medication use, which both increase with age and are more prevalent in older women (Ausman & Russell, 1990; Vestal & Cusack, 1990). GH restores T-cell proliferative responses and IL-2 synthesis in aged rats, augments the activity of NK cells and cytotoxic T cells, and increases the growth rate of macrophages (Kelley, 1991). It is possible that declining GH levels in older people, especially women, may place them at greater risk of immunosuppression (Dilman & Blumenthal, 1981).

Prolactin has important effects on immunity that may be differentially gender related. Prolactin has been shown to restore both the cell-mediated and humoral immune responses in hypophysectomized female rats, as measured by antibody production and delayed hypersensitivity skin responses. Moreover, elevated immune response in females may relate to the fact that estrogen stimulates prolactin secretion, which is immunostimulatory (Bernton, Bryant, & Holaday, 1991; Grossman, 1990). In animals, acute stress evokes a rapid increase in prolactin release, this is followed by decreased prolactin secretion and then refractoriness to further stimulation with repetition of the acute stress (Tache, Du Ruisseau, Ducharme, et al., 1978).

Estrogens have been shown generally to depress cell-mediated immunity (Ablin, Bartkus, & Gonder, 1988) but can elevate antibody responses to T-dependent antigens (Stimson & Hunter, 1990). That sex hormones may be involved in autoimmune disease is suggested by differential incidence and severity of rheumatoid arthritis in women using oral contraceptives. In limited research studies, it has been found that proliferative response to PHA mitogen is decreased in women taking oral contraceptives derived from progesterone or estrogen (Vandenbrouke, Boersma, Festin, et al., 1982). Animal studies have found that B-cell mitogens can elicit rheumatoid factor antibody production in female rats (Schuurs & Verheul, 1990), and this effect is inhibited by estradiol but not testosterone.

Menopause is associated with increased IL-1 production that is reversed with estrogen replacement (Regelson, Loria, & Mohanned 1988). There are receptors on lymphoid cells for estrogen and androgens (McCruden & Stimson, 1991). Estrogen may contribute to the increased incidence of autoimmune diseases in women (Lahita 1984; Sthoeger, Chiorzzi, & Lahita, 1989).

GENDER, DEPRESSION, IMMUNITY, AND AGING

Depressive illness and symptoms, unrelated to bereavement, affect more than 15% of the geriatric population. Rates of depression and anxiety are higher among older women than men. These differences may be related to women more readily admitting to psychological distress, greater social acceptance of these emotions in women, or possibly a greater number of losses among older women compared with older men. Several studies have found a relationship between stressful life events and onset of depression in women (Harris, 1991).

Studies addressing the issue of depression, immunity, and age are often contradictory in their findings (Stein, Miller, & Trestman, 1991). These differences are often due to methodologic problems such as sample size, immunologic tests used, and lack of control for sex, age, hospitalization status and diagnosis. A recent metaanalytic review (Herbert & Cohen, 1992) suggests that when all these factors are accounted for, there remains a reliable association between decreased cellular immune function and depression. In addition, this relationship is significantly impacted by the severity of the depression and by age.

In a study with age and sex-matched controls, depressed patients did not significantly differ from controls in NK cell activity mitogen-induced lymphocyte stimulation responses to PHA, Con A, and pokeweed mitogen (PWM). However, when response to mitogen was analyzed looking at age differences, depressed older patients did not show an increased lymphocyte response with age compared with age-matched controls (Stein, 1989). Decreased lymphocyte response to mitogens appears to occur only in old and not in young, depressed, male patients, the youngest depressives even showing increases (Schleifer, Keller, Camerino, et al., 1983). In contrast, NK activity is decreased in patients with major depressive disorder of all ages (Irwin, Daniels, Smith, et al., 1987). In most of these studies gender differences were either not reported, or only males were used in the study sample.

Women are better represented in studies of bereavement, marital status, caregiving, and immunity. Research suggests that the lymphocyte stimulation response to mitogens is significantly lower following the death of a spouse compared with prebereavement responses or those after the loss has been worked through (Bartrop, Luckhurst, Lazarus, et al., 1977; Irwin, et al., 1987; Schleifer et al., 1983). This phenomenon has been demonstrated in both men and women. The study by Irwin et al. (1987) included older women (mean age 57, SD=7) and that of Bartrop et al. (1977) had an age range up to the age of 65. Age differences were not analyzed in either group. It would have been interesting to look at the relationship between age and immune suppression as did a study by Guidi, Bartoloni, Frasca, et al., (1991), which found that both age and depression were negatively related to PHA stimulation of lymphocytes and Il-2 stimulation of NK cells. It seems depression in the elderly can be immunosuppressive.

A recent study has suggested that there may be different immune responses between depressed patients and patients anticipating bereavement but who are not depressed (Spurrell & Creed, 1993). This study of a 11 depressed females (mean age, 36 years) and 8 women (mean age, 55 years) whose husbands had cancer found that PHA response in the depressed patients was negatively correlated with depression and enhanced PHA responses seemed to be associated with anticipatory grief. The finding of immunoenhancement in the spousal group may be a reflection of good coping response, emotional expressiveness, or social support.

As previously mentioned, caregiving is associated with increased health impairments. Female caregivers to Alzheimer's disease patients are not only at risk for depression (Crook & Miller, 1985) but also for immunosuppression (Kennedy, Kiecolt-Glaser, & Glaser, 1988; Kiecolt-Glaser, Glaser, Shuttleworth, et al., 1987). These studies found that caregivers had generally poorer immune functions as evidenced by lower percentages of total T lymphocytes and helper T lymphocytes, lower helper/suppressor ratios, and higher antibody levels of Epstein-Barr virus (indicative of viral activation) compared with age matched controls. It has been emphasized that the distress-related immunosuppression may have its most detrimental health consequences in older adult caregivers (Kiecolt-Glaser & Glaser, 1991). Because women tend more often to provide caregiving, these potential health problems place older female caregivers in double jeopardy.

Marital status has been associated with increased risk for psychiatric disorders such as depression (Bloom, Asher, & White, 1978), wheras marital satisfaction is significantly related to psychological well-being (Glenn &

Weaver, 1981). Separated and divorced persons suffer more acute and chronic illnesses, and have significantly greater mortality rates from diseases including pneumonia, tuberculosis, and some types of cancer (Bloom et al., 1978). Kennedy et al. (1988) looked at the effects of marital disruption (divorce or separation) on the immune system in 38 women, who were matched with 38 controls. Results showed that single and divorced women had lowered blastogenic response to mitogens (Con A and PHA), lower percentages of T-helper lymphocytes and NK cells, and higher antibody titers to Epstein-Barr virus. Unfortunately, ages for the group were not presented, but it can be speculated, based on the research showing the negative interaction among depression, immunity, and age, that marital disruption would be more immunosuppressive in older women. This likelihood is enhanced because divorce or separation in the elderly might be expected to have more negative psychological impact.

GENDER, IMMUNITY, STRESS, AND PSYCHOLOGICAL DISTRESS

Some stressors have been shown to suppress immune activity in humans (Workman & La Via 1987). However, the conditions under which this occurs are related to the nature, context, timing, intensity, and duration of the stressor. In addition, research suggests that psychological factors of control, coping style, and social support are important modulators of the stressor and, in turn, the immune reaction (Kemeny et al., 1992).

Several animal studies have show that uncontrollable stress has more immunosuppressive consequence than stress that can be controlled (Shavit, Lewis, Terman et al., 1984). Similarly, in humans, it has been found that perceived low control over significant life stressors predicts T-cell responses to mitogenic (PHA) and antigenic challenge in older males and females (Rodin, 1986). Additionally, in this study, a pessimistic explanatory style was associated with a lower T4/T8 ratio and low response to stimulation by PHA. This association was not related to age, and gender differences were not analyzed (Kamen-Siegel, Rodin, Seligman et al., 1991). In a younger sample (ages 18–26), subjects who perceived that they had no control over a stressor showed reduced NK activity.

Another study looked at the relationship among coping style, stress, social support, and immunity. Thirty-three elderly women (mean age, 73 years) were classified as either having experienced marked adversity in the past year or no major stress. These women were compared both immunologically and in terms of coping style. The investigators reported that women who had experienced high-stress women had significantly lower ratios of $CD4^+$ to $CD8^+$ cells than did women experiencing low-stress. Further analysis showed that a significant portion of the difference was ac-counted for by differences in coping style and satisfaction with social support. Specifically, it appeared that lower CD4/CD8 ratio was related to dissatisfaction with social supports and emotion-focused coping in older women (McNaughton, Smith, Patterson, & Grant 1990).

In our own unpublished research, we predicted that anticipated life stress, that is, a concern about negative events that might occur in the next 3 months ("worry") in older and younger women, would be related to im-munologic measures. Twenty-eight young and 48 older, healthy, commu-nity-dwelling women were tested both immunologically and psycho-logically. Results suggested that despite no significant age differences in NK activity and numbers between young and old women, there were dif-ferences in the relationship of these immune variables and anticipated life stress (ALS) and distress. Specifically, anger and ALS were positively cor-related with NK cytotoxic activity in the young, whereas there appeared to be no such relationship in the elderly. Similarly, our study of brief laborato-ry mental stress (time-pressured mental arithmetic) in collaboration with Naliboff, Benton, Solomon (1991), found increases in NK activity following the stress in young but not old subjects. These studies suggest that exper-imentally induced down-regulation is more difficult in older persons.

This review suggests that more research is needed regarding the effects of gender, age, and psychological distress on immunity. Particularly, re-search that examines how positive psychological factors or interventions effect immune function in older women would be important. At least one study has looked at the relationship between relaxation and immune func-tion in an older population (Kiecolt-Glaser, Glaser, Williger, et al., 1985) and found that relaxation was immunoenhancing for participants. How-ever, most studies looking at positive emotions or psychological factors have focused on a younger population (Hall & O'Grady, 1991; Martin & Dobbin, 1988; Zachariae, Kristensen, Hokland, et al., 1990). It is unfortu-nate that so few of the human studies on naturalistic and experimental ex-periential effects on immunity have been done only in young persons and generally neglect gender as well as age effects. Studies of gender, age, psy-chological factors, and immunity may lead to interventions to help reduce morbidity and enhance life satisfaction in the largely female older popula-tion.

REFERENCES

Ablin, R. J., Bartkus, J. M., & Gonder, J. J. (1988). In vitro effects of diethylstilbestrol and the LHRH analogue leuprolide on natural killer cell activity. *Immunophar-macology, 15,* 95–101.

Ausman, L. M., & Russell, R. M. (1990). Nutrition and age . In E. Schneider & J. Rowe (Ed.), *Handbook of the biology of aging* (3rd ed.). San Diego: Academic Press.

Barr, J., Johnson, K., & and Warshaw, L. (1992). Supporting the elderly: Work place programs for employed caregivers. *The Milbank Memorial Fund Quarterly, 70,* 509–533.

Bartrop, R., Luckhurst, E., Lazarus, L., Kiloh, L. G., & Penny, R. (1977, April 16). Depressed lymphocyte function after bereavement. *Lancet, II,* 834–836.

Baum, A., & Grunberg, N. E. (1991). Gender, stress, and health. *Health Psychology, 10,* 80–85.

Bernton, E. W., Bryant, H. U., & Holaday, J. W. (1991). Prolactin and immune function. In R. Ader, D. Felton, & N. Cohen (Ed.), *Psychoneuroimmunology* (2nd ed., pp. 403–428). San Diego: Academic Press.

Bloom, B. L., Asher, S., & White, S. (1978). Marital disruption as a stressor: A review and analysis. *Psychological Bulletin, 85,* 867–894.

Brock, D. B., Guralnik, J. M., & Brody, J. A. (1990). Demography and epidemiology of aging in the United States. In E. Schneider & J. Rowe (Ed.), *Handbook of the biology of aging* (3rd ed., pp. 3–23). San Diego: Academic Press.

Brocklehurst, J., Morris, P., Andrews, K., Richards, B., & Laycock, P. (1981). Social effects of stroke. *Social Science and Medicine, 15A,* 35–39.

Chopra, R. K. (1990). Mechanism of impaired T-cell function in the elderly. *Reviews of Biological Research in Aging, 4,* 83–104.

Cleary, P. (1987). Gender differences in stress-related disorders. In R. Barnett, L. Biener, & G. Banich (Eds.), *Gender and stress* (pp. 39-72). New York: Free Press.

Clipp, E. C., & George L. K. (1990). Psychotropic drug use among caregivers of patients with dementia. *Journal of the American Geriatric Society, 38,* 227–235.

Cohen, D., Luchins, D., Eisdorfer, C. P., Ashford, W., Gorelick, P., Hirschman, R., Freels, S., Levy, P., Semla, T., & Shaw, H. (1990). Caring for relatives with Alzheimer's disease: the mental health risks to spouses, adult children, and other family cargivers. *Behavior, Health, and Aging, 1,* 171–182.

Crook, T. H., & Miller, N. E. (1985). The challenges of Alzheimer's disease. *American Psychology, 40,* 1245–1250.

Dilman, V., & Blumenthal, H. (1981). *The law of deviation of homeostasis and disease of aging.* Boston: John Wright PSG.

Ershler, W., Moore, A., Roessner, K., & Ranges, G. (1985). interleukin-2 and aging-ing: Decreased Interleukin-2 production in healthy old people does not correlate with reduced helper cell numbers of antibody response to influenza vaccine and is not corrected in i=vitro by thymosin alpha-1. *Immunopharmacology, 10,* 11–17.

Fabris, N. (1991). Neuroendocrine–immune interactions: A theoretical approach to aging. *Archeological Gerontological Geriatrics, 12,* 219–230.

Ferro, S., & Salit, I. E. (1992). HIV infection in patients over 55 years of age. *Journal of Acquired Immune Deficiency Syndromes, 5,* 348–353.

Fiatarone, M. A., Morly, J. E., Bloom, Eda T., Benton, D., Solomon, G. F., & Makinodan, T. (1989). The effect of exercise on natural killer cell activity in young and old subjects. *Journal of Gerontology: Medical Sciences, 44,* M37–M45.

Gardner, L. I. J., Grundage, J. F., McNeil, J. G., Milazzo, M. J., Redfield, R. R., Aronson, N. E., Craig, D. B., Davis, C., Gates, R. H., Levin, L. I., Michael, R. A., Oster, C. N., Ryan, W. C., Burke, D. S., Tramont, E. C., & the Military Medical Consortium for Applied Retrovirology. (1992). Predictors of HIV-1 disease progression in early- and late-stage patients: The U.S. Army Natural History Cohort. *Journal of Acquired Immune Deficiency Syndromes, 5*, 782–793.

Glenn, N., & Weaver, C. (1981). The contribution of marital happiness to global happiness. *Journal of Marriage and Family, 43*, 151–168.

Goodman, M., Rosenblatt, M. M., Gottlieb, J., Miller, J., & Chen, C. (1963). Effect of age, sex and schizophrenia on thyroid autoantibody production. *Archives of General Psychiatry, 8*, 114–122.

Grossman, C. J. (1990). Are there underlying immune-neuroendocrine interactions responsible for immunological sexual dimorphism? *Progress in Neuroendocrinimmunology, 3*, 75–82.

Guidi, L., Bartoloni, C., Frasca, D., Antico, L., Pili, R., Cursi, F., Tempesta, E., Rumi, C., Menini, E., Carbonin, P., Doria, G., & and Gambassi, G. (1991). Impairment of lymphocyte activities in depressed aged subjects. *Mechanisms of Ageing and Development, 60*, 13–24.

Gupta, S., & Good, R. A. (1979). Subpopulations of human T lymphocytes. X. Alterations in T, B, third population cells, and T cells with receptors for immunoglubulin M (T mu) or g (T gamma) in aging humans. *Journal of Immunology, 122*, 1214–1219.

Haddock, R., Kibler, R., Matrisian, L., Larson, D., Poulos, B., & and Magun, B. (1985). Prolactin receptors on human T and B lymphocytes: Antagonism of prolactin binding by cyclosporine. *Journal of Immunology, 134*, 3027–3031.

Hall, N. R., & O'Grady, M. P. (1991). Psychosocial interventions and immune function. In R. Ader, D. L. Felten, & N. Cohen (Eds.), *Psychoneuroimmunology* (2nd ed., pp. 1067–1080). San Diego: Harcourt Brace Jovanovich.

Hallgren, H. M., & Yunis, E. (1977). Suppressor lymphocytes in young and aged humans. *Journal of Immunology, 118*, 2004–2008.

Harris, T. (1991). Life, stress and illness: the question of specificity. *Annals of Behavioral Medicine, 13*, 211–219.

Hashimoto, M., & Wakabayashi, Y. (1990, July). Differentiation and proliferation of T-cells in the elderly. *Acta Haematologica Japonica, 53*, 717–724.

Herberman, R. R., Ortaldo, J. R., & Bonnard, G. D. (1979). Augmentation by interferon of human natural and antibody-dependent cell-mediated cytotoxicity. *Nature, 277*, 221–223.

Herbert, T. B., & Cohen, S. (1992). Depression and immunity: a meta-analytic review. *Psychological Bulletin, 113*, 1–49.

Inman, R. (1978). Immunologic sex differences and the female preponderance in systemic lupus erythematosus. *Arthritis and Rheumatology, 21*, 849–852.

Irwin, M., Daniels, M., Smith, T. L., Bloom, E., & and Weiner, H. (1987). Impaired natural killer cell activity during bereavement. *Brain, Behavior, and Immunity, 1*, 98–104.

Kamen-Siegel, L., Rodin, J., Seligman, M. E. P., & Dwyer, J. (1991). Explanatory style and cell-mediated immunity in elderly men and women. *Health Psychology, 10*, 229–235.

Kelley, K. W. (1991). Growth hormone in immunobiology. In R. Ader, D. Felton, &

N. Cohen (Eds.), *Psychoneuroimmunology* (2nd ed., pp. 377–402). San Diego: Academic Press.

Kemeny, M., Solomon, G., Morley, J. E., & and Herbert, T. L. (1992). Psychoneuroimmunology. In C. B. Nemeroff (Ed.), *A comprehensive textbook of neuroendocrinology* (pp. 563–591). Boca Raton, FL: CRC Press.

Kennedy, S., Kiecolt-Glaser, J. K., & Glaser, R. (1988). Immunological consequences of acute and chronic stressors: mediating role of interpersonal relationships. *British Journal of Medical Psychology, 61*, 77–85.

Kiecolt-Glaser, J. K., & Glaser, R. (1991). Stress and immune function in humans. In R. Ader, D. Felten, & N. Cohen (Ed.), *Psychoneuroimmunology,* (2nd ed., pp. 849–867). San Diego: Harcourt Brace Jovanovich.

Kiecolt-Glaser, J., Glaser, R., Shuttleworth, E., Dyer, C., Ogrocki, P., & Spieicher, C. (1987). Chronic stress and immunity in family caregivers of Alzheimer's disease victims. *Psychosomatic Medicine, 49*, 523-535.

Kiecolt-Glaser, J. K., Glaser, R., Williger, D.. Messick, G., Sheppard, S. Ricker, D. Romisher, S. C., Briner, W., Bonnell, G., & Donnerberg, R. (1985). Psychosocial enhancement of immunocompetence in a geriatric population. *Health Psychology, 4*, 25–41.

Kiess, W., & Butenandt, O. (1985). Specific growth hormone receptors on human peripheral mononuclear cells: Reexpression, identification and characterization. *Journal of Clinical Endocrinological Metabolism, 60*, 740–746.

Kroemer, G., & Marinez-A. C. (1992). Mechanisms of self-tolerance. *Immunology Today, 13*: 401–404.

Lahita, R. G. (1984). Effects of sex hormones, nutrition, & aging on the immune response. In D. P. Stites, J. D. Stobo, H. H. Fudenberg, & J. V. Wells (Eds.), *Basic and clinical immunology* (pp. 288–311). Los Altos, CA: Lange Medical.

Manton, K. G. (1989). Epidemiological, demographic, and social correlates of disability among the elderly. *The Milbank Memorial Fund Quarterly, 67*(Part. 1), 13–58.

Martin, R. A., & Dobbin, J. P. (1988). Sense of humor, hassles, and immunoglobulin A: evidence for a stress-moderating effect of humor. *International Journal of Psychiatry in Medicine, 18*, 93–105.

Matour, D., Melnicoff, M., Kaye, D., & Murasko, D. M. (1989). The role of T cell phenotypes in decreased lymphoproliferation of the elderly. *Clinical Immunology and Immunopathology, 50*, 82–99.

McCruden, A., & Stimson, W. H. (1991). Sex hormones and immune function. In R. Ader, D. Felton, & N. Cohen (Eds.), *Psychoneuroimmunology* (2nd ed.., pp. 475–494). San Diego: Academic Press.

McNaughton, M. E., Smith, L. W., Patterson, T. L., & Grant, I. (1990). Stress, social support, coping resources, and immune status in elderly women. *Journal of Nervous & Mental Disease, 38*, 460–461.

Miller, R. (1990). Aging and the immune response. In E. Schneider & J. Rowe (Ed.), *Handbook of the biology of aging* (pp. 157–180). San Diego, CA: Academic Press.

Moos, R. I., & Solomon, G. F. (1964). Personality correlates of the rapidity of progression of rheumatoid arthritis. *Annals of Rheumatic Diseases, 23*, 145–151.

Moos, R. I., & Solomon, G. F. (1965). Personality correlates of the degree of functional incapacity of patients with physical disease. *Journal of Chronic Disease*, *18*, 1019–1038.

Naliboff, B. D., Benton, D., Solomon, G. F., Morley, J. E., Fahey, J. L., Bloom, E. T., Makinodan, T., & Gilmore, S. L. (1991). Immunological changes in young and old adults during brief laboratory stress. *Psychosomatic Medicine*, *53*, 121–132.

Pieri, C., Recchioni, R., Moroni, F., Marcheselli, F., & Damianovich, S. (1992). The response of human lymphocytes to phytohemagglutinin is impaired at different levels during aging. In N. Fabris, D. Harman, D. L. Knook, E. Steinhagen-Thiessen, & I. Zs.-Nagy (Eds.), *Physiopathological processes of aging* (pp. 110–119). New York: Annals of the New York Academy of Sciences.

Prinz, P., Weitzman, E., Cunningham, G., & Karakan, I. (1983). Plasma growth hormone during sleep in young and aged men. *Journal of Gerontology*, *38*, 519–524.

Regelson, W., Loria, R., & Mohanned, K. (1988). Hormonal intervention: "buffer hormones" or "state dependency" The role of dehydroepiandrosterone (DHEA), thyroid hormone, estrogen and hypophysectomey in aging. In W. Pierpaoli & N. Spector (Eds.), *Neuroimmunomodulation: Interventions in aging and cancer* (pp. 260–273). New York: Annals of the New York Academy of Sciences.

Repetti, R., Matthews, K., & Waldron, I. (1989). Effects of paid employment on women's mental and physical health. *American Psychologist*, *44*, 1394–1401.

Rodin, J. (1986). Aging and health: Effects of the sense of control. *Science*, *233*, 1271–1276.

Sainsbury, P., & Grad de Alarcon, J. (1970). The psychiatrist and the geriatric patient: The effects of community care on the family of the geriatric patient. *Journal of Geriatric Psychiatry*, *4*, 23–41.

Schleifer, S., Keller, S., Camerino, M., Thornton, J., & Stein, M. (1983). Suppression of lymphocyte stimulation following bereavement. *Journal of the American Medical Association*, *250*, 374–377.

Schuurs, A. H., & Verheul, H. M. (1990). Effects of gender and sex steroids on the immune response. *Journal of Steroid Biochemistry*, *35*, 157–172.

Shavit, Y., Lewis, J., Terman, G., Gale, R., & Leibeskind, J. (1984). Opioid peptides mediate the suppressive effect of stress on natural killer cell cytotoxicity. *Science*, *223*, 188–190.

Solomon, G. (1981a). Emotional and personality factors in the onset and course of autoimmune disease, particularly rheumatoid arthritis. In R. Ader (ed.), *Psychoneuroimmunology*, pp. 159–192. New York Academic Press.

Solomon, G. (1981b). Immunologic abnormalities in mental illness. In R. Ader (Ed.), *Psychoneuroimunology* (pp. 259–178). New York: Academic Press.

Solomon, G. (1989). Psychoneuroimmunology and human immunodeficiency virus infection. *Psychiatric Medicine*, *7*, 47–57.

Solomon, G. F. (1992). Response to Richard Lazarus's 'can we demonstrate important psychosocial influences on healths." *Advances*, *8*, 32–36.

Spurrell, M., & Creed, F. H. (1993). Lymphocyte response in depressed patients and subjects anticipating bereavement. *British Journal of Psychiatry*, *162*, 60–64.

Stein, M. (1989). Stress, depression, and the immune system. *Journal of Clinical Psychiatry*, *50*, 35–42.

Stein, M., Miller, A. H., & Trestman, R. L. (1991). Depression and the immune system. In R. Ader, D. L. Felten, & N. Cohen (Eds.), *Psychoneuroimmunology* (pp. 897–930). San Diego: Academic Press.

Sthoeger, Z., Chiorzzi, N., & Lahita, R. (1988). Regulation of the immune response by sex hormones: In vitro effects of estradiol and testosterone on pokeweed mitogen-induced human B cell differentiation. *The Journal of Immunology, 141,* 91–98.

Stimson, W. H., & Hunter, J. C. (1990). Oestrogen-induced immuno- regulation mediation through the thymus. *Journal of Clinical and Laboratory Immunology, 4,* 27–33.

Strickland, B. (1988). Sex related differences in health and illness. *Psychology of Women, 12,* 381–399.

Tache, Y., Du Ruisseau, P., Ducharme, J., & Collu, R. (1978). Pattern of adenohypo-physeal hormone changes in male rats following chronic stress. *Neuroendocrinology, 26,* 208–219.

Thoman, M. (1985). Role of interleukin-2 in the age-related impairment of immune function. *Journal of the American Geriatrics Society, 33,* 781–788.

Thompson, J. S., Wekstein, D. R., Rhoades, J. L., Kirkpatrick, C., Brown, S. A., Roszman, T., Straus, R., & Tietz, N. (1984). The immune status of healthy centenarians. *Journal of the American Geriatrics Society, 32*(4), 274-281.

U.S. Bureau of the Census. (1991). *Statistical data.* Washington, DC: U.S. Government Printing Office.

Vandenbrouke, J., Boersma, J., Festin, J., Valkenburg, H., Cats, A., Huber-Bruning, O., & Rasher, J. (1982). Oral contraceptives and rheumatoid arthritis: Further evidence for a preventive effect. *Lancet, 2,* 839–842.

Verbrugge, L. (1985). Gender and health. *Journal of Health and Social Behavior, 26,* 156–182.

Vestal, R. E., & Cusack, B. J. (1990). Pharmacology and aging. In E. Schneider & J. Rowe (Eds.), *Handbook of the biology of aging* (3rd ed., pp. 349–383). San Diego: Academic Press.

Vidalon, C., Khurana, R., Chae, S., Gegick, C. G., Stephan, T., Noaln, S., & Danowski, T. S. (1973). Age-related changes in growth hormone in non-diabetic women. *Journal of American Geriatrics Society, 21,* 253–255.

Weksler, M. (1981). The senescence of the immune system. *Hospital Practice, 16,* 53–64.

Workman, E. A., & La Via, M. F. (1987). Immunological effects of psychological stressors: a review of the literature. *International Journal of Psychosomatics, 34,* 35–40.

Zachariae, R., Kristensen, J., Hokland, P., Ellegaard, J., Metze, E., & Hokland, M. (1990). Effect of psychological intervention in the form of relaxation and guided imagery on cellular immune function in normal healthy subjects. *Psychotherapy Psychosomatic, 54,* 32–39.

The Pineal Aging Clock:

13

An Approach to Age-Delaying Strategies

Walter Pierpaoli

We have demonstrated recently that administration of the pineal hormone melatonin (indoleamine N-acetyl-5-methoxy-tryptamine) to aging mice produces an aging-postponing effect (Pierpaoli, Dall'Ara, Pedrinis, et al., 1991; Pierpaoli & Maestroni, 1987; Pierpaoli & Yi, 1990a). These early findings suggested that the neurohormone could influence the course of aging. In rodents, melatonin is secreted to a large extent by the pineal gland. However, no evidence was available that the life-prolonging effects of melatonin administration were directly related to a specific function of the pineal gland or to an age-related decay of pineal melatonin-secreting capacity. Therefore we decided to evaluate whether in rodents there is an intrinsic progressive inability of the aging pineal gland to maintain functions typical of a juvenile state. These experiments started by implanting the intact pineal gland from young donor mice into the thymus of aging, genetically identical, nonpinealectomized recipients. The rationale and methods for this intervention have been described elsewhere (Pierpaoli et al., 1991; Pierpaoli & Regelson, 1992). The life-prolonging or aging-postponing effects of this intervention confirmed our assumption that, whether or not pineal melatonin was responsible for the delay of aging observed earlier

(Pierpaoli & Yi, 1990b), certainly the pineal gland possesses the true character of a primary, central "aging clock" (Pierpaoli & Yi, 1990b). This latter model suggested that melatonin as well as other pineal-derived components can influence and maintain a great variety of adaptive functions (endocrine, sexual, metabolic, immune, etc.) that are related to juvenile performance.

We describe a relatively simple and reproducible method to study the pathogenesis of aging along with the more invasive techniques of prolonged food restriction (low caloric diet) and hypophysectomy, which had shown an aging-postponing or even aging-reversing effect (Everitt, Syedsman, & Jones, 1980). We propose further interventions that may help to clarify the relevance of the pineal clock better, and propose a general hypothesis on the mechanism by which the pineal gland controls ontogeny, reproduction, and aging. Three main questions are discussed: (a) Is the pineal gland a logical outcome of adaptive processes? (b) Is there a metabolic clock whose expiration precedes but is linked to the "genetic clock"? (c) Can we propose a general mechanism for the operation of the "pineal aging clock"?

PINEAL GLAND IS LOGICAL OUTCOME OF ADAPTIVE PROCESSES

In every species, it is inevitable that the progressive phylogenetic and ontogenetic adaptation to environmental variables is a prerequisite for survival and is thus selected for by any living and self-reproducing creature. Adaptability means the selective capacity to adopt new tasks. This refers not only to cells, tissues, and organs, but also to *molecules* (see later discussion on multifunctional peptide). In the evolutionary construction of the living world as it is now, two external natural aspects are considered to be pre-eminent in the species-selective process, namely, periodical (daily and seasonal) variations of light and temperature.

These interconnected undulatory and rhythmic physical elements, which depend on variations of solar light and heating energy, are the breeders of life on this planet. Even the selective, but repetitive models of nature are reflected in the close mechanistic similarity of the physiologic changes occurring in a circadian or seasonal fashion, namely, sleep (night) and hibernation (winter). Simply stated, physiologic sleep can be described, from the hormonal, neural, thermoregulatory viewpoint, as a "small hibernation," repeated every 24 hours. Sleep patterns are closely related to the pineal gland and hormonal changes (Arendt, 1991; Berger & Philips, 1991; Borbely, 1985; Lieberman, 1985). In addition to light and temperature, there exists a third, almost neglected and underestimated element, which constitutes an integral part of the "pineal complex"–driven regulation and which is responsible for the selective pressure of the environment on developing molecules, cells, and organs in the different species. This element is the *circumlunar rhythms* (the moon phases), with their powerful effects on electromagnetism and gravity. It is possible that the evolution of primeval, originally marine species into terrestrial species was largely influenced by cyclical lunar high and low tide, which allows periodical exposure to air and its many components (gas, ultraviolet light, sounds, odors etc.). The photoreceptive sensors of the primeval "pineal complex" have thus developed in phylogeny in concomitance with synchronous changes of temperature, light, gravity, and electromagnetism. In fact, detection and regulation of all these main physical elements are attributed to the pineal gland (Erlich & Aduzza, 1985; Hastings, Vance, & Maywood, 1989).

Evolutionary development of a "general adaptive device" to all these physical variables was thus a *sine qua non* for coping with the constant threat to survival. It was also required for generation of "resistance" (natural immunity) and species reproduction (Pierpaoli, 1981). Genetic pressure was not a primary factor for species selection but a concomitant adaptation of those individuals who could adopt a *new capacity in a changing environment*. Through time, they were selected by the environment to survive and reproduce.

The later evolution of the "regulator of the regulators" to the present shape and structure in animal species does not constitute a backward step. Eventually, other structures and sensory organs assumed the tasks of the "primeval eye," but it was in *addition* to preexisting and preserved functions of the pineal gland, and not a radical mutation to different, non-preexisting structures. For example, the harderian gland, the gut, the retina, and the CNS are evolutionary steps for location and maintenance of indoleamine functions from its original "third eye" location in invertebrates and more primitive species. It is logical to assume that the necessity for a regulator of primary body functions (feeding, thermoregulation, and sexual and immune capacity) in relation to external variables forced the elaboration of a primitive and later sophisticated "pineal complex" that integrates *all* endogenous and exogenous stimuli into a finely tuned, afferent regulatory response. This is represented in higher species by modification of sensory organs and central, neuroendocrine feedback mechanisms, such as hormones, cytokines, and neurotransmitters. It is for the benefit of the survivors that the "aging clock" emerged in phylogeny and was maintained and constantly improved. This "pineal clock," however, is responsible for scanning the time, not only for death, but for the genetically programmed maturation of reproductive functions (puberty in humans) and for maintenance of identity-defense capacity (Gupta, Riedel, Frick, et al., 1983; Karsch, Bittman, Foster, et al., 1984; Pierpaoli, 1981; Waldhauser & Steger, 1986). Its decay initiates the cascade of negative adaptive and compensatory events known as "metabolic aging," which is a manifestation, not of a program, but of the diseases of aging. Aging is thus an amenable process, and correction of pineal dysfunction during senescence may prolong the state of youth and "add good years to a long and healthy life."

METABOLIC CLOCK LINKED TO GENETIC CLOCK

The discovery of methods suitable to retard aging and thus prolong life of animals, such as caloric restriction, hormonal supplementation, and hypophysectomy (Regelson, 1983; Regelson, Loria, Kalimi, 1988), demonstrates unequivocally that a basic deterioration of neuroendocrine regulation is the common denominator of senescence. An unlimited number of side effects related to this CNS-hormonal decay has been disclosed in the literature. In my view, these are not relevant to understanding *why* we age but only illustrate *how* we age. Dilman's proposals and his theories on aging processes are still valid and fit the "pineal aging clock" hypothesis (Dilman, 1991). In fact, his original discovery of pineal peptides (Dilman, Anisimov, Ostroumova, et al., 1979) indicates that we still do not know how many pineal agents may affect aging. Also his definitions of "hyperadaptosis" and "metabolic immunosuppression" are appropriate to describe those compensatory alterations of endocrine and immune functions that are a consequence of a decay of hormonal-regulatory, pineal activity. In fact, there is no contradiction in the immense gerontologic and geriatric literature now available on the fact that we can prolong life via "pineal interventions" at the time when the attrition of age is visible (Pierpaoli & Regelson, 1992). However, the models reported with melatonin administration and pineal grafting seem to support the concept that avoidance or postponement or aging-related aesthetic and organic alterations would be feasible only *if a central aging clock did exist.* Even if some documented deficiencies could be corrected with genetic or pharmacologic interventions such as control of free radicals, gene modification, cell membrane rigidity, ionic imbalances, hormonal deficiencies, autosensitization, autoimmune processes and so on, the perspective for long-lasting and curative therapy is weak indeed (Pierpaoli & Fabris, 1991). The addition of *one* missing element in the decaying body would not eliminate the cause and would not be able to stop a retrograde cascade of beneficial events. On the contrary, ad hoc interventions on one severe deficiency during aging may alleviate the symptoms temporarily but will certainly be ineffective over the long range. Experimental interventions may even accelerate aging (e.g., the intriguing, paradoxical effects of somatotropic hormone). Such strategies may be relevant to specific cases when alleviation of aging discomfort is more urgent than hypothetical "radical" intervention. The problem lies in the existence, even during aging, of many rebound and feedback mechanisms that do not obey the simplistic logic of medical "correction." Senescence of the body is a slow process and any genuine prophylactic action to postpone aging must result in a clear-cut and reproducible life-prolonging treatment in animals and humans. Any temporary correction of aging parameters is illusory and misleading without long-term observation.

The remarkable maintenance and reconstitution of juvenile conditions in aging mice using a method that does not contradict any present hypothesis on the course of aging, offers a possibility to investigate the genesis, progression, and role of all those alterations considered to be relevant to aging. Certainly there may be an interdependence between the genomic changes and anomalies occurring during aging (Cutler, 1991; Vijg, Gossen, DeLeeuw, et al., 1991) and a pineal-related aging. Our method will serve to establish whether such events can be prevented or corrected with melatonin or pineal grafting. In other words, pineal cells could be primarily affected by intrinsic genomic changes as a prelude to aging. Conversely, neuroendocrine-hormonal alterations may be the cause of the genomic changes and the consequent subversion of cellular functions. In fact, hormones (e.g., thyroxine or steroids) are ultimately activators of specific genes by binding to enhancer proteins and may be themselves responsible for genetic alterations within target cells (Bradshaw & Gill, 1983; Hollenberg, Weinberger, Ong, et al., 1985; Sap, Munoz, Damm, et al., 1986). It is at the level of gene expression that hormones may alter cell function during aging.

GENERAL MECHANISM FOR OPERATION OF PINEAL AGING CLOCK

Evidence that the thyroid gland mediates the effects of pineal melatonin (Pierpaoli et al., 1991) led us to the unanticipated and surprising observation that thyrotropin releasing hormone (TRH), a ubiquitous tripeptide, may be a major effector for the varied pineal regulatory functions (Griffith, 1985; Holaday, D'Arnato, & Fadar, 1981; Jackson, 1982; Martino, Seo, Lernmark, et al., 1980; Nemeroff, Loosen, Bissett, et al., 1979; Vriend, 1978; Youngblood , Humm, Krizer, et al., 1979). Our data have shown that TRH, whose production in the retina depends on light (Martino et al., 1980), is a potent immunostimulatory, thymotropic agent and can antagonize the thymolytic effects of corticosteroids via a nonthyroid-dependent effect (Lesnikov, Korneva, Dall'Ara, et al., 1992; Pierpaoli & Regelson, 1992; Pierpaoli & Yi, 1990b). By using the thymus and the "immune model" for proposing that the thymus is a simple "amplifier" of antigen-selected lymphocytes, we have shown that certain hormones (thyroxine, growth hormone, insulin, prolactin) can modulate the expression of the immune reaction (Pierpaoli, 1981; Pierpaoli & Besedovsky, 1975; Pierpaoli, Fabris, & Sorkin, 1970; Pierpaoli, Kopp, & Bianchi, 1976; Pierpaoli, Kopp, Mueller, et al., 1977; Pierpaoli & Sorkin, 1972). It is thus at the level of *activation-amplification* that we propose TRH as a major vehicle for the targeted amplification of the pineal-melatonin central messages (Pierpaoli & Regelson, 1992; Pierpaoli & Yi, 1990b). This phylogenetically ancient molecule (Jackson, 1982) has acquired in evolution the character of "multifunctional peptide" by complying with the complex task of targeted, local adaptation of cells, tissues, and organs to light and temperature-dependent processes. It is at the level of rapid energy production that TRH may exert its most ancient tasks. The epithelial cells in frog skin and the insulin-producing β-cells of the pancreas (Jackson & Reichlin, 1977; Martino et al., 1980; Youngblood et al., 1979) both illustrate that TRH presence is needed in large amounts when immediate intervention for life-saving, oxygen-dependent, high-energy phosphate-bond production is needed. Local synthesis of energy allows the expression of specificity as *it is via amplication that function can be exerted and becomes measurable, leading to the full manifestation of specific cell functions.*

How can TRH be considered a key effector molecule for the pineal regulation of thermoregulation, reproduction, immunity, and for the fundamental adaptive role to circadian and seasonal environmental changes? This ubiquitous peptide has no toxic side effects even at very high pharmacologic doses, (Holaday, Long, Martinez-Arizala, et al., 1989) and may have a basic function in the *burst* activation of tyrosine kinase activity. This facilitates insulin activity on its cell receptors (Ebina et al., 1985) with consequent acceleration of anabolic processes (e.g., synthesis of glycogen, fatty acids, proteins) and inhibition of catabolic ones (e.g., the breakdown of glycogen and fat). Phosphorylation of proteins by PKC decreases the tyrosine kinase activity of the insulin receptor and regulates glucose consumption and cell respiration. A normal PKC function controls neural excitability, whereas cell degeneration is associated with high levels of PKC function (Nishizuka, 1986). Thus, it my be at the level of the PKC-transducing system that exogenous TRH *directly* affects the aging process by repairing the inability of aging cells to *amplify* their specific function through a "burst" of TRH-induced activity modulating other hormones (Albert & Tashjian, 1985). This adaptive function of TRH may constitute a key element in the oxidative cascade. In fact, TRH may be also related to the effects of IL-1 β on thyroid function (Dubuis, Dayer, Siegrist-Kaiser, et al., 1988). TRH, a physiologic regulator of pituitary hormone secretion, induces a "burst" phase of acute hormone secretion by activation of PKC via diacylglycerol and a simultaneous spike in $[Ca^{2+}]$ (Albert & Tashjian, 1985). The effects of TRH on the secretion of prolactin, a main immunomodulating agent (Hall, 1984; Pierpaoli, 1981) is further evidence for the postulated key role of TRH as mediator of pineal function through a "burst" of hormones that maintain body homeostasis (temperature, ovarian cycle, immunity, etc.) and provide constant adaptation of daily and seasonal modifications in all species.

We propose that melatonin and other pineal-derived agents exert their activity by targeted activation and oxidative, energetic amplification of local functions through TRH-induced activation of hormonal effects on gene expression enzyme activity, and transport processes (Ebina, Ellis, Jarnagin, et al., 1985; Hollenberg et al., 1985; James & Bradshaw, 1984; Sap et al., 1986). Corrective interventions on key, metabolic or defense (immunity) functions are feasible. A *seasonal* correction of these aging-related diseases by administration of melatonin (Pierpaoli, 1991) or by "rapid intervention" with TRH may thus initiate a positive cascade of energy-providing events to CNS-decaying functions (e.g., memory, sleep, concentration, attention, etc.) that would provide relief to manifestations of senescence. As an example, TRH and related peptides may constitute a natural remedy to the typical hypercortisolism of aging by antagonizing the elevated corticosteroid level that blocks the memory-enhancing effects of nootropics and cholinomimetics (Mondadori, Ducret, & Häusler, 1992). TRH alone may also enhance memory or facilitate the activity of nootropics. Ad hoc interventions in "metabolic aging" may allow us to understand if a separation exists between the "pineal aging clock" and the "genetic clock." To attain this goal, we may acquire longevity either by losing the capacity to "count" our years (Spector, 1988) or by learning to wait for the end of those endless in vivo experiments that are the final answer to any hypothesis on the causes of aging. This will be a most arduous task.

REFERENCES

Albert, P. R., & Tashjian, A. H., Jr. (1985). Dual actions of phorbol esters on cytosolic free Ca^{2+} concentrations and reconstitution with ionomycin of acute thyrotropin-releasing hormone responses. *Journal of Biological Chemistry, 260*, 8746–8759.

Arendt, J. (1991). Melatonin in humans: Jet-lag and after. In J. Arendt & P. Pevet (Eds.), *Advances in pineal research* (Vol. 5, pp. 229–302). London: John Libbey & Co.

Berger, R. J., & Phillips, N. H. (1991). Suppression of slow wave sleep and circadian rhythms of body temperature in the pigeon by continuous bright light, and their reinstatement by daily melatonin infusions. In J. Arendt & P. Pevet (Eds.), (Vol. 5, pp. 275–278). London: John Libbey & Co.

Borbely, A. A. (1985). Endogenous sleep substances and sleep regulation. In R. J. Wurtman & F. Waldhauser (Eds.), *Melatonin in humans* (pp. 219–229). Cambridge, MA: Center for Brain Sciences.

Bradshaw, R. A., & Gill, G. N. (Eds.). (1983). *Evolution of hormone-receptor systems.* New York: Alan R. Liss.

Cutler, R. G. (1991). Human longevity and aging: Possible role of reactive oxygen species. *Annals of the New York Academy of Science, 621,* 1–28.

Dilman, V. M. (1991). Pathogenetic approaches to prevention of age-associated increase of cancer incidence. *Annals of the New York Academy of Sciences, 621,* 385–400.

Dilman, V. M., Anisimov, V. N., Ostroumova, M. N., Khavinson, V. Kh., & Morozov, V. G. (1979). Study of the anti-tumor effect of popypeptide pineal extract. *Oncology, 36,* 274–280.

Dubuis, J. M., Dayer, J. M., Siegrist-Kaiser, C. A., & Burger, A. G. (1988). Human recombinant interleukin-1 decreases plasma thyroid hormone and thyroid stimulating hormone levels in rats. *Endocrinology, 123,* 2175–2181.

Ebina, Y., Ellis, L., Jarnagin, K., Edery, M., Graf, L., Clauser, E., Ou, J., Masiarz, F., Kan, Y. W., Goldfine, I. D., Roth, R. A., & Rutter, W. J. (1985). The human insulin receptor cDNA: The structural basis for hormone-activated trans-membrane signalling. *Cell, 40,* 747–758.

Erlich, S. S., & Aduzza, M. L. J. (1985). The pineal gland: Anatomy, physiology and clinical significance. *Journal of Neurosurgery, 63,* 321–341.

Everitt, A. V., Syedsman, N. J., & Jones, F. (1980). The effects of hypophysectomy and continuous food restriction, begun at ages 70 and 400 days, on collagen aging, proteinuria, incidence of pathology and longevity in the male rat. *Mechanisms of Aging and Development, 12,* 161–172.

Griffith, E. C. (1985). Thyrotropin releasing hormone: Endocrine and central effects. *Psychoneuroendocrinology, 10,* 225–235.

Gupta, D., Riedel, L., Frick, H. J., Attanasio, A., & Ranke, M. B. (1983). Circulating melatonin in children in relation to puberty, endocrine disorders, functional tests and racial origin. *Neuroendocrinology Letter, 5,* 63–78.

Hall, T. R. (1984). Control of prolactin secretion in vertebrates—a comparative study. *General Pharmacology, 15,* 189–195.

Hastings, M. H., Vance, G., & Maywood, E. (1989). Phylogeny and function of the pineal. *Experientia, 45,* 903–1008.

Holaday J. W., D'Amato, R. J., & Faden, A. I. (1981). Thyrotropin-releasing hormone improves cardiovascular function in experimental endotoxic and hemmorrhagic shock. *Science, 213,* 216–218.

Holaday, J. W., Long, J. B., Martinez-Arizala, A., Chen, H. S., Reynolds, D. G., & Gurll, N. J. (1989). Effects of TRH in circulatory shock and central nervous system ischemia. *Annals of the New York Academy of Sciences, 553,* 370–379.

Hollenberg, S. M., Weinberger, C., Ong, E. S., Cerelli, G., Oro, A., Lebo, R., Thompson, E. B., Rosenfeld, M. G., & Evens, R. M. (1985). Primary structure and expression of a functional human glucocorticoid receptor cDNA. *Nature, 318,* 635–641.

Jackson, I. M. D. (1982). Thyrotropin-releasing hormone. *New England Journal of Medicine, 306,* 145–155.

Jackson, I. M. D., & Reichlin, S. (1977). Brain thyrotropin-releasing hormone is independent of the hypothalamus. *Nature, 267,* 853–854.
James, R., & Bradshaw, R. A. (1984). Polypeptide growth factors. *Annals of the Review of Biochemistry, 53,* 259–292.
Karsch, F. J., Bittman, E. L., Foster, D. L., Goodman, R. L., Legan, S. J., & Robinson, J.
E. (1984). Neuroendocrine basis of seasonal reproduction. *Records of Progress
in Hormone Research, 40,* 185–232.
Lesnikov, V. A., Korneva, E. A., Dall'Ara, A., & Pierpaoli, W. (1992). The involvement of pineal gland and melatonin in immunity and aging: II. Thyrotropin
releasing hormone and melatonin forestall involution and promote reconstitution of the thymus in anterior hypothalamic area (AHA)-lesioned mice. *International Journal of Neuroscience, 62,* 141–153.
Lieberman, H. R. (1985). Behavior, sleep and melatonin. In R. J. Wurtman & F.
Waldhauser (Eds.), *Melatonin in humans* (pp. 209–218). Cambridge, MA: Center for Brain Sciences.
Martino, E., Seo, H., Lernmark, A., & Refetoff, S. (1980). Ontogenetic patterns of
thyrotropin-releasing hormone-like material in rat hypothalamus, pancreas
and retina: Selective effect of light deprivation. *Proceedings of the National Academy of Sciences USA, 77,* 4345–4348.
Mondadori, C., Ducret, T., & Häusler, A. (1992). Elevated corticosteroid levels
block the memory-improving effects of nootropics and cholinomimetics.
Psychopharmacology, 108, 11–15.
Nemeroff, C. B., Loosen, P. T., Bissette, G., Manberg, P. J., Wilson, I. C., Lipton, M. A.
& Prange, A. J. Jr. (1979). Pharmaco-behavioral effects of hypothalamic peptides in animals and man: Focus on thyrotropin-releasing hormone and
neurotensin. *Psychoneuroendocrinology, 3,* 279–310.
Nishizuka, Y. (1986). Studies and perspectives of protein kinase C. *Science, 233,*
305–312.
Pierpaoli, W. (1981). Integrated phylogenetic and ontogenetic evolution of neuroendocrine and identity-defence, immune functions. In R. Ader. (Ed.), *Psychoneuroimmunology* (pp. 575–606). New York: Academic Press.
Pierpaoli, W. (1991). The pineal gland: A circadian or seasonal aging clock? [Edito-
rial] *Aging, 3,* 99–101.
Pierpaoli, W., & Besedovsky, H. O. (1975). Role of the thymus in programming of
neuroendocrine functions. *Clinical and Experimental Immunology, 20,* 323–338.
Pierpaoli, W., Dall'Ara, A., Pedrinis, E., & Regelson, W. (1991). The pineal control of
aging: The effects of melatonin and pineal grafting on the survival of older
mice. In W. Pierpaoli & N. Fabris (Eds.), Physiological senescence and its postponement: Theoretical approaches and rational interventions. *Annals of the
New York Academy of Science, 621,* 291–313.
Pierpaoli, W., & Fabris, N., (Eds.). (1991). Physiological senescence and its postponement: Theoretical approaches and rational interventions. (Second
Stromboli Conferences on Aging and Cancer). *Annals of the New York Academy
of Science, 621,* 291–313.
Pierpaoli, W., Fabris, N., & Sorkin, E. (1970). Developmental hormones and
immunological maturation. In G. E. W. Wolstenholme & J. Knight (Eds.), *Hor-*

mones and the immune response (Ciba Foundation Study Group No. 36, pp. 126–143). London: Churchill.

Pierpaoli, W., Kopp, H. G., & Bianchi, E. (1976). Interdependence of thymic and neuroendocrine functions in ontogeny. *Clinical and Experimental Immunology, 24,* 501–506.

Pierpaoli, W., Kopp, H. G., Müller, J., & Keller, M. (1977). Interdependence between neuroendocrine programming and the generation of immune recognition in ontogeny. *Cellular Immunology, 29,* 16–27.

Pierpaoli, W., & Maestroni, G. (1987). Melatonin: A principal neuroimmunoregulatory and anti-stress hormone: Its anti-aging effects. *Immunology Letter, 16,* 355–362.

Pierpaoli, W., & Regelson, W. in press. Pineal control of aging: Melatonin or pineal grafting prolong survival of older mice. *Proceedings of the National Academy of Science, USA.*

Pierpaoli, W., & Sorkin, E. (1972). Alterations of adrenal cortex and thyroid in mice with congenital absence of the thymus. *Nature New Biology, 238,* 282–285.

Pierpaoli, W., & Yi, C. X. (1991a). The involvement of pineal gland and melatonin in immunity and aging: I. Thymus-mediated, immunoreconstituting and antiviral activity of thyrotropin releasing hormone (TRH). *Journal of Neuroimmunology, 27,* 99–109.

Pierpaoli, W., & Yi, C. X. (1990b). The pineal gland and melatonin: The aging clock? A concept and experimental evidence. In G. Nappi, E. Martignoni, A. R. Genazzani, & F. Petraglia (Eds.), *Stress and the aging brain* (Aging Series, Vol. 37, pp. 171–175). New York: Raven Press.

Regelson, W. (1983). The evidence for pituitary and thyroid control of aging: Is age reversal a myth or reality? The search for a "death hormone." In W. Regelson & F. M. Sinex (Eds.), *Interventions in the aging process* (Part B, pp. 3–52). New York: Alan R. Liss.

PART III
Infectious Syndromes in the Elderly: Cause, Course, and Treatment

Urinary Tract Infection in the Elderly

14

Steven L. Berk

Urinary tract infection is the most common infectious disease problem in the elderly (Berk & Smith, 1983). The spectrum of illness ranges from benign asymptomatic bacteriuria to life-threatening pyelonephritis with septic shock. Advancing age is a risk factor for urinary tract infection. Increasing risk is explained by a combination of physiological and social factors. Table 14.1 lists some of the processes most likely to explain the high incidence of bacteriuria in the elderly.

PATHOGENESIS OF URINARY TRACT INFECTION

In both older and younger adults, infection of the urinary tract usually occurs by an ascending route of infection. The anterior urethra is colonized by bacteria. In elderly women, the urethra is close to the heavily colonized vagina and perineum and is easily contaminated, particularly when fecal incontinence or poor hygiene is present. Low-dose oral estrogens have been shown to change vaginal flora from gram-negative enterics to lactobacilli, thereby decreasing the incidence of urinary tract infection (Brandenburg, Mellstrom, Samsioe, et al., 1987).

TABLE 14.1 Factors Predisposing to Urinary Tract
Infections in Old Age

- •Prostate hypertrophy in men

- •Perineal soiling in women

- •Bladder dysfunction

- •Genitourinary instrumentation

- •Fecal incontinence

- •Loss of bactericidal prostatic secretions in men

- •Loss of hormone-dependent protection against introital
  colonization in postmenopausal women

Virulence factors of bacteria play a role in the pathogenesis. Most important is the ability of the etiologic agent to adhere to uroepithelium. Some
bacteria are more able to adhere to the uroepithelium of older compared
with younger men.

Physiologic changes in old age also predispose to bacteriuria and infection (Baldassarre & Kaye, 1991). Urine itself does have some antibacterial
activity, and this activity appears to decrease with age (Kaye, 1968). Renal
function declines with aging causing less ability to acidify urine. The high
incidence of glycosuria in the older person may induce bacterial growth
(Ascher, Sussman, & Weiser, 1968). Prostatic secretions in elderly men may
be less bactericidal (Meares, 1991). Inability to completely empty the bladder because of prostatic disease, neurogenic bladder, or bladder prolapse
in women also encourages bacteriuria.

MICROBIOLOGY

Organisms known to cause urinary tract infection are similar in young and
old patient populations. *Escherichia coli* is by for the most common pathogen in both groups (Nicolle, Bjornson, & Harding, 1983). Elderly patients
are more likely to have resistant gram-negative bacilli such as Enterobac-
ter, Serratia and Pseudomonas, but this probably reflects factors such as
prior antibiotic therapy and institutionalization (Turck & Stamm, 1981).
Staphylococcus saprophyticus, commonly seen as a cause of dysuria in
younger women, is not common in older women. In some studies a high

TABLE 14.2 Bacteriuria in Older Persons

	% bacteriuria	
	Men	Women
Elderly persons living at home	2 - 13%	1.5 - 4.3%
Elderly persons living in nursing home or long-term geriatric care facility	15 - 37%	18 - 31%
Elderly, hospitalized patients	30 - 59%	30 - 55%

incidence of gram-positive cocci, such as *S. epidermis* and *Enterococcus faecalis* have been reported in elderly men (Lipsky, 1989).

INCIDENCE OF BACTERIURIA

The incidence of bacteriuria varies with the patient population studied. Table 14.2 summarizes data on bacteriuria from several studies (Dontas, 1990). The incidence of bacteriuria in elderly men and women is similar. The incidence of bacteriuria increases with the degree of debility and institutionalization from 2% in some ambulatory elderly to 59% in some hospitalized patient series (Boscia, Kobasa, & Knight, 1986). The geriatric population with bacteriuria is not a stable one. In one study 17% of women and 6% of men with initial negative cultures had positives ones on the second or third culture. Forty percent of women and 75% of men became culture negative on subsequent surveys (Boscia et al., 1986).

Asymptomatic Bacteriuria

Patients without symptoms of urinary tract infection who have significant bacteriuria (defined as greater than 10^5 of the same bacterial species per milliliter of urine on two consecutive, aseptically collected urine cultures) are categorized as having asymptomatic bacteriuria. Because of the high incidence of asymptomatic bacteriuria in older persons, the value of antibi-

otic therapy in this setting has become a critical issue. In at least two studies, those elderly nursing home patients with asymptomatic bacteriuria
died earlier than those with sterile urine (Dontas, Kasviki-Charvati, &
Papanayiotou, 1981; Sourander, 1966). Some studies have failed to confirm
this association. (Nicolle et al., 1983; Nordenstam, Brandberg, Oden, et al.,
1986). In addition, randomized controlled trials of antibiotic therapy for
asymptomatic bacteriuria in both elderly males and elderly females have
failed to demonstrate that treatment has an effect on mortality (Nicolle,
Henderson, Bjornson, et al., 1987; Nicolle, Mayhew, & Bryant, 1987). Moreover patients with asymptomatic bacteriuria treated with antibiotics do
not maintain urine sterility. Antibiotics, then, are not generally recommended for this condition in the elderly patient. Such therapy will be associated with antibiotic side effects and development of resistant organisms.
Patients undergoing urinary tract surgery, such as transurethral prostatectomy, should be treated with short-course therapy directed at the particular pathogen grown from the urine. Asymptomatic bacteriuria is not in
itself an indication for anatomic assessment of the urinary tract. Patients
with bacteriuria and obstructive uropathy, however, should be considered
for antibiotic therapy.

Recently Nicolle, Muir, Harding, et al. (1988) studied asymptomatic
bacteriuria in elderly institutionalized women. Sixty-seven percent of
bacteriuria was localized to the kidney by Fairley bladder washout technique.

CYSTITIS VERSUS PYELONEPHRITIS

Distinguishing cystitis from pyelonephritis is a critical first step in managing the elderly patient. Pyelonephritis requires a longer duration of
treatment and usually necessitates parenteral therapy. Hence, management clearly depends on localization of the infection as best as is practical.
Unfortunately, recent studies have shown clinical signs and symptoms to
be unreliable in differentiating upper and lower tract infection (Pappas,
1991; Sheldon & Gonzales, 1984). Table 14.3 describes some of the clinical
and laboratory parameters that have been used in older persons. Fever
may not always occur with pyelonephritis, and vague abdominal pain is
more common than classical flank pain. In one study, 21% of elderly patients with acute pyelonephritis were initially misdiagnosed owing to
presence of gastrointestinal or pulmonary symptoms (Gleckman, Blagg,
Hilbert, et al., 1982). Bacteremia (61%) and shock (21%) were much more
common than in younger adults. White blood cell casts are usually absent
in pyelonephritis and, when present, could be a manifestation of other renal disease. Peripheral leukocytosis is often absent in older people. De-

TABLE 14.3 Clinical Distinction Between Cystitis and Pyelonephritis

Cystitis	Pyelonephritis
dysuria, urgency, frequency	nausea, rigors, fever
suprapubic tenderness	CVA tenderness
normal peripheral WBC count	elevated WBC count
WBC's in urine	WBC's in urine may have WBC casts
without bacteremia	60% bacteremic
negative ACB test	positive ACB test

finitive diagnosis can be made by ureteral catheterization and bladder wash-out methods, but these are invasive procedures and of no practical value in most clinical settings. Hence the physician must act often with some uncertainty in assessing a urinary tract focus of infection. In addition, the clinician may find it difficult to exclude pyelonephritis in the septic elderly patient with no definite focus of infection (Eposito, Gleckman, Cram, et al., 1980).

ACUTE PROSTATITIS

Prostatitis is a common but poorly understood inflammatory process in adult males. The clinical diagnosis of acute bacterial prostatitis is usually straightforward. Patients develop an acute illness with chills, fever, and local symptoms of back or perineal pain. Symptoms of frequency and dysuria are also present. Malaise, generalized myalgias, and prostration have been described. On rectal examination the prostate is tender, swollen, and indurated. Urinary retention resulting from bladder outlet obstruction may be recognized by bladder percussion. Laboratory data will show an elevated peripheral white blood cell count. A midstream urine sample will show white blood cells and greater than 10^5 bacteria. In the setting of acute bacterial prostatitis, prostatic massage is contraindicated as it may lead to bacteremia. (In chronic prostatitis, prostatic massage and collection of prostatic secretions for examination for bacteria and white blood cells is diagnostic.)

TREATMENT OF URINARY TRACT INFECTION

The treatment of urinary tract infection will depend on whether the infection involves kidney, bladder, or prostate. Basic principles in the management of pyelonephritis are listed in Table 14.4. The antibiotic of choice will vary from one practitioner to another and will depend on susceptibility patterns at one's own institution. Table 14.5 lists antibiotics of particular value in the initial management of urosepsis in the elderly. Because of the many new β-lactams available with excellent activity to most gram-negative bacilli, therapy with aminoglycosides is rarely necessary (File & Tan, 1989). Elderly patients are more likely to have aminoglycoside-induced nephrotoxicity and ototoxicity. Hence aminoglycosides should be used cautiously with dosing based on calculation of patients creatinine clearance and only when a multiple antibiotic resistant organism is suspected. The antibiotic of choice will be dependent on several factors. Antibiotic studies should be evaluated with the following parameters in mind: (a) effect of therapy on clinical symptoms; (b) ability to eradicate initial infecting organism; (c) likelihood of drug resistance; and (d) side effect profile (Rubin, Beam, & Stamm, 1992). If gram-positive cocci in chains are seen on gram stain, enterococcus is most likely, and ampicillin or piperacillin will be suitable antibiotics of choice. The patients' underlying disease process may play a role in antibiotic selection. Imipenem-cilastin should be avoided in patients with seizures; similarly, ticarcillin or timentin should be avoided in patients with congestive heart failure. Aztreonam may be useful in patients who have had anaphylaxis to penicillin.

TREATMENT OF CYSTITIS

Many studies have confirmed that short course therapy for lower urinary tract infection (3 days or even one dose) is as effective as a 7- to 14-day course (Kunin, 1981; Souney & Polk, 1982). These studies have generally been performed in young women with symptoms of cystitis. Many different oral regimens have been used including trimethoprim-sulfamethoxazole, norfloxacin, ciprofloxacin, cephalexin and amoxicillin, with or without clauvulanic acid. Cystitis in elderly women has not been as well studied. Long-term eradication of bacteriuria is less likely to be seen in the elderly women, particularly if functional status is poor. It is recommended that elderly women with typical symptoms of cystitis be treated for 3 days with a quinolone or trimethoprim. Relapse after 3 days should be considered evidence for upper tract disease, and treatment guidelines, as previously described, should be followed (Baldassarre & Kaye, 1991).

TABLE 14.4 Treatment of Upper Tract Infection in the Elderly

1. Initial treatment based on gram stain of urine;

2. Parenteral antibiotic will usually be necessary;

3. Antibiotic choice will depend on suspicion of resistant organism. Patients having received prior antibiotic therapy, those with structural abnormalities of the urinary tract will need antipseudomonal coverage initially.

4. Failure to respond to 48-72 hours of therapy suggests obstruction, intrarenal or perinephric abscess. Obtain ultrasound.

5. Length of treatment 10-21 days.

6. Relapse or reinfection requires longer term therapy. Evaluate for the presence of a non-sterilized nidus of infection as well as for anatomic or functional abnormalities of the urinary tract.

TABLE 14.5 Antibiotics Useful in the Initial
Management of Pyelonephritis or Urosepsis

1. Third generation cephalosporins

2. Newer penicillins

3. Aztreonam

4. Imipenem-cilastatin

5. Quinolones

6. Avoid aminoglycosides, if possible

Low-dose oral or intravaginal estrogens may be useful in managing recurrent urinary tract infections in women. Estrogen preserves glycogen
stores in vaginal epithelium and promotes the growth of lactobacilli,
thereby preventing atrophic vaginitis and fecal overgrowth (Privette,
Cede, Peterson, et al., 1988).

Men with lower urinary tract infection symptoms should be treated for 7
to 10 days. Patients should be evaluated for prostatic disease or structural
abnormality. Both acute and chronic prostatitis occur commonly in elderly
men, but the special features of the disease in the elderly are not well defined.

TREATMENT OF ACUTE PROSTATITIS

Patients with acute bacterial prostatitis should have blood cultures and
urine gram stain and culture before antibiotic therapy (Becopoulos, Georgoulias, Constantimides, et al., 1990). Gram-positive cocci seen in chains
suggest enterococcal infection, for which ampicillin plus an aminoglycoside is a suitable regimen. Most patients will have gram-negative bacilli on
smear. Trimethoprim-sulfamethoxazole is commonly used for community-acquired infection. Although only lipid-soluble and basic antibiotics
penetrate the normal prostate gland, diffusion into an acutely inflamed
prostate is less of a problem (Meares, 1982). Quinolones, particularly
ciprofloxacin, the monobactam aztreonam, aminoglycosides, and third-
generation cephalosporins have been used successfully. Antibiotic doses
should attain therapeutic levels in the serum. Response is usually dramatic. Analgesia, hydration, bed rest, and stool softener are also recom-

mended. Complications of acute bacterial prostatitis include septicemia, prostatic abscess, and epididymitis. Chronic prostatitis may occur after infection in some patients. Prostatic abscess may occur secondary to anaerobic bacteria. Treatment requires transurethral prostatectomy.

CATHETER-RELATED URINARY TRACT INFECTION

The urinary tract is the most common source of nosocomial infection. Most of these hospital-acquired infections are related to catheterization and urinary tract manipulation (Turck & Stamm, 1981). Long-term catheterization may be necessary in the elderly patient who has an anatomically or functionally obstructed urinary tract. More than 15% of elderly patients admitted to community hospitals require urinary catheterization. The frequency of urinary catheterization in the nursing home is even higher (Dontas, 1990).

Urinary catheterization carries an increasing risk of bacteriuria over time and can result in pyelonephritis, urosepsis, urethral abscess, and epididymitis. The urinary or Foley catheter predisposes to infection for several reasons. The catheter bypasses normal mucosal defense mechanisms, serves as a foreign body, and may prevent complete bladder emptying. Bacteria may enter the bladder through the catheter lumen or by ascending between the outside of the catheter and the urethral mucosa. Bacteria may be introduced during the catheter insertion or may have already been present in the patient with asymptomatic bacteriuria. The offending agent may also ascend from the drainage bag. In most instances, *Escherichia coli* and other gram-negative bacilli from the perineum or rectal surface will cause infection ascending from outside the catheter along the mucosal sheath. More resistant organisms such as *Pseudomonas aeruginosa* and *Serratia marcescens* tend to come from the hands of hospital personnel and reach the bladder through the catheter lumen.

The clinical suspicion of catheter-related infection is based on signs and symptoms previously described in discussion of cystitis and pyelonephritis. Quantitative cultures must be obtained by aseptic needle aspiration of the distal catheter or sampling port. Although most infections will result in greater than 10^5 bacteria per milliliter of urine, well-documented cases of urosepsis can occur with counts of 10^2 to 10^3 (Gleckman, Shannon, & Crowley, 1978). Catheter urine specimens may not always reflect the microbiology of the bladder. Some authors have suggested that in patients with catheter-related infections, the old catheter should be removed and urine collected and cultured from the newly placed catheter (Grahn, Norman, White, et al., 1985).

Prevention

Measures recommended to minimize infectious complications of indwelling catheters are as follows:

1. Indwelling catheters should be used only when absolutely necessary. Incontinence clothing or condom catheters may be preferable to indwelling catheters in many patients.
2. Catheterization should be performed by trained personnel using aseptic technique. Postcatheterization urine culture should be obtained.
3. A sterile drainage system must be kept closed. Those that come open or leak must be replaced immediately.
4. Perineum and urethral meatus should be kept clean.
5. Downhill flow must be maintained, and the drainage bag should be emptied as necessary.

A closed drainage system is recommended. The meatal surface should be kept clean with soap and water. Antibiotic creams or ointments have not been shown to be of routine benefit. Impregnation of the catheter with antibiotics has also not been successful. Catheters will usually need to be changed monthly. However, catheter change should be based on encrustation of the catheter or blocked flow more than on any particular schedule. Catheter and drainage tubes should not be disconnected.

In addition to the prevention of bacteriuria and urosepsis, patients with valvular heart disease and indwelling catheters are at risk for endocarditis, particularly with the enterococcus. Prophylactic antibiotics should be used at the time of catheter insertion and removal in these patients.

Condom catheters are useful alternatives to the Foley catheter to maintain dryness of the incontinent patient or prevent irritation of adjacent wounds. However, bacteriuria, local skin maceration, and bladder distention does occur (Johnson, 1983; Ouslander, Greengod, & Chen, 1987).

Treatment

Principles of antibiotic therapy in the treatment of catheter-related infection are not different from these for other urinary tract infections. Bacteremia and urosepsis can occur at any time and will often require the rapid institution of empiric antibiotic therapy. Urine gram stain will be helpful particularly in directing therapy to gram-positive cocci. The antibiotic sensitivity pattern of gram-negative bacilli in one's own hospital will form the basis of antibiotic selection in this setting. In hospitals where resistant *P. aeruginosa* is a problem, aminoglycoside therapy will often be necessary. A third-generation cephalosporin, aztreonam, and imipenem-cilastatin provide adequate empiric coverage for gram-negative bacilli at many institutions. Once culture results and antibiotic susceptibility is available one may switch to a safer, less broad-spectrum antibiotic.

REFERENCES

Ascher, A. W., Sussman, M., & Weiser, R. (1968). Bacterial growth in human urine. In F. O'Grady & W. Brumfitt (Eds.), *Urinary tract infection* (pp. 3–13). London: Oxford University.

Baldassarre, J. S., & Kaye, D. (1991). Special problems of urinary tract infection in the elderly. *Medical Clinics of North America, 75*, 375–387.

Becopoulos, T., Georgoulias, D., Constantinides, C., Stathakis, H., & Koamisia, J. (1990). Acute prostatitis: Which antibiotic to use first. *Journal of Chemotherapy, 2*, 244–246.

Berk, S. L., & Smith J. K. (1983). Infectious diseases in the elderly. *Medical Clinics of North America, 66*, 273–293.

Boscia, J. A., Kobasa, W. D., Knight, R. A., et al. (1986). Epidemiology of bacteriuria in an elderly ambulatory population. *American Journal of Medicine, 80*, 208–214.

Brandenberg, A., Mellstrom, D., Samsioe, G., et al. (1987). Low dose oral estriol treatment in elderly women with urogenital infections. *Acta Obstetrical Gynecologia Scandinavia, 140* (suppl.), 33–38.

Dontas, A. (1990). Urinary-tract infection in nursing-home residents. In A. Verghese & S. L. Berk (Eds.), *Infections in the nursing home and long term care facilities* (pp. 126–140). Switzerland: S. Karger.

Dontas, A. S., Kasviki-Charvati, O., Papanayiotou, P. C., et al. (1981). Bacteriuria and survival in old age. *New England Journal of Medicine, 304*, 939–943.

Esposito, A. L., Gleckman, R. A., Cram, S., et al. (1980). Community-acquired bacteremia in the elderly: Analysis of one hundred consecutive episodes. *Journal of the American Geriatrics Society, 28*, 315–319.

File, T. M., Jr., & Tan, J. S. (1989). Urinary tract infections in the elderly. *Geriatrics, 44*, 15–19.

Gleckman, R., Blagg, N., Hibert, D., et al. (1982). Acute pyelonephritis in the elderly. *Southern Medical Journal, 75*, 551–554.

Gleckman, R., Shannon, R. J., & Crowley, M. (1978). Symptomatic bacterial urinary tract infections in men: Limitations of quantitative urine cultures. *Journal of Urology, 120*, 645–646.

Grahn, D., Norman, D. C., White, M. L., Cantrell, M., & Yoshikawa, T. (1985). Validity of urinary catheter specimen for diagnosis of urinary tract infection in the elderly. *Archives of Internal Medicine, 145*, 1858–1860.

Johnson, E. T. (1983). The condom catheter: Urinary tract infection and other complications. *Southern Medical Journal, 76*, 597–582.

Kaye, D. (1968). Antibacterial activity of human urine. *Journal of Clinical Investigation, 47*, 2374–2390.

190 Infectious Syndromes in the Elderly

Kunin, C. M. (1981). Duration of treatment of urinary tract infections. *American Journal of Medicine, 71*, 849–854.

Lipsky, B. A. (1989). Urinary tract infection in men: Epidemiology, pathophysiology, diagnosis and treatment. *Annals of Internal Medicine, 110*, 138–150.

Meares, E. M., Jr. (1982). Prostatitis: Review of pharmacokinetics and therapy. *Review of Infectious Diseases, 4*, 475.

Meares, E. M., Jr. (1991). Prostatitis. *Medical Clinics of North America, 75*, 405–424.

Nicolle, L. E., Bjornson, J., Harding, G. K. M., et al. (1983). Bacteriuria in elderly institutionalized men. *New England Journal of Medicine, 309*, 1420–1425.

Nicolle, L. E., Henderson, E. Bjornson, J., et al. (1987). The association of bacteriuria with resident characteristics and survival in elderly institutionalized men. *Annals of Internal Medicine, 106*, 682–686.

Nicolle, L. E., Mayhew, W. J., & Bryan, L. (1987). Prospective, randomized comparison of therapy and no therapy for asymptomatic bacteriuria in institutionalized elderly women. *American Journal of Medicine, 83*, 27–33.

Nicolle, L. E., Muir, P., Harding, G. K. M., et al. (1988). Localization of UTI in elderly institutionalized women with asymptomatic bacteriuria. *Journal of Infectious Diseases, 157*, 65–70.

Nordenstam, G. R., Brandberg, C., Oden, A. S., et al. (1986). Bacteriuria and mortality in an elderly population. *New England Journal of Medicine, 314*, 1152–1156.

Ouslander, J. G., Greengod, B., & Chen, S. (1987). External catheter use and urinary tract infections among incontinent male nursing home patients. *Journal of the American Geriatrics Society*, 1063–1070.

Pappas, P. (1991). Laboratory in the diagnosis and management of urinary tract infections. *Medical Clinics of North America, 75*, 313–327.

Privette, M., Cade, R., Peterson, J., et al. (1988). Prevention of recurrent UTI in postmenopausal women. *Nephron, 50*, 24–27.

Rubin, R. H. Beam, T. R., & Stamm, W. E. (1992). An approach to evaluating antibacterial agents in the treatment of urinary tract infection. *Clinical Infectious Diseases, 13*(Suppl. 2), S246–S251.

Sheldon, C. A., Gonzalez, R. (1984). Differentiation of upper and lower urinary tract infections: How and when? *Medical Clinics of North America, 68*, 321–333.

Souney, P., & Polk, B. F. (1982). Single-dose antimicrobial therapy for urinary tract infections in women. *Review of Infectious Diseases, 4*, 29–32.

Sourander, L. B. (1966). Urinary tract infection in the aged—an epidemiological study. *Annals of Medicine of Internal Fenn, 55*(Suppl. 45), 7–55.

Turck, M., & Stamm, W. E. (1981). Nosocomial infection of the urinary tract. *American Journal of Medicine, 70*, 651–654.

Pneumonia in the Elderly $\boxed{15}$

Donald J. Kennedy

Infection is a significant medical problem in older persons. It is one of the most frequent causes of hospital admission and identifiable causes of death in this age group. Influenza and pneumonia are the leading cause of death secondary to infection in patients older than age 65. Delayed clinical recognition, problems in determining the precise microbiological diagnosis, and the presence of other underlying illness contribute to the physician's difficulty in managing pneumonia in the elderly (Gleckman 1991; Marrie, Haldane, Vanora, et al., 1985). Initial antimicrobial therapy is directed at likely pathogens based on underlying host factors, the clinical presentation, and the place of acquisition of the pneumonia.

ACQUISITION OF INFECTIOUS PNEUMONIA

Tuberculosis and influenza can be acquired by direct contact with infected individuals by inhalation of infectious material. Hematogenous spread of bacterial infection from a distant source including septic thrombophlebitis, tricuspid or pulmonic endocarditis, or pyelonephritis can also result in bacterial pneumonia.

However, the most common method of acquiring pneumonia is by aspiration of oropharyngeal contents that contain respiratory pathogens. The upper airway of normal individuals can be colonized by a variety of bacterial organisms that are potential pathogens including *Streptococcus pneumoniae, Haemophilus influenza,* and *Moraxella catarrhalis.* The inoculum of bacteria, the virulence of the organism, and the underlying host defense mechanisms are major determinants not only of whether clinical infection will be established, but of the severity and consequences of the pneumonia.

The types and amounts of bacterial flora in the upper respiratory tract of an individual are variable. If the patient is presently or recently in an institution or has received antimicrobial therapy, there is an alteration of the normal respiratory flora. Within a few days of admission to the hospital, there is a gradual and progressive likelihood of a change in colonization of the patient from normal respiratory organisms to the flora of the particular institution, primarily gram-negative rods. Use of antibiotics for the prophylaxis or treatment of infectious diseases other than pneumonia can select for organisms that may not be inhibited by an antibiotic selected to treat community-acquired infection. The elderly patient who is institutionalized or on antibiotics may develop pneumonia with organisms that are very different from patients who live independently and, therefore, may require selection of different antimicrobial therapy (Stein, 1990).

COMMUNITY ACQUIRED PNEUMONIA

An important consideration in the clinical presentation of respiratory tract infections in the elderly is differentiating the acute from chronic course. Respiratory and systemic symptoms of a few days' duration are associated with acute bacterial or viral infections and are likely to require immediate evaluation and treatment. When complaints are of longer duration, a more complete evaluation should be performed to establish a precise diagnosis and guide specific therapy. Evaluation for mixed aerobic-anaerobic lung abscesses, tuberculosis, and other slow-growing organisms should be undertaken including invasive procedures if adequate sputum examination is unsuccessful (Gleckman, 1985). In the elderly patient with a chronic clinical presentation, the differential diagnosis also includes many other noninfectious conditions such as neoplasia, pulmonary infarction, or allergic lung disease.

Acute bacterial pneumonia is referred to as typical when characterized by the presence of fever, chills, cough with purulent sputum production, leukocytosis, and localized infiltrates. Presumptive identification of the etiologic agent can be made by the morphology of the organisms on gram stain and empiric treatment begun. Diagnostic evaluation should also include blood cultures as well as an evaluation to exclude other causes of the patient's symptoms. Underlying systemic disease such as congestive heart failure may enhance the risk of pneumonia. Multiple myeloma and chronic lymphocytic leukemia are associated with defects in immunoglobulin production and predispose to infections with encapsulated bacteria, especially *Streptococcus pneumoniae*.

Atypical pneumonia is characterized by a nonproductive cough, diffuse or patchy infiltrates on x-ray film, lack of leukocytosis, and no organism on gram strain. Although *Mycoplasma pneumoniae* is the most common etiology of this presentation in adolescents and young adults, it is rare in older persons. Common causes of this symptom complex in older persons include *Chlamydia pneumoniae*, respiratory viruses, and *Legionella pneumophilia*. Recommended initial treatment is with a macrolide antibiotic, such as erythromycin, which will include coverage for the preceding pathogens as well as for *Streptococcus pneumoniae*.

Important aspects of evaluation on physical examination include the level of consciousness, cough reflex and intact swallowing mechanisms, and local anatomic or physiological abnormalities involved in the clearance of respiratory secretions. Depression of consciousness and respiratory secretion clearance problems predispose the patient to large volumes of aspiration and increase the likelihood of a mixed pulmonary infection with oropharyngeal flora. Focal adventitious sounds on chest examinations are useful in following the response of infection to therapy.

Radiographic evaluation for pneumonia should be obtained whenever the presenting complaints or physical examination suggest lower respiratory tract infection. In older persons, the classic presentation of bacterial pneumonia may not be present resulting in a lack of fever or leukocytosis, absence of adventitious lung sounds, or no recognizable cough (Fox, 1988; Harper & Newton, 1988). Therefore, elderly patients with deterioration in their ability to perform activities of daily living should be evaluated for the presence of underlying infection in general and specifically for pneumonia.

The chest x-ray film is necessary to confirm the clinical diagnosis of pneumonia and is helpful in determining the likely microbiologic etiology. Typical acute bacterial pneumonia is localized to a focal segment or lobe of the lung. Atypical pneumonia has a diffuse, patchy, or interstitial pattern on chest x-ray film (Gleckman & Bergman). The presence of a pleural effusion at the time of diagnosis of bacterial pneumonia requires sampling of the effusion to exclude the presence of an emphysema, which, if present, would require drainage for successful management.

Influenza virus is easily communicable, capable of spread within an institution, and can cause lower respiratory infection. It is clinically recognized by its epidemic pattern in the winter months, widespread presence in the community, and its production of an atypical pneumonia when it involves the lower respiratory tract. Because of the associated morbidity and mortality with influenza infection, vaccination should be used in the fall preceding each influenza season.

HOSPITAL ACQUIRED BACTERIAL PNEUMONIA

Because the primary mechanism of acquisition of acute bacterial pneumonia in the hospitalized patient is aspiration, knowledge of the common nosocomial pathogens in a particular institution is useful in predicting the likely causative organism. National surveys of nosocomial pneumonia pathogens report that up to 70% of these infections are due to gram-negative rod bacteria including *Pseudomonas aeruginosa*. There are a variety of *Enterobacteriaceae* isolates that can be the responsible pathogens and empiric antimicrobial coverage should include coverage for these organisms. After gram-negative rods, the next most likely group of pathogens are gram-positive cocci including *Staphylococcus aureus* in 10% to 15% and *Steptococcus pneumoniae* in 5% of reported cases of nosocomial pneumonia. Penicillin is the drug of choice for pneumococcal infection and selection of antibiotics for staphylococci will depend on the resistance pattern in a given institution. A semisynthetic penicillin or first- or second-generation cephalosporin will be adequate for staphylococci unless methicillin or oxacillin resistance is likely. Presently, vancomycin is the drug of choice for methicillin-resistant staphylococci. Although not reported in most surveys of nosocomial infections, an important component of aspiration pneumonia is the normal mouth flora that is aspirated along with the gram-negative rods. The antibiotic regimen for nosocomial pneumonia should include adequate coverage for mouth flora as well as the identified pathogen. Poor clinical response to treatment as well as suprainfection with streptococci have been documented when drugs with a narrow spectrum of activity against gram-negative rods only have been used.

Isolation of *Legionella pneumophilia* in nosocomial pneumonia is being reported with increasing frequency in selected hospitals. Diagnosis can be established by culture, genetic probe, Dieterle silver tissue stain, or paired serology. Presence of the organism in the environment or significant background incidence of infection in a given location should lead to appropriate diagnostic testing and possibly initial therapy directed at this organism.

TREATMENT

Proper selection of initial therapy is based on the clinicians judgment of likely pathogens. These can be predicted based on the onset of symptoms (acute vs. chronic), setting of acquisition (community vs. hospital or nursing home), clinical findings (typical bacterial vs. atypical), and initial gram stain (Norman, 1991).

Acute atypical pneumonia can be treated with erythromycin, which will cover the common respiratory pathogens found in that syndrome. Newer antibiotics that are similar to erythromycin, such as azithromycin and clairithromycin, provide extended activity against *Haemophilus influenza* and *Moraxella catarrhalis* as well as decreased gastrointestinal toxicity. However, these agents are presently available only in oral formulation, are much more expensive, and offer little therapeutic gain compared with erythromycin.

Therapy for acute bacterial pneumonia is based on the sputum gram stain if a predominant organism is apparent. When gram-positive, lancet-shaped diplococci are present, penicillin should be used. If a reliable sputum gram stain is not available, an antibiotic with an extended spectrum should be selected. Choices would include a second- or third-generation cephalosporin (cefuroxine, ceftriaxone) or a penicillin plus a β-lactamase inhibitor or (ampicillin sulbactam or ticarcillin clavulanate).

A variety of antibiotics are presently available for the management of nosocomial pneumonia in the elderly. Although aminoglycosides have excellent activity against gram-negative rods, their toxicity in the elderly, the availability of other agents, and the poor clinical response seen when used as single agents usually warrants selection of alternative agents. Their use should be reserved for critically ill patients or organisms resistant to other drugs.

Because hospital-acquired bacterial pneumonia is usually due to gram-negative rods or *Staphylococcus aureus*, selection of a third-generation cephalosporin, or extended spectrum penicillin with a β-lactamase inhibitor would provide coverage unless methicillin-resistant *Staphylococcus aureus* is likely. Knowledge of recent clinical isolates and susceptibility data from organisms in a particular institution will help select an individual agent and whether therapy with vancomycin should be used to cover for methicillin-resistant *Staphylococcus aureus*. Although Primaxin, a carbapenem antibiotic, has an appropriate spectrum of coverage for the organisms associated with nosocomial bacterial pneumonia, it has been associated with the lowering of seizure threshold in patients predisposed to seizures. Patients at greatest risk are those who would be placed on full doses of the drug, have even mild renal impairment, and have underlying structural or functional CNS disease. These factors are present in many elderly patients who are treated for hospital-acquired bacterial pneumonia. Aztreonam combines good gram-negative rod coverage with the overall toxicity profile of a cephalosporin or penicillin. In addition, because it is a monobactam, there is no immediate hypersensitivity cross-reactivity with the penicillins, and, therefore, it can be used in the penicillin-allergic patient. Because of its lack of coverage for gram-positive and anaerobic organisms, it should not be used as a single agent for lower respiratory tract infections that occur by aspiration of mouth flora.

Recent release of quinolone antibiotics has given physicians agents with excellent activity against many gram-negative rods. In addition, the serum levels achieved by oral administration are similar to levels obtained by intravenous infusion for both ciprofloxacin and ofloxacin. This permits oral therapy for a variety of serious gram-negative infections, especially after an adequate clinical response has been documented to parenteral therapy. However, the quinolone antibiotics lack sufficient activity to treat anaerobes and have limited activity against streptococcal organisms. Reports of streptococcal bacteremia in patients receiving quinolone therapy for gram-negative infections should be a warning that additional coverage for streptococci and anaerobes be included if there is pneumonia secondary to aspiration of mouth flora.

Macrolide antibiotics such as erythromycin and clindamycin have been useful agents for lower respiratory tract infections because of their coverage of gram-positive organisms. Erythromycin is also the drug of choice for a community-acquired atypical pneumonia because it is active against mycoplasmas, *Legionella, species,* and chlamydiae. Clindamycin has excellent activity against mouth organisms, including anaerobes, and has been useful for treatment of community-acquired aspiration pneumonia when enteric gram-negative bacilli are not likely to be present.

Amantadine can reduce the duration and severity of acute infection with influenza A (but not B) virus if therapy is initiated at the time of the initial manifestations of infection. However, the drug does have side effects including alterations of mental function that are more pronounced in the elderly and specifically in patients with renal insufficiency. The incidence and severity of side effects can be reduced by properly adjusting the dose.

PREVENTION

Annual immunization against influenza A and B is recommended for all elderly individuals as well as younger patients with significant medical illness (Besdine, 1986). Although local reactions can occur in up to one third of the recipients, they are usually mild. Because the vaccine components are made from egg-grown viruses, patients with a history of anaphylactic reactions or signs of immediate hypersensitivity to eggs or egg products should not receive the vaccine. In a host who responds to a vaccination that contain appropriate antigens, protection from serious illness is about 75%.

Because of the continued variability of the surface antigens of the influenza viruses, yearly vaccination before influenza season is recommended.

Pneumococcal infection can be caused by a variety of serotypes of the bacterium. The presently available pneumococcal vaccine contains antigens from the 23 different serotypes that are most frequently isolated in invasive disease. A single injection has been associated with an overall efficacy rate of greater than 50% against bacteremic illness, in both high-risk young as well as elderly patients. Revaccination should be considered for patients who were vaccinated 6 or more years previously. Because the indications in older persons for influenza and pneumococcal vaccination are similar, the two vaccinations can be given simultaneously at separate sites with no increase in side effects or decreased antibody responses.

During epidemics of influenza A, unimmunized patients can benefit from preventive therapy with oral amantadine (Besdine, 1986). The agent must be taken daily during the epidemic or for at least 2 weeks following vaccination to provide time for immunity from the vaccine to develop. However, CNS side effects of amantadine can occur, particularly in patients with mild renal insufficiency. Because of its toxicity, need for prolonged administration, lack of activity against influenza B, and ability to promote the emergence of drug-resistance strains of virus, amantadine should not be used as a substitute for immunization in older persons.

Avoidance of treatment with drugs that will decrease the level of consciousness will help prevent aspiration and the subsequent development of pneumonia. Patients with anatomic and physiologic abnormalities of swallowing should be carefully evaluated for evidence of aspiration and steps taken to reduce that risk.

SUMMARY

Management of lower respiratory tract infections in the elderly will remain a challenge to the practicing physician. An accurate assessment of the patient should permit predicting likely pathogens and subsequent selection of appropriate antimicrobial therapy. Recent developments made in antibiotics have increased the spectrum of covered pathogens, permitted less frequent doses of parenteral drugs, reduced the incidence of significant toxic side effects, and expanded options for oral therapy.

REFERENCES

Besdine, R. W. (1986). Pneumonia and influenza: Vaccination of elderly is justified. *Geriatrics, 41*, 13–16.

Fox, R. A. (1988). Atypical presentation of geriatric infections. *Geriatrics, 43*, 58–68.

Gleckman, R. A. (1985). Community-acquired pneumonia in the geriatric patient. *Hospital Practice*, 57–71.

Gleckman, R. A. (1991). Pneumonia: Update on diagnosis and treatment. *Geriatrics, 46*, 49–56.

Gleckman, R. A., & Bergman, M. M. (1987). Bacterial pneumonia: Specific diagnosis and treatment of the elderly. *Geriatrics, 42*, 29–41.

Harper, C., & Newton, P. (1989). Clinical aspects of pneumonia in the elderly veteran. *Journal of American Geriatrics Society, 37*, 867–872.

Marrie, T. J., Haldane, E., Vanora, F. Ruth, S., Durant, H., & Kwan, C. (1985). Community-acquired pneumonia requiring hospitalization: Is it different in the elderly? *Journal of the American Geriatrics Society, 33*, 671–680.

Norman, D. C., (1991). Pneumonia in the elderly: Empiric antimicrobial therapy. *Geriatrics, 46*, 26–32.

Stein, D. (1990). Managing pneumonia acquired in nursing homes: Special concerns. *Geriatrics, 45*, 39–47.

Methicillin-Resistant *Staphylococcus aureus* (MRSA): Epidemiology and Control in the Long-Term Care Setting

16

Suzanne F. Bradley

Following the introduction of penicillin, staphylococci typically developed resistance to many antibiotics within several years. It was not surprising, therefore, that resistance developed shortly after the development of penicillinase-resistant pencillins, such as methicillin. Methicillin-resistant staphylococci did not spread rapidly, and, in fact, it was initially hypothesized that these organisms were less virulent than their susceptible counterparts. Presumably because of increased antibiotic use, MRSA emerged in epidemic proportions in Europe and Australia in the late 1960s and in the United States a decade later. In acutely ill patients in tertiary care hospitals, MRSA organisms proved to be at least as virulent as methicillin-susceptible strains, and the development of newer antibiotic classes was required to combat these strains (Brumfitt & Hamilton-Miller, 1989). Only much later did MRSA spread from medical centers to smaller hospitals and in some parts of the country MRSA infection now is community acquired (Saravolatz, Pohlod, & Arking, 1982). In 1990, it was estimated that 95% of all U.S. hospitals had taken care of at least one patient with MRSA, and methicillin-resistance occurred in 11% to 15% of all *S. aureus* isolates (Boyce, 1991; Panililio, Culver, Gaynes, et al., 1992; Wenzel, Nettleman, Jones, et al., 1991).

SIGNIFICANCE OF MRSA

Acute Care Institutions

Great effort has been made to limit the spread of MRSA in acute care settings for several reasons. Initially, many felt that these organisms might be more virulent than methicillin-susceptible *S. aureus* (MSSA). With increased recognition of the problem and early use of appropriate antibiotics, there has been little evidence in laboratory or clinical studies that MRSA causes more serious infection than MSSA (Boyce, Landry, Deetz, et al., 1981; Crossley, Landesman, & Zaske, 1979; Hershow, Kayre & Smith, 1992; Lentino, Hennein, Krause, et al., 1985; Peacock, Moorman, Wenzel, et al., 1981). Aside from the issue of increased virulence, there is also a concern that the introduction of MRSA into a facility will cause an overall increase in the rate of serious staphylococcal infections (Wenzel et al., 1991). Most persons colonized with *S. aureus* seem to carry a single strain that inhibits the acquisition of other strains, a process called bacterial interference (Verhof & Verbrugh, 1981). Therefore, MRSA appears to replace methicillin-susceptible strains rather than increase the overall rate of staphylococcal carriage in long-term care (Strausbaugh, Jacobsen, Sewell, et al., 1991). However, it is clear that the introduction of MRSA does increase costs in terms of the use of expensive, often toxic antibiotics and infection control measures that place greater demands on the time of health care workers and increase supply expenditures (Boyce, 1992). Great debate is still ongoing between acute care centers whether intensive infection control policies directed against MRSA are effective or even necessary.

Aged Patient

Both MSSA and MRSA appear to have an equal propensity to cause serious infections such as pneumonia, wound infection, endocarditis, bacteremia, and urinary tract infections (Bradley, 1992). Although a great many people carry staphylococci transiently during their lives, patients with underlying diseases, such as diabetes mellitus or significant renal impairment requiring dialysis, are more likely to have persistent carriage and may have greatly increased risks of infection (Chow & Yu, 1989; Tuazon, Perez, Kishaha, et al., 1974). The institutionalized elderly are more likely to become colonized with *S. aureus* than younger adults perhaps because of an increased frequency of predisposing chronic disease rather than a specific age-related defect (Noble et al., 1967; Phair, Kauffman, & Bjornson, et al., 1978). In hospitalized patients, it has been shown that most nosocomial infections, especially those resulting from *S. aureus*, occur in the elderly (Brumfitt & Hamilton-Miller, 1989; Craven, Reed, Kolish, et al., 1981; Emori, Banerjee, Culver, et al., 1991; Ward, Winn, Hartstein, et al., 1981), and these patients are also more likely to die of *S. aureus* infection than persons of other age groups (Locksley, Cohen, Quinn, et al., 1982). Although aging may be a significant risk factor for staphylococcal infection in acutely ill hospitalized patients, it is not clear that elderly persons who are residents of long-term care facilities and who are relatively well but have stable chronic illnesses have the same degree of risk.

MRSA AND THE ROLE OF NURSING HOMES

The history of MRSA in acute care hospitals in the United States has been closely linked with nursing homes. The earliest introduction of MRSA into acute care facilities was traced to colonized, debilitated residents of long-term care facilities (Barrett, McGee, & Finland, 1968; Haley, Hightower, Khabboz, et al., 1982; O'Toole, Drew, Dahlgren et al., 1970; Ward et al., 1981). Residents of nursing homes were more likely to be colonized with MRSA on admission to hospital than patients admitted from the community (Hsu & Macaluso, 1988). In hospital-based studies it has been well appreciated that the most debilitated, often elderly, patients were most likely to harbor MRSA (Boyce et al., 1981; Craven et al., 1981; Locksley et al., 1982; Ward et al., 1981). On the basis of these findings, many assumed that nursing homes were "reservoirs" of MRSA that perpetuated the problem in hospitals.

PREVALENCE OF MRSA IN LONG-TERM CARE

Although the concept of nursing homes as "MRSA reservoirs" is well accepted by many, it is clear from the literature that little is truly known about the prevalence and significance of MRSA in long-term care facilities (Boyce, 1991; Kauffman, Bradley, & Terpenning, 1990). In a questionnaire survey of Minnesota nursing homes, few facilities (12%) knew if they had MRSA-positive residents, fewer regarded it as a problem (8%), and even fewer still routinely reviewed cultures obtained for clinical reasons for the presence of MRSA. Yet, a majority (69%) had sought consultative help, and

TABLE 16.1 Studies Assessing the Prevalence of Methicillin-Resistant *Staphylococcus aureus* in Chronic Care Facilities

Author/Date	No. Beds	Facility Type	Affiliation	Surveillance/Sites/Duration
Aeilts (1982)	600	rehabilitation hospital	university referral center	prospectively assess pts with (+) clinical cultures in response to an outbreak/N,T,W,P,U/32 mo.
Bradley (1991)	120	geriatric evaluation rehabilitation skilled LTCF	VAMC university	prospectively assess all pts monthly/N,W,P,R/12 mo.
Hsu (1991)	150	skilled LTCF unskilled LTCF psychiatry	community	prospectively survey 117-129 pts on 8 occasions/N/15 mo.
Muder (1991)	432	intermediate care skilled LTCF	VAMC university	prospectively assess all pts monthly or bimonthly/N or other sites as clinically indicated/36 mo.
Murphy (1992)	233	intermediate care skilled LTCF chronic med care rehabilitation	university	point prevalence survey, then screen all new admissions/N,W,U,S/4 mo.
Mylotte (1992)	N/A	75 private, public, or non-profit LTCF in NY state	hospital-based free-standing	questionnaire survey

O'Toole (1970)	unknown	4 skilled LTCF	unknown	point prevalence survey of pts and some staff from 4 nursing homes following a hospital outbreak/variable sites cultured
Pennington (1982)	340	rehabilitation/ extended care hospital	unknown	prospectively assess all pts on admission/N,T,W,P/12 mo.
Storch (1987)	182	skilled LTCF	university	prospective and retrospective assessment of (+) clinical cultures in response to an MRSA outbreak, point prevalence survey of nasal carriage in some pts and all staff/13 mo.
Strausbaugh (1991)	120	skilled LTCF	VAMC university	prospectively assess pts with (+) clinical cultures and their roommates in response to an outbreak, 3 targeted surveys of some pts and staff during 1988, one survey of all pts and staff in 3/89, screen all new admissions since 4/89/N,W,U/36 mo.
Thomas (1989)	170	skilled LTCF	unknown	two point prevalence surveys of all pts and staff in response to an outbreak/N,W/3 mo.
Thum (1991)	N/A	345 skilled & intermediate care facilities in Minnesota	unknown	questionnaire survey

N=nares, W=wound, P=perineum, T=throat, U=urine
LTCF=long-term care facility
VAMC=Department of Veterans Affairs

many (43%) would not accept colonized patients with or without provisions for special care (Thurn, Belongia, & Crossley, et al., 1991). In western New York, 72% of nursing homes responding to a questionnaire surveyed clinical cultures for MRSA, 81% reported colonized or infected patients in their facility, and 21% considered this to be a problem. These facilities tended to be large, accepted acute care admissions frequently, and 92% had at least a part-time active infection control program (Mylotte, Karuza, & Bentley, 1992). In Minnesota and New York, differences in MRSA prevalence may reflect true regional differences or differences in infection control resources.

Humans may commonly harbor *S. aureus*, including resistant strains, asymptomatically in a variety of different body sites (nares, skin, rectum, and others) for variable periods (Verhof & Verbrugh, 1981). It is not surprising, therefore, that if one screens for MRSA using only cultures obtained for clinically suspected infection, many asymptomatic carriers might be missed (Boyce, 1992). Few studies directly assessing the prevalence of MRSA colonized or infected patients in long-term care facilities have been done, and the methods employed have been quite variable (see Table 16.1). Most information about the epidemiology of MRSA in the long-term care setting has been obtained by point prevalence surveys in response to outbreaks of MRSA infection. Few studies about the transmissibility of MRSA in nursing homes have been done in a longitudinal fashion in the absence of an epidemic. The institutions in question have also varied widely in patient demographics, size, types of chronic care services offered, and affiliations with large, tertiary acute care facilities affiliated with universities or the Department of Veterans Affairs. It is, therefore, difficult to generalize these few experiences from facilities where patients are predominantly male veterans or from regions where MRSA is endemic to small, community-based nursing homes that care for a predominantly female population, and where the problem of MRSA is perceived to be rare.

MRSA AS AN ENDEMIC ORGANISM IN LONG-TERM CARE

Most long-term prospective studies of MRSA epidemiology have been performed, out of necessity, in long-term care facilities where the organism is endemic. In the endemic setting, 8% to 34% of long-term care patients were colonized with MRSA (Bradley, Terpenning, Ramsey, et al., 1991; Hsu, 1991; Muder, Brennan, Wagener, et al., 1991; Murphy, Denman, Bennett, et al., 1992). Overall, MRSA carriers had significantly poorer functional status and were more likely to require increased nursing care because of limited mobility, wounds, feeding tubes, or urinary catheters (Bradley et al., 1991; Hsu, 1991; Muder et al., 1991; Murphy et al., 1992). Debilitated patients tended to remain colonized with large numbers of the same MRSA strain isolated from multiple body sites over a period of months and therefore accounted for the greatest proportion of carriers. However, some very functional patients tended to carry small numbers of one of several MRSA strains, usually in a single site, such as the nares, for a brief period during their stay (Bradley et al., 1991). As patients are admitted to nursing homes from various institutions, each carrying his own MRSA strain, it is not surprising to find many different strains circulating within one nursing home (Bradley et al., 1991; Hsu, 1991; Muder et al., 1991). Despite the high prevalence of MRSA within a facility, roommates rarely shared the same strain, suggesting that transmission between patients was low (Bradley et al., 1991; Hsu et al., 1988).

Patients who carried MRSA did not necessarily develop infection with that organism. In facilities where 13% to 23% of patients carried MRSA, 3% to 4% of patients developed infection with that organism (Bradley et al., 1991; Muder et al., 1991). In our long-term care facility, of the 9 MRSA infections that developed in 341 patients during a 1-year period, 7 occurred in known carriers, and no mortality was seen (Bradley et al., 1991). In Muder's study (1991), 15 MRSA infections occurred in 197 patients followed over 3 years, and 11 of those infections occurred in MRSA carriers. MRSA carriers were more likely to die from infection because of staphylococci than noncarriers. Although these findings could suggest that MRSA is more virulent than MSSA, it was also found that MRSA carriers were significantly more likely to die than noncarriers from all causes, both infectious and noninfectious. They also tended to be patients that required dialysis or intermediate care. It would appear that MRSA carriage is a marker for increased debility, infection with the same strain, and death. It is not clear that the presence of MRSA carriers in a long-term care facility increases the risk of MRSA infection for noncarriers, who are not debilitated.

MRSA AS AN EPIDEMIC ORGANISM IN LONG-TERM CARE

The epidemiology of MRSA in long-term care has been described much more frequently following an outbreak of actual infection, usually with a single strain (Aeilts, Sapico, Canawati, et al., 1982; Strausbaugh et al., 1991; Storch, Radcliff, Meyer et al, 1987; Thomas, Bridge, Waterman et al., 1989). One outbreak occurred following an outbreak of influenza, an infection that is commonly complicated by staphylococcal pneumonia (Storch et al., 1987). As in the endemic setting, patient debility appeared to influence patterns of MRSA colonization and infection greatly. In one large rehabilitation hospital where MRSA was widely spread, infections were perceived to be of low severity in areas caring for patients requiring more intensive care and virtually absent in areas providing rehabilitation (Aeilts et al., 1982). In other studies, MRSA colonization was predicted by the presence of wounds, invasive devices, prior antibiotic treatment, or need for assistance (Strausbaugh et al., 1991; Thomas et al., 1989). MRSA did not increase an institution's infection rate nor did the introduction of this organism increase patient mortality from infection (Strausbaugh et al., 1991).

ROUTINE MANAGEMENT OF THE MRSA CARRIER IN LONG-TERM CARE

Healthy persons carry or come in contact with staphylococci on a daily basis without developing serious illness, and in some parts of the United States MRSA has become part of normal community flora (Saravolatz et al., 1982). In the long-term care setting, great effort has been made to protect the majority of residents from the MRSA carrier (see Table 16.2). If MRSA carriers are at greatest risk of infecting themselves, then the identification and protection of persons at significant risk of becoming persistently colonized and infected would be the most prudent use of infection control resources. However, until specific criteria are available to identify patients at risk of infection, then more conventional infection control methods must be relied on to limit the spread of MRSA infection. Unfortunately, there is little agreement among acute care facilities, let alone long-term care facilities, about which infection control methods are effective in the containment of MRSA (Boyce, 1992).

Relatively few nursing homes appear to have specific policies regarding admission of MRSA-positive patients. In Minnesota 13% to 21% of facilities and 69% of facilities in western New York had such policies (Mylotte et al., 1992; Thurn et al., 1991). In Minnesota, only 6% of institutions would accept MRSA-colonized patients, and 3% would accept MRSA-infected patients without restriction or special care. Forty-two percent and 43% of facilities would not accept known MRSA colonized or infected patients under any circumstances, and 47% and 44% of institutions accepted colonized or infected patients with restrictions for special care. These facilities dealt with MRSA-colonized or -infected patients by applying some type of isolation procedure (18% to 19%), cohorting residents together (2% to 3%), placing them in private rooms (8% to 10%), or by discharging them back to hospital (8% to 10%) (Thurn et al., (1991).

Other studies in individual nursing facilities show even less agreement regarding the most effective means to control MRSA in the long-term care setting (see Table 16.2). The lack of concensus on control of MRSA may be due to the failure to prove that the use of one or more infection control method(s) is clearly superior to another. The prevalence of staphylococci in an institution normally waxes and wanes over months to years, so that conclusions drawn from relatively short-term studies of infection control methods may be erroneous (Goetz & Muder, 1992).

Most methods of MRSA control are based on observations that staphylococci are spread primarily by direct contact between individuals. Airborne and environmental sources of MRSA are less likely methods of transmission (Boyce et al., 1981; Casewell & Hill, 1986; Peacock, Marsik, & Wenzel, 1980; Thompson, Cabezudo, & Wenzel, 1982). It is possible that patients, staff, or maybe visitors, might carry MRSA and introduce it into the facility. Therefore, a facility with a very strict MRSA policy might suggest that all persons should be screened on admission to the facility and on a routine basis thereafter to assure that they did not acquire the organism at any time during their stay. Such frequent screening for asymptomatic carriage of MRSA at multiple sites is extremely labor intensive and costly. Ideally, all colonized patients would have to remain in strict isolation in a private room or MRSA ward (requiring gowns, gloves, and masks) until multiple negative cultures were obtained on separate occasions. Similarly, colonized staff might remain off duty or work only in a restricted MRSA ward until their cultures became negative. A strict approach to MRSA control is not practical for most nursing homes, even those that have access to a full-time infection control practitioner (Kauffman et al., 1990).

For most facilities, it is impossible to know the MRSA carrier status of all residents and staff at any given moment. If MRSA colonization is known from hospital records or clinical cultures, then the following infection control procedures can be initiated. For most MRSA-colonized patients, spread of MRSA can be controlled if colonized or infected wounds are covered by a bandage, gloves and gowns are only used when contact is made with moist body surfaces, and good handwashing is enforced (Boyce 1991; Cohen, Morita, & Bradford, 1991; Cookson, 1991; Linnemann, Morre, Stanek, et al., 1991; Thompson et al., 1982). If patients have MRSA-infected tracheostomies, pneumonia, or large wounds that cannot be easily contained by simple contact measures, then strict isolation of the patient is recommended (Boyce, 1991; Kauffman et al., 1990, Thompson et al., 1982). Recent studies in acute care suggest that contact isolation might be as effective as strict isolation in the control of MRSA (Goetz & Muder, 1992; Linnemann et al., 1991). For long-term care facilities, contact isolation is more easily performed and is less expensive. In addition, most of colonized patients are not restricted to their rooms and are able to participate in rehabilitation and social programs.

MANAGEMENT OF MRSA INFECTION OUTBREAKS IN LONG-TERM CARE

Institutions should monitor their normal rate of MRSA infections. If a rise over that baseline rate is detected for MRSA infections, then a possible outbreak may be in progress. Even if an increase in the number of MRSA infections is detected, not all known carriers should be implicated because many carry organisms that are different from the infecting strain. Only persons having contact with the infected patients (patients and staff) need to be screened for the presence of asymptomatic MRSA carriage and isolated if they are positive for the infecting organism in question. Patients should remain in strict isolation (private room, cohort, or ward), and staff should remain off duty until their cultures of nares and any cutaneous wounds are negative on several occasions, the outbreak has abated, or it has been determined that their strain is different from the infecting strain.

Determination of the epidemic strain, by phage typing or other methods, can be helpful in identifying persons carrying strains of MRSA unrelated to the outbreak who may be kept in isolation unnecessarily. Most microbiology laboratories cannot differentiate MRSA strains, so that isolates may need to be sent to state, federal, or other research laboratories. While determination of MRSA strains may result in additional cost initially, it would limit the expenses incurred in trying to identify, isolate, and, perhaps, eliminate MRSA cases that might be epidemiologically unrelated (Boyce, 1992; Bradley, 1992, Kauffman et al., 1990).

ROLE OF ANTIMICROBIAL DECOLONIZATION IN LONG-TERM CARE

Many disinfectants and antimicrobial agents active against MRSA have been used alone or in combination with various isolation procedures in an attempt to eliminate the organism from acute and chronic care facilities. In recent surveys, 13% to 81% of long-term care facilities attempted to eradicate MRSA carriage in their patients by various means (Mylotte et al., 1992; Thurn et al., 1991). Unfortunately, there is no single agent that has been shown to be effective in permanently ridding a facility of MRSA.

Agents such as chlorhexidine, triclosan, phenol, and hexachlorophene have been used to disinfect environmental surfaces even though there is little evidence that fomites are a significant source of outbreaks. In addition to iodine, chlorhexidine, hexachlorophene, and triclosan have also been used to disinfect the skin of colonized patients and staff with variable success (Bradley, 1992) (Table 16.2). Topical antibiotics (bacitracin, tetracycline, vancomycin, mupirocin, and others) and oral agents (trimethoprim-sulfamethoxazole, ciprofloxacin, novobiocin, minocycline, and fusidic acid alone or in combination with rifampin) have been tried to eradicate the carrier state (Bradley, 1992). Topical therapy limited to the nares is often only transiently effective in eliminating MRSA from that site. Patients are recolonized from other untreated sites within weeks of treatment (Aeilts et al., 1982). Systemic antibiotics are more effective in decolonizing all sites of carriage, but drug toxicity and antibiotic resistance are common complications, and beneficial effects are often transient (Storch et al., 1987; Strausbaugh, Jacobsen, Sewell, et al., 1992).

Most recently, mupirocin ointment has been a very promising agent for the treatment of the nasal MRSA carrier state (Bradley, in press). In one study, after 5 to 7 days of therapy, mupirocin transiently eliminated MRSA from nares in virtually all persons treated (Cederna, Terpenning, Ensberg, et al., 1990). However, the carrier state soon returned within weeks of discontinuation of the drug. Chronic therapy with mupirocin for 3 months was effective in eliminating MRSA colonization in long-term care patients, but only if wounds were treated in addition to nares (Kauffman, Terpenning, He, et al., 1993). Despite chronic mupirocin therapy, relapses occurred that required an increased frequency in administration of the drug. Constant culture-surveillance of all patients was necessary to identify new carriers or patients that relapsed while on therapy. The development of mupirocin resistance was also a significant sequelae of chronic mupirocin therapy (Bradley, in press; Kauffman et al., 1993).

On the basis of these studies, one should not treat long-term care patients with a brief course of antibiotics and assume that they have been cleared of their carrier state or that MRSA has been eliminated from a facility. Brief antibiotic treatment of carriers might be justified during an outbreak of MRSA infection where reduction of the amount of circulating bacteria within the facility could lead to termination of the epidemic. Intermittent treatment of staphylococcal carriage in dialysis patients has been effective in reducing the number of infections in this population at risk (Yu, Goetz, Wagener, et al., 1986). Intermittent treatment of very debilitated long-term care patients persistently colonized with many of organisms might be justified to reduce their risk of self-infection, but this hypothesis has not been studied.

TABLE 16.2 Methods of MRSA on Studies of Chronic Care Facilities

Author/Date	Isolation	Infection Control Procedure	Decolonization Procedures	Environmental Disinfection
Aeilts (1982)	private room or cohort	wound/skin, strict isolation trach pts only	bacitracin ointment hexaclorophene (pt wash, staff hands)	staphene
Bradley (1991)	private room for trach pts	contact strict isolation trach pts	mediscrub (hands only)	none
Kauffman (1993)	private room for trach pts	contact strict isolation trach pts	mupirocin mediscrub (hands only)	see above
Murphy (1992)	unknown	universal precautions	unknown	unknown
Pennington (1982)	separate bays	wound/skin	hibiclens/hexol (hands only)	safsol, hexol

Storch (1987)	separate wards & staff	contact	rifampin (staff)	separate linen
Strausbaugh (1991)	cohort	contact body substance	chlorhexidine (hands only)	unknown
Strausbaugh (1992)	cohort	body substance	rifampin ± TMP/SMX or clindamycin; chlorhexidine (hands only)	Wex-cide
Thomas (1989)	separate wards & staff	unknown	unknown	unknown

pt(s) = patients
TMP/SMX = trimethoprim/sulfamethoxazole

SUMMARY

Recent studies suggest that the epidemiology and significance of MRSA in long-term care differs from that reported for acute care hospitals. Presumably differences in host factors account for differences in risk of infection with MRSA between acute and chronic care populations. Some chronic care patients appear to be at greater risk of colonization and infection from MRSA than other long-term care patients. If risk factors for MRSA infection can be identified, then perhaps more emphasis should be placed on prevention of infection in this subgroup of patients. Until more is understood about the epidemiology of MRSA, limited but effective infection control procedures are feasible even in the long-term care setting.

REFERENCES

Aeilts, G. D., Sapico, F. L., Canawati, H. N., Malik, G. M. & Montgomerie, J. Z. (1992). Methicillian-resistant *Staphylococcus aureus* colonization and infection in a rehabilitation facility. *Journal of Clinical Microbiology, 16,* 218-223.

Barrett, F. F., McGehee, R. F., & Finland, M. (1968). Methicillin-resistant *Staphylococcus aureus* at Boston City Hospital. *New England Journal of Medicine, 279,* 441–448.

Boyce, J. M. (1991). Methicillin-resistant *Staphylococcus aureus* in nursing homes: Putting the problem in perspective. *Infection Control and Hospital Epidemiology, 12,* 413–415.

Boyce, J. M. (1992). Methicillin-resistant *Staphylococcus aureus* in hospitals and long-term care facilities: Microbiology, epidemiology, and preventive measures. *Infection Control and Hospital Epidemiology, 13,* 725–737.

Boyce, J. M., Landry, M., Deetz, T. R., & DuPont, H. L. (1991). Epidemiologic studies of an outbreak of nosocomial methicillin-resistant *Staphylococcus aureus* infections. *Infection Control and Hospital Epidemiology, 2,* 110–116.

Bradley, S. F. (1992). Methicillin-resistant *Staphylococcus aureus* infection. *Geriatric Clinics of North American, 8,* 853–868.

Bradley, S. F. (in press). Effectiveness of mupirocin in the control of methicillin-resistant *Staphylococcus aureus. Infections in Medicine.*

Bradley, S. F., Terpenning, M. S., Ramsey, M. A., Zarins, L. T., Jorgensen, K. A., Sottile, W. S., Schaberg, D. R., & Kauffman, C. A. (1991). Methicillin-resistant *Staphylococcus aureus*: Colonization and infection in a long-term care facility. *Annals of Internal Medicine, 115,* 417–422.

Brumfitt, W., & Hamilton-Miller, J. (1989). Methicillin-resistant *Staphylococcus aureus.New England Journal of Medicine, 320,* 1188–1196.

Casewell, M. W., & Hill, R. L. R. (1986). The carrier state: Methicillin-resistant *Staphylococcus aureus. Journal of Antimicrobial Chemotherapy, 18A,* 1–12.

Cederna, J. E., Terpenning, M. S., Ensberg, M., Bradley, S. F., & Kauffman, C. A.

(1990). *Staphylococcus aureus* nasal colonization in a nursing home: Eradication with mupirocin. *Infection Control and Hospital Epidemiology, 11,* 13–16.

Chow, J. W., & Yu, V. L. (1989). Staphylococcus nasal carriage in hemodialysis patients: Its role in infection and approaches to prophylaxis. *Archives of Internal Medicine, 149,* 1258–1262.

Cohen, S. H., Morita, M. M., & Bradford, M. (1991). A seven-year experience with methicillin-resistant *Staphylococcus aureus. American Journal of Medicine, 91,* 233S–237S.

Cookson, B. D. (1991). Epidemiology and control of nosocomial methicillin-resistant *Staphylococcus aureus. Current Opinion on Infections Diseases, 4,* 530–535.

Craven, D. E., Reed, D., Kollisch, N., DeMaria, A., Lichtenberg, D., Shen, K., & McCabe, W. R. (1981). A large outbreak of infections caused by strains of *Staphylococcus aureus* resistant to oxacillin and aminoglycosides. *American Journal of Medicine, 71,* 53–58.

Crossley, K., Landesman, B., & Zaske, D. (1979). An outbreak of infections caused by strains of *Staphylococcus aureus* resistant to oxacillin and aminoglycosides: II. Epidemiologic studies. *Journal of Infection Diseases, 139,* 280–287.

Emori, T. G., Banerjee, S. N., Culver, D. H., Gaynes, R. P., Horan, T. C., Edwards, J. R., et al. (1991). Nosocomial infections in elderly patients in the United States, 1986–1990. *American Journal of Medicine, 91,* 289S–293S.

Goetz, A. M., & Muder, R. R. (1992). The problem of methicillin-resistant *Staphylococcus aureus*: A critical appraisal of the efficacy of infection control procedures with a suggested approach for infection control programs. *American Journal of Infection Control, 20,* 80–84.

Haley, R. W., Hightower, A. W., Khabbaz, R. F., Thornsberry, C., Martone, W. J., Allen, J. R., & Hughes, J. M. (1982). The emergence of methicillin-resistant *Staphylococcus aureus* infections in United States hospitals: Possible role of the house-staff-patient circuit. *Annals of Internal Medicine, 97,* 297–308.

Hershow, R. C., Khayr, W. F., & Smith, N. L. (1992). A comparison of clinical virulence of nosocomially acquired methicillin-resistant and methicillin-sensitive *Staphylococcus aureus* infections in a university hospital. *Infection Control and Hospital Epidemiology, 13,* 587–593.

Hsu, C. C. S. (1991). Serial survey of methicillin-resistant *Staphylococcus arueus* nasal carriage among residents in a nursing home. *Infection Control and Hospital Epidemiology, 12,* 416–421.

Hsu, C. C. S., Macaluso, C. P., Special, L., & Hubble, R. H. (1988). High rate of methicillin resistance of *Staphylococcus aureus* isolated from hospitalized nursing home patients. *Archives of Internal Medicine, 148,* 569–570.

Kauffman, C. A., Bradley, S. F., & Terpenning, M. S. (1990). Methicillin-resistant *Staphylococcus aureus* in long-term care facilities. *Infection Control and Hospital Epidemiology, 11,* 600–603.

Kauffman, C. A., Terpenning, M. S., He, X., Zarins, L. T., Ramsey, M. A., Jorgensen, K. A., Sottile, W. S., & Bradley, S. F. (1993). Attempts to eradicate methicillin-resistant *Staphylococcus aureus* from a long-term care facility with the use of mupirocin ointment. *American Journal of Medicine, 94,* 371–378.

Lentino, J. R., Hennein, H., Krause, S., Pappas, S., Fuller, G., Schaaff, D., & DiConstanzo, M. B. (1985). A comparison of pneumonia caused by gentamicin, methicillin-resistant and gentamicin, methicillin-sensitive *Staphylococcus aureus*: Epidemiologic and clinical studies. *Infection Control and Hospital Epidemiology, 6*, 267–272.

Linneman, C. C., Morre, P., Stanek, J. L., & Pfaller, M. A. (1991). Reemergence of epidemic methicillin-resistant *Staphylococcus aureus* in a general hospital associated with changing staphylococcal strains. *American Journal of Medicine, 91*, 238S–244S.

Locksley, R. M., Cohen, M. L., Quinn, T. C., Tompkins, L. S., Coyle, M. B., Kirihara, J. M., & Counts, G. W. (1992). Multiply antibiotic-resistant *Staphylococcus aureus*: Introduction, transmission, and evolution of nosocomial infection *Annals of Internal Medicine, 97*, 317–324.

Muder, R. R., Brennen, C., Wagener, M. M., Vickers, R. M., Rihs, J. D., Hancock, G. A., Yee, Y. C., Miller, J. M., & Yu, V. L. (1991). Methicillin-resistant staphylococcal colonization and infection in a long-term care unit. *Annals of Internal Medicine, 114*, 107–112.

Murphy, S., Denman, S., Bennett, R. G., Greenough, W. B., Lindsay, J., Zelesnick, L. B. (1992). Methicillin-resistant *Staphylococcus aureus* colonization in a long-term care facility. *Journal of the American Geriatrics Society, 40*, 213–217.

Mylotte, J. M., Karuza, J., & Bentley, D. W. (1992). Methicillin-resistant *Staphylococcus aureus*: A questionnaire survey of 75 long-term care facilities in western New York. *Infection Control and Hospital Epidemiology, 13*, 711–718.

Noble, W. C., Valenburg, H. A., & Wolters, C. H. (1967). Carriage of *Staphylococcus aureus* in random samples of a normal population. *Journal of Hygiene, 65*, 567–573.

O'Toole, R. D., Drew, W. L., Dahlgren, B. J., & Beaty, H. N. (1970). An outbreak of methicillin-resistant *Staphylococcus aureus* infection: Observations in hospital and nursing home. *Journal of the American Medical Society, 213*, 257–263.

Panlilio, A. L., Culver, D. H., Gaynes, R. P., Banerjee, S., Henderson, T. S., Tolson, J. S., & Martone, W. J. (1992). National nosocomial infections surveillance systems: Methicillin-resistant *Staphylococcus aureus* in U.S. hospitals, 1975–1991. *Infection Control and Hospital Epidemiology, 13*, 582–586.

Peacock, J. E., Marsik, F. J., & Wenzel, R. P. (1980). Methicillin-resistant *Staphylococcus aureus*: Introduction and spread within a hospital. *Annals of Internal Medicine, 93*, 526–532.

Peacock, J. E., Marsik, F. J., & Wenzel, R. P. (1980). Methicillin-resistant *Staphylococcus aureus*: Introduction and spread within a hospital. *Annals of Internal Medicine, 93*, 526–532.

Peacock, J. E., Moorman, D. R., Wenzel, R. P. & Mandell, G. L. (1981). Methicillin-resistant *Staphylococcus aureus*: Microbiologic characteristics, antimicrobial susceptibilities, and assessment of virulence of an epidemic strain. *Journal of Infectious Diseases, 144*, 575–582.

Phair, J. P., Kauffman, C. A., & Bjornson A. (1978). Investigation of host defense mechanisms in the aged as determinants of nosocomial colonization and pneumonia. *Journal of the Reticuloendothelial Society, 23*, 397–405.

Saravolatz, L. D., Pohlod, D. J., & Arking, L. M. (1982). Community-acquired methicillin-resistant *Staphylococcus aureus* infections: A new source for nosocomial outbreaks. *Annals of Internal Medicine, 97*, 325–329.

Storch, G. A., Radcliff, J. L., Meyer, P. L., & Hinrichs, J. H. (1987). Methicillin-resistant *Staphylococcus aureus* in a nursing home. *Infection Control and Hospital Epidemiology, 8*, 24–29.

Strausbaugh, L. J., Jacobson, C., Sewell, D. L., Potter, S., & Ward, T. T. (1992). Antimicrobial therapy for methicillin-resistant *Staphylococcus aureus* colonization in residents and staff of a Veterans Affairs nursing home care unit. *Infection Control and Hospital Epidemiology, 13*, 151–159.

Strausbaugh, L. J., Jacobson, C., Sewell, D. L., Potter, S., & Ward, T. T. (1991). Methicillin resistant *Staphylococcus aureus* in extended-care facilities: Experiences in a Veterans Affairs nursing home and a review of the literature. *Infection Control and Hospital Epidemiology, 12*, 36–45.

Thomas, J. C., Bridge, J., Waterman, S., Vogt, J., Kilman, L., & Hancock, G. (1989). Transmission and control of methicillin-resistant *Staphylococcus aureus* in a skilled nursing facility. *Infection Control and Hospital Epidemiology, 10*, 106–110.

Thompson, R. L., Cabezudo, I., & Wenzel, R. P. (1982). Epidemiology of nosocomial infections caused by methicillin-resistant *Staphylococcus aureus*. *Annals of Internal Medicine, 97*, 309–317.

Thurn, J. R., Belongia, E. A., & Crossley, K. (1991). Methicillin-resistant *Staphylococcus aureus* in Minnesota nursing homes. *Journal of the American Geriatrics Society, 39*, 1105–1109.

Tuazon, C. U., Perez, A., Kishaba, T. et al. (1975). *Staphylococcus aureus* among insulin-injecting diabetic patients. *Journal of the American Medical Society, 231*, 1272.

Verhof, J., & Verbrugh, H. A. (1981). Host determinants in staphylococcal disease. *Annual Review of Medicine, 32*, 107–122.

Ward, T. T., Winn, R. E., Hartstein, A. L., & Sewell, D. L. (1981). Observations relating to an interhospital outbreak of methicillin-resistant *Staphylococcus aureus*: Role of antimicrobial therapy in infection control. *Infection Control, and Hospital Epidemiology, 2*, 453–459.

Wenzel, R. P., Nettleman, M. D., Jones, R. N., & Pfaller, M. A. (1991). Methicillin-resistant *Staphylococcus aureus*: Implications for the 1990s, and effective control measures. *American Journal of Medicine, 91*, 221S–227S.

Yu, V. L., Goetz, A., Wagener, M., Smith, P. B., Rihs, J. D., & Hanchett, M. D. (1986). *Staphylococcus aureus* nasal carriage and infection in patients on hemodialysis: Efficacy of antibiotic prophylaxis. *New England Journal of Medicine, 315*, 91–96.

Clostridium 17

difficile Infection
in the Elderly

Richard G. Bennett

Clostridium difficile infection is diagnosed frequently in elderly patients treated in hospitals, and therefore this infection is increasingly encountered by clinicians caring for older individuals at home or in a nursing home. Like younger patients, most older individuals with symptomatic *C. difficile* infection have recently been treated with antibiotics and will present with diarrhea and perhaps fever. However, *C. difficile* infection in the elderly may lead more frequently to less common symptoms including toxic megacolon, high fever without obvious source, fever with a leukemoid reaction, and relapsing infection over many months. Additionally, *C. difficile* results in protein-losing enteropathy, which may worsen the nutritional state in vulnerable older patients. In this chapter, these special considerations are reviewed and current approaches to diagnosis, treatment, and infection control in long-term care facilities are presented.

HISTORICAL PERSPECTIVE

C. difficile was originally described by investigators who were studying the commensal gastrointestinal flora in infants and identified an elongated, spore-producing, obligate anerobe that was difficult to culture (Hall & O'Toole, 1935). Because the infants from whom these organisms were cultured were healthy and asymptomatic, *Bacillus difficilis*, as they called the organism, was not believed to be a human pathogen even though the bacteria was recognized as producing a potent toxin that was lethal when injected into guinea pigs.

The increasing use of antibiotics in the 1940s and 1950s led to the recognition of antibiotic-associated diarrhea. Several patients during this time who were treated with antibiotics also developed a severe diarrheal illness with high fevers. Some of these patients died, and autopsies revealed fibrinous "pseudomembranes" and severe inflammation of the colon (Reiner, Schlesinger, & Miller, 1952). Although *Staphylococcus aureus* was cultured from some patients with pseudomembranous colitis in the 1960s, the etiology of this syndrome, and of antibiotic-associated diarrhea in general, remained obscure.

With the introduction of clindamycin in the 1970s, a tremendous increase in the number of cases of postantibiotic pseudomembranous colitis was observed (Tedesco, Stanley, & Alpers, 1974). Intensive investigation in several laboratories led to the identification in 1978 of *C. difficile* as the cause of almost all cases of pseudomembranous colitis as well as the agent responsible for 15% to 25% of cases antibiotic-associated diarrhea (Bartlett, Chang, Gurwith, et al., 1978; George, Symonds, Dimock, et al., 1978). Through the present time, no other bacteria are routinely diagnosed as causing diarrhea following administration of antibiotics.

During the last 15 years, *C. difficile* has become recognized not only as an enteropathogen but also as an infectious agent that can cause outbreaks. When outbreaks of *C. difficile* diarrhea occur in hospitals, age is typically a major risk factor for becoming symptomatically infected (Brown, Talbot, Axelrod, et al., 1990; McFarland, Surawicz, & Stamm, 1990). *C. difficile* has also emerged as a frequent problem among nursing home patients, and the need for more creative approaches to treating this infection in the elderly has become apparent.

DIAGNOSIS OF *C. difficile* INFECTION

To appreciate fully the epidemiology of *C. difficile* among the elderly, as well as the approach to treatment and infection control, the current methods for identifying the presence of *C. difficile* and its toxins in stool specimens must be understood. *C. difficile* only infects the colon and perhaps the distal ileum, and neither the organism nor its toxins is believed to enter the bloodstream even with severe infections. Currently only analysis of stool specimens is needed to confirm the diagnosis of *C. difficile* disease.

C. difficile remains a difficult organism to culture. Anaerobic techniques using special selective media must be used to recover the organism, even from diarrheic specimens from individuals with known infection. Growth of the organism on agar plates takes up to 48 hours, and additional testing that can take 4 to 7 days is required to show that the recovered isolates produce toxins. Because culturing stool to identify toxigenic *C. difficile* is labor intensive and time-consuming, virtually no hospital laboratories rely on stool culture for making clinical diagnoses. However, because culturing stool or rectal swabs is currently the most sensitive method for identifying the presence of *C. difficile* in an individual, culture methods are regularly employed in epidemiologic studies of *C. difficile* infection. Culturing stool in a research laboratory can routinely identify carriers of *C. difficile* among hospital and nursing home patients who are asymptomatic and cannot be recognized with available clinical tests for *C. difficile* toxins. This important observation underlies the development of rational approaches to infection control within long-term care facilities that will be considered subsequently.

The standard test for diagnosing *C. difficile* remains a tissue culture assay that detects toxins produced by the organism. This assay arose from the original studies that were used to identify *C. difficile* as the cause of pseudomembranous colitis in the 1970s. In brief, a well of a microtiter plate in which fibroblasts are growing is exposed to a small amount of a cell-free filtrate made from the stool of a patient with diarrhea or from a broth culture supernatant in which putative *C. difficile* was grown. A similar amount of cell-free filtrate is added to another well along with anticlostridial antibody. If *C. difficile* toxins are present in the filtrate, the fibroblasts in the first well will undergo characteristic actinomorphic changes, that is, the fibroblasts that are typically long, thin, and confluent will become round, develop sharp projections, and separate. The presence of antibody in the companion well will prevent these changes, providing confirmation that *C. difficile* toxins are present in the specimen. It is imperative to remember that a *C. difficile* assay of stool typically must be ordered as a separate test for a patient with diarrhea (i.e., ordering a "stool culture" will not identify *C. difficile*), and most laboratories only perform a *C. difficile* assay when this test is ordered specifically.

The major problem with the *C. difficile* tissue culture assay is that several days are required before a result is reported as positive. By convention this assay is allowed to progress for 48 hours before a positive result is confirmed. Because many laboratories only set up this test daily, 3 to 4 days can easily pass between ordering a *C. difficile* assay and obtaining the final result. Until recently this problem was often even worse because many clinical laboratories did not have tissue culture facilities and relied on reference laboratories for these tests. Fortunately in the last several years commercially prepared tissue culture plates are more widely available, and these assays are being carried out in more hospitals.

The tissue culture assay remains the "gold standard" for diagnosing *C. difficile* infection. Virtually every patient with pseudomembranous colitis confirmed endoscopically will have a positive stool assay. Because the assay is good for confirming the diagnosis of this severe infection, most authorities do not recommend routine colonoscopy for patients with the typical symptoms of pseudomembranous colitis, and will begin presumptive treatment and wait for the confirmatory test result. For patients with diarrhea during or following a course of antibiotics, 20% to 30% will typically have a positive assay for *C. difficile* and by definition have *C. difficile* diarrhea. An additional 10% to 15% might have a negative toxin assay, but a positive stool culture in a research laboratory. Thus *C. difficile* is responsible for less than half of the cases of antibiotic-associated diarrhea.

Since the late 1980s new tests for *C. difficile* have been developed and marketed. The first introduced was a latex agglutination test that provides reasonable sensitivity and specificity compared with the tissue culture toxin assay, as well as the added advantage of yielding results in as little as 30 minutes (Bennett, Laughon, Mundy, et al., 1989). Newer tests relying on enzyme immunoassays have been introduced recently that are also reliable and take only several hours (Doern, Coughlin, & Wu, 1992). Both types of tests usually are as sensitive as the tissue culture assay for diagnosing *C. difficile* infection in symptomatic patients, and less sensitive than stool or rectal swab culture for identifying carriers. Such tests are being used increasingly in hospital and commercial laboratories, and their popularity and acceptance should continue to rise in coming years. In the future, new approaches to diagnosis and identification of carriage may rely on amplification of sequences of the toxin gene. These potentially extremely sensitive methods may necessitate a reevaluation of our current understanding of the epidemiology of this organism.

SPECTRUM OF *C. difficile* DISEASE AMONG THE ELDERLY

In the largest epidemiologic study of *C. difficile* published, investigators in Sweden determined that the carriage rate of *C. difficile* was 3% among 600 healthy volunteers who had not been treated with antibiotics within the previous 6 weeks (Aronsson, Mollby, & Nord, 1985). In our own investigations of the prevalence of *C. difficile* across the life-span, more than 700 specimens from participants in the Baltimore Longitudinal Study on Aging were analyzed. There was no age-related increased prevalence rate identified, as only 4 subjects had a positive stool culture, and none had a positive toxin assay (Bennett R., unpublished data). Currently there is no evidence that age alone is a risk factor for being asymptomatically colonized with this organism. In other words, because C. *difficile* cannot be recovered from most adults using current culture methodologies, a positive stool culture or toxin assay for C. *difficile* should always be regarded as abnormal regardless of the patient's age.

The risks of carriage have not been established. Intuitively, individuals who harbor this organism should be at higher risk for becoming symptomatic following exposure to antimicrobials and should also contribute to environmental contamination. Most interestingly in the elderly, however, is the association that has been seen between carriage and subsequent mortality. In two separate studies, an association between carriage and death has been observed (Bender, Bennett, Laughon, et al., 1986; Thomas, Bennett, Laughon, et al., 1990). However, because few of the subsequent deaths were obviously related to infection with C. *difficile*, carriage should be viewed simply as a marker for subsequent increased mortality. In other words, carriage of C. *difficile* is not being touted as an occult lethal infection, and only an occasional patient who is known to be colonized with C. *difficile* appears to die from the infection.

In both younger and older adults, C. *difficile* diarrhea typically occurs only in individuals who have been treated with antibiotics. However, analysis of almost 5,000 specimens from individuals with diarrhea in Sweden showed that the incidence of C. *difficile* diarrhea increased dramatically from less than 30 cases per million in the third decade of life to 250 cases per million in the eighth (Aronsson et al., 1985). Besides age, other explanations for this increase are that older people with diarrhea might be more likely to visit a physician and be tested for C. *difficile* than younger people, or alternatively, that older people are more likely to be treated for other infections with antibiotics and thereby be placed at increased risk for C. *difficile* infection. However, retrospective investigations of hospital outbreaks of C. *difficile* (Brown et al., 1990) and a prospective study of C. *difficile* infection among hospitalized patients (McFarland et al., 1990) consistently show that age is a risk factor for this infection. Because age does not appear to be a risk factor for carriage, other comorbid conditions that predispose the elderly to infections generally, and especially the frequency with which antibiotics are prescribed to older patients, probably explain these observations.

Pseudomembranous colitis is a life-threatening infection caused by C. *difficile*. The syndrome involves diarrhea that can be copious and watery, high fever (even of 103 °F to 105 °F in nursing home patients), and abdominal distention and pain. Classically the diagnosis is confirmed when pseudomembranes are identified with colonoscopy. Because clinicians have become more aware of this diagnosis in the last decade, endoscopic procedures are less frequently pursued in such patients, and the diagnosis is confirmed following receipt of a positive *C. difficile* assay. These severe infections often occur in elderly patients, and a high index of suspicion should be maintained for this diagnosis whenever an older patient has a high unexplained fever or develops a distended abdomen. It is also imperative to remember that pseudomembranous colitis can present without diarrhea. Such patients can have marked abdominal distention with radiographic evidence of toxic megacolon (see Figure 17.1), and leukemoid reactions with white blood cell counts of 25,000 to 50,000/mm^3. Considering the diagnosis of pseudomembranous colitis in these individuals and beginning treatment promptly can prevent exploratory laparotomy or even death in an affected patient.

In older patients who are diagnosed with *C. difficile* diarrhea or pseudomembranous colitis, the risk of a recurrent bout of diarrhea may be higher than in younger patients. Although only 5% to 10% of adults who develop symptomatic *C. difficile* will have a relapse, relapses among elderly nursing home patients are not unusual. Studies using typing methods have shown that recurrent diarrhea can result from the same organism (i.e., a true relapse) or from a different strain (i.e., reinfection leading to new symptoms) (Bobo, Gaydos, Bennett, et al., 1987; McFarland, Mulligan, Kwok, et al., 1989). Unusual older patients may have many bouts of recurrent diarrhea over many months, and it is this group of patients who remain the most difficult to manage.

Finally, the elderly also may be at increased risk for the nutritional consequences of *C. difficile* infection. If serial bouts of diarrhea and fever occur, these recurrent illnesses can clearly worsen the nutritional state. In addition, *C. difficile* results in protein-losing enteropathy. Significant loss of serum proteins into the gut with pseudomembranous colitis can result in anasarca, and based on the identification of α_1-antitrypsin[1] in stool specimens, protein-losing enteropathy also occurs in patients with positive *C. difficile* stool cultures without diarrhea as well as in patients with *C. difficile* diarrhea and normal colonoscopy (Rybolt, Bennett, Laughon, et al., 1989). In one case report, long-standing carriage of *C. difficile* was associated with poor weight gain and low serum albumin despite aggressive nutritional support over many months, and these problems improved following weeks of treatment with oral vancomycin (Bennett & Greenough, 1990).

C. difficile Infection Among Nursing Home Patients

The problem of *C. difficile* infection in long-term care facilities has received increasing attention in recent years following the first report of this infection in a nursing home (Bender et al., 1986). In this study, an initial point prevalence survey using stool culture found that 33% of patients on one

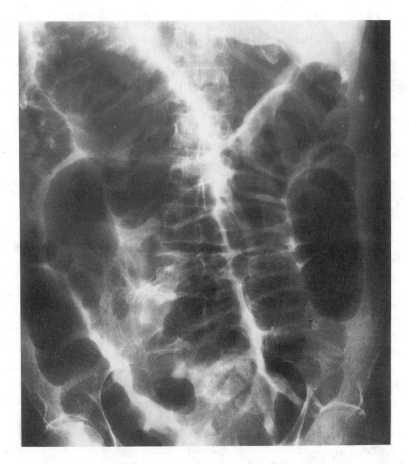

FIGURE 17.1   An abdominal radiograph of a nursing home patient with a history of recurrent *C. difficile* diarrhea who developed toxic megacolon. This condition was precipitated by the prescription of diphenoxylate, which was given
over a several-day period after one *C. difficile* assay was negative. A high fever
and abdominal distention developed, and this radiograph was obtained. The
patient was admitted to the hospital for intravenous hydration and responded
to treatment with oral vancomycin. (Radiograph originally published in *Geriatrics* and reprinted with permission; Bennett & Greenough, 1990.)

ward of a 233-bed facility were colonized with *C. difficile* versus less than
10% of residents on the other wards. The affected ward housed the most
debilitated residents in the facility including patients with severe pressure
ulcers, closed-head trauma, and end-stage renal failure on dialysis. Serial
surveys were carried out on this ward over the following 6 months, and the

point prevalence rates remained high (33% to 47%) despite interventions including initial treatment with metronidazole or vancomycin of all patients with positive stool toxin assays, prescription of modified enteric isolation for all patients with positive stool toxin assays, and recommendations to the attending physicians to avoid specific classes of antibiotics thought to be most likely to predispose to *C. difficile* infection. This study raised the question of whether *C. difficile* infection was endemic in long-term care facilities.

In the years since this investigation, other studies and reports have shown that although *C. difficile* can be a significant problem among residents of nursing homes, this organism is not typically an endemic pathogen in long-term care facilities. Clusters of cases of *C. difficile* in nursing homes have been reported in Baltimore, Philadelphia, and Chicago (Bennett, Laughon, Greenough, et al., 1989), but true epidemic outbreaks of infection with rapid spread among nursing home patients might be best characterized as a scenario that includes occasional spread of infection from resident to resident, particularly to residents recently treated with antibiotics, and frequent admission to the faculty of individuals who are infected with *C. difficile*. These latter patients may have had a previously treated bout of *C. difficile* diarrhea in the hospital, or may simply have been infected in the hospital and may develop symptoms for the first time in the nursing home. With the identification of one or two cases of confirmed *C. difficile* diarrhea in a facility, nursing and physician concern is heightened and more frequent testing for *C. difficile* is ordered. Testing often occurs for all patients with any loose stools, and so individuals with *C. difficile* diarrhea that might be only minimal and self-limited are identified as infected. Thus, nursing homes with a "problem" with *C. difficile* infection may be as likely to have increased vigilance, as an actual increased incidence and prevalence of infection.

Whether or not *C. difficile* is perceived as a problem in a long-term care facility, rigorous and rational attention to infection control in all nursing homes is necessary to minimize the morbidity from this infection. Strict adherence to universal precautions for all residents, and regular in-service training for all staff members on the importance of handwashing will provide the foundation for infection control generally and for *C. difficile* infection specifically. In addition, rational prescription of antibiotics must be assured by the medical director and nursing quality control officer to minimize the risk that susceptible individuals are made more vulnerable to this potentially lethal infection. Although "sterilization" of the environment is an ideal, given the ubiquity of this organism and the hardiness of the spores it produces, a false sense of security will be engendered by those who rely on soap and germicidals for infection control. Special consideration should also be given to the communal use of electronic thermometers as some investigators believe that infection can be spread using this new technology (Brooks, Veal, Kramer, et al., 1992).

Perhaps the most crucial component of an infection control system is maintaining a high index of suspicion for *C. difficile* disease. In a nursing home where many doctors may care for residents, the medical director and infection control nurse must often provide education to the physician staff about the approach to diagnosing and treating this infection. With respect to the degree of "isolation" required for patients with *C. difficile* infection, because many patients have unrecognized carriage of this organism, a rational approach is recommended regarding the need of isolating those few patients who are known to be infected. A positive test for *C. difficile* should *not* be a basis for denying admission to a nursing home. Patients admitted to a facility who are asymptomatic and only have a positive test should be treated like an uninfected resident, except perhaps in a rare case where stool is unable to be contained within a diaper in a demented patient. For patients who develop *C. difficile* diarrhea in the nursing home, treatment within the patient's room is appropriate (i.e., isolation in a private room is not necessary); soiled linens should be bagged at the bedside to minimize environmental contamination; and treatment in the room can be discontinued once the patient feels well, again unless fecal soiling of the environment is thought likely. This rational approach to infection control in a long-term care facility differs from the stricter approach advocated by the Centers for Disease Control for hospital patients but has been adopted by the Maryland State Department of Health (Maryland State Department of Health, 1989).

TREATMENT OF *C. difficile* INFECTION

Whether caring for patients in a hospital, nursing home, or office, prevention remains the key for minimizing the incidence of *C. difficile* disease. Although prevention involves attention to infection control as discussed earlier, avoiding the use of antibiotics is the most important single method for reducing the incidence of this infection generally. Because the establishment of *C. difficile* in the colon requires the disruption of the normal flora by antibiotics, the use of systemic antibiotics should be avoided whenever possible. For example, a patient with an episode of vomiting with aspiration and a fever several hours later might be treated with aerosolized broncodilators and chest percussion, one with an infected pressure sore and a low-grade fever might be treated with debridement and betadine wet-to-dry dressings, and another patient with a fever without obvious source who is otherwise clinically stable might be monitored and given extra fluids for 12 to 24 hours. If such patients become afebrile, as will often be the case, the need to prescribe antibiotics is obviated and the risk of a frail patient developing *C. difficile* diarrhea is avoided.

Whenever a patient who is a being treated with antibodies develops diarrhea, the antimicrobial agent should be discontinued if possible. Antibiotics are often arbitrarily ordered for 7 to 14 days for nursing home patients with dysuria, bronchitis, or unexplained fevers, and when diarrhea develops after the 5th or 6th day of therapy serious consideration should be given to discontinuing antibiotic therapy. Although theoretical concerns regarding incompletely treating an infection or predisposing to the emergence of resistant bacteria can be raised, discontinuation of the antibiotic will often be followed by cessation of diarrhea in 1 to 2 days with no return of the original symptoms for which antibiotics were prescribed. If the antibiotic regimen cannot be discontinued, additional therapy directed against *C. difficile* may be needed.

The initial approach to the treatment of a patient with symptomatic *C. difficile* infection should be based on the severity of disease as defined by the volume of diarrheal stool losses (minimal [<1 L/day], moderate [1 to 2 L/day], or severe [>2 L/day]; the extent of fever (minimal (<99.9 °F), moderate [100 °F to 101 °F], or severe [>101 °F]); the presence or absence of abdominal pain and distention; the ability to replace diarrheal fluid losses volitionally using prescribed oral rehydration therapy; and the elevation of the white blood cell count (minimal [<12,000/mm^3], moderate [12,000 to 25,000/mm^3], or severe [>25,000/mm^3]). Relying on this simple approach to patient assessment, therapy for an elderly patient with *C. difficile* diarrhea can be prescribed. Therapy always includes careful attention to volume status and prescription of oral rehydration therapy, prescription of an agent with anti–*C. difficile* activity, and absolute avoidance of antiperistaltic drugs (e.g., diphenoxylate or loperamide), which might precipitate the development of pseudomembranous colitis.

Patients with minimal symptoms simply require supportive therapy including oral rehydration and bismuth subsalicylate. Commercial oral rehydration therapy solutions includes packets with premeasured glucose and salts (e.g., Oral Rehydration Salts, Jianas Bros., Kansas City, MO) or premixed solutions (e.g., Pedialyte, Ross Laboratories, Columbus, OH; Ricelyte, Mead Johnson, Evansville, IN). As with any patient with gastroenteritis, those with *C. difficile* diarrhea typically require 1 to 2 L to replace diarrheal losses and intraluminal fluid once symptoms are identified, and additional 1 to 2 L each day to replace ongoing losses. Sports drinks (e.g., Gator Ade) may have too little salt and too much sugar to be appropriate oral rehydration therapy solution.

Besides Oral Rehydration Therapy, prescription of bismuth subsalicylate to patients with minimal illness from *C. difficile* should be considered. Bismuth subsalicylate has antibacterial activity against *C. difficile* in vitro (Cornick, Silva, & Gorbach, 1990) and is protective in an animal model of this infection (Chang, Dong, & Gorbach, 1990). There are no published clinical trails employing bismuth subsalicylate for individuals with *C. difficile* infection, but this mediation can be safely given to elderly patients and appears to be effective in reducing diarrheal symptoms. Bismuth subsalicylate can be prescribed 30 mL every 2 hours up to 8 doses, and then 30 to 60 mL every 6 hours as needed for diarrhea over the following 3 to 4 days. Because *C. difficile* is often a self-limited illness, there is currently no rigorous proof that this regimen is more effective than oral rehydration alone. However, while awaiting clinical trails to establish whether or not bismuth subsalicylate is truly effective, this medication is recommended for older patients based on the available in vitro and in vivo studies and our own experience.

The two most frequently prescribed antibiotics to combat *C. difficile* infection are vancomycin and metronidazole. Because oral vancomycin is so expensive, most experts agree that metronidazole can be prescribed for patients who are clinically stable and have no severe symptoms as described earlier. For patients with moderate symptoms, metronidazole 500 mg every 6 hours for 7 to 10 days can be prescribed. In a comparison trial of metronidazole and vancomycin, both antibiotics were effective in alleviating symptoms of diarrhea over 3 to 5 days, and in preventing relapse that occurred in only 5% to 15% of subjects (Teasley, Gerding, Olson, et al., 1983). Although this study showed similar therapeutic efficacy, most specialists believe that oral vancomycin should always be used for patients with severe symptoms and for patients with confirmed pseudomembranous colitis. For patients with severe symptoms, vancomycin 500 mg every 6 hours for 10 to 14 days should be ordered. If symptoms improve quickly, the dose of vancomycin can be decreased to 250 mg after 4 to 5 days, and then to 125 mg after 10 days to minimize pharmacy costs. Although other antibiotics are available that have activity against *C. difficile* (e.g., bacitracin), their use is limited because antibiotic resistance does not underlie treatment failure (i.e., spores in the gut are thought to germinate and lead to another bout of illness), and therefore either metronidazole or vancomycin can also be used treating relapses.

Treating recurrent infection remains one of the challenges of dealing with *C. difficile* infection among elderly. This is particularly true among the frailest nursing home patients who may develop recurrent disease over many months. Current approaches to treating these patients include careful attention to the overall nutritional state and creative use of the available antibiotics. For patients with intermittent but minimal diarrhea (e.g., loose stools 2 to 4 days each week) and persistently positive *C. difficile* laboratory tests, standing orders for bismuth subsalicylate as needed can be considered. For patients with deteriorating nutritional status or more troubling symptoms, prescription of tapering doses of vancomycin over many weeks may prove necessary. In the future, the efficacy of treating such patients with microbial replacement, for example, *Lactobacillus* GG (Gorbach, Chang, & Goldin 1987), or *Saccharomyces boulardii* (Kimmey, Elmer, Surawicz, et al., 1990), may be established.

SUMMARY

C. difficile infection is likely to become an increasing problem in clinical practice as the number of older patients in the population increases. Older patients are most likely to develop *C. difficile* diarrhea without systemic symptoms following treatment with antibiotics for another infection. However, atypical presentations with severe systemic illness and colitis without diarrhea can be seen in the elderly. Diagnosis of infection continues to rely on detecting toxin in stool specimens with a tissue culture assay. In coming years, the increasing use and acceptance of immunologic assays will decrease the time required for making the diagnosis of *C. difficile* infection. The approach to treatment of the elderly patient should be based on careful attention to replacement of diarrheal fluid losses, the prescription of antibiotics based on the severity of symptoms, and the avoidance of antiperistalic drugs. In long-term care facilities, a rational approach to infection control can minimize the spread of infection without unnecessarily burdening an individual patient by requiring strict adherence to isolation within a private room.

NOTE

1. α_1-Antitrypsin is a serum protein not usually found in the stool that is resistant to enzymatic and bacterial degradation. Presence of α_1-antitrypsin in stool is a marker for protein-losing enteropathy.

REFERENCES

Aronsson, B., Mollby, R., & Nord, C. E. (1985). Antimicrobial agents and *Clostridium difficile* in acute enteric disease: Epidemiological data from Sweden, 1980–1982. *Journal of Infectious Diseases, 151*, 476–481.

Bartlett, J. G., Chang, T. W., Gurwith, M., Gorbach, S. L., & Onderdonk, A. B. (1978). Antibiotic-associated pseudomembranous colitis due to toxin-producing clostridia. *New England Journal of Medicine, 298*, 531–534.

Bender, B. S., Bennett, R. G., Laughon, B. E., Greenough, W. B., Gaydos, C., Sears, S.,

Forman, M., & Bartlett, J. G. (1986). Is *Clostridium difficile* endemic in chronic-care facilities? *Lancet, 2,* 11–13.

Bennett, R., & Greenough, W. (1990). *C. difficile* diarrhea: A common and over-looked nursing home infection. *Geriatrics, 45,* 77– 87.

Bennett, R., Laughon, B., Greenough, W., & Bartlett, J. (1989). *Clostridium difficile* in elderly patients [Letter]. *Age & Aging, 18,* 354–355.

Bennett, R. G., Laughon, B. E., Mundy, L. M., Bobo, L., Gaydos, C., Greenough, W., & Bartlett, J. (1989). Evaluation of a latex agglutination test for *Clostridium difficile* in two nursing home outbreaks. *Journal of Clinical Microbiology, 27,* 889–893.

Bobo, L., Gaydos, C., Bennett, R., Laughon, B., & Bartlett, J. (1987). Comparison of methods for typing *Clostridium difficile*. *Abstracts of the Annual Meeting of the American Society of Microbiology,* C–10.

Brooks, S. E., Veal, R. O., Kramer, M., Dore, L., Schupf, N., & Adachi, M. (1992). Reduction in the incidence of *Clostridium difficile*-associated diarrhea in an acute care hospital and a skilled nursing facility following replacement of electronic thermometers with single-use disposables. *Infection Control and Hospital Epidemiology, 13,* 98–103.

Brown, E., Talbot, G. H., Axelrod, R., Provencher, M., & Hoegg, C. (1990). Risk factors of *Clostridium difficile* toxin-associated diarrhea. *Infection Control and Hospital Epidemiology, 11,* 283– 290.

Chang, T. -W., Dong, M. -Y., & Gorbach, S. L. (1990). Effect of bismuth subsalicylate on *Clostridium difficile* colitis in hamsters. *Review of Infectious Diseases,* 12(Suppl. 1), S57–S58.

Cornick, N. A., Silva, M., & Gorbach, S. L. (1990). In vitro activity of bismuth subsalicylate. *Review of Infectious Diseases,* 12(Suppl. 1), S9–S10.

Doern, G. V., Coughlin, R. T., & Wu, L. (1992). Laboratory diagnosis of *Clostridium difficile*-associated gastrointestinal disease: Comparison of a monoclonal antibody enzyme immunoassay for toxins A and B with a monoclonal antibody enzyme immunoassay for toxin A only and two cytotoxicity assays. *Journal of Clinical Microbiology, 30,* 2042–2046.

George, R. H., Symonds, J. M., Dimock, F., Brown, J. D., Arabi, Y., Shinagawa, N., Keighley, M. R. B., Alexander-Williams, J., & Burdon, D. W. (1978). Identification of *Clostridium difficile* as a cause of pseudomembranous colitis. *British Medical Journal, 1,* 695.

Gorbach, S. L., Chang, T. -W., & Goldin, B. (1987). Successful treatment of relapsing *Clostridium difficile* colitis with *Lactobacillus* GG [Letter]. *Lancet, 2,* 1519.

Hall, I. C., & O'Toole E. (1935). Intestinal flora in new-born infants. *American Journal of Disabled Children, 49,* 390–402.

Kimmey, M. B., Elmer, G. W., Surawicz, C. M., & McFarland, L. V. (1990). Prevention of further recurrences of *Clostridium difficile* colitis with *Saccharomyces boulardii*. *Digestive Diseases and Sciences, 35,* 897–901.

Maryland Department of Health and Mental Hygiene. (1989). Clostridium difficile *in long-term care facilities: Recommendations for control and for admission of residents*. Baltimore, MD: Author.

McFarland, L. V., Mulligan, M. E., Kwok, R. Y. Y., & Stamm, W. E. (1989). Nosocomial acquisition of *Clostridium difficile* infection. *New England Journal of Medicine, 320,* 204–210.

McFarland, L. V., Surawicz, C. M., & Stamm, W. E. (199). Risk factors for *Clostridium difficile* carriage and *C. difficile*-associated diarrhea in a cohort of hospitalized patients. *Journal of Infectious Diseases, 162,* 678–684.

Reiner, L., Schlesinger, M. J., & Miller, G. M. (1952). Pseudomembranous colitis following aureomycin and chloramphenicol. *Archives of Pathology, 54,* 39–67.

Rybolt, A. H., Bennett, R. G., Laughon, B. E., Thomas, D. R., Greenough, W. B., & Bartlett, J. G. (1989). Protein-losing enteropathy associated with *Clostridium difficile* infection. *Lancet, 1,* 1353–1355.

Teasley, D. G., Gerding, D. N., Olson, M. M., Peterson, L. R., Gebhard, R. L., Schwartz, M. J., & Lee, J. T. (1983). Prospective randomised trial of metronidazole versus vancomycin for *C. difficile*-associated diarrhea and colitis. *Lancet, 2,* 1043–1046.

Tedesco, F. J., Stanley, R. J., & Alpers, D. H. (1974). Diagnostic features of clindamycin-associated pseudomembranous colitis. *New England Journal of Medicine, 290,* 841–843.

Thomas, D. R., Bennett, R. G., Laughon, B. E., Greenough, W. B., Bartlett, J. G. (1990). Postantibiotic colonization with *Clostridium difficile* in nursing-home patients. *Journal of the American Geriatrics Society, 38,* 415–420.

PART IV
Preventive and Therapeutic Strategies

Aging, Nutrition, and Immunity $\boxed{18}$

James S. Goodwin and Edith L. Burns

This chapter considers how the interactions between aging and immune function are modulated by nutrition. We begin with a review of the immunologic effects of nutritional deficiencies, followed by a review of nutritional changes with aging. We then consider the possibility that some of the well-described age-related changes in immunity may be secondary to age-related changes in nutritional status. One point to make at the outset is the exceptionally small database on which to draw when addressing this issue. This is illustrated by the results of a literature search of the topics aging/nutrition/immunity. Of the 46 articles published from 1986 through the present, more than 80% were review articles. As all too frequently occurs in geriatrics and gerontology, once a potentially important area is identified, far more effort is expended on reviewing how little we know than in expanding the body of knowledge.

IMMUNOLOGIC CONSEQUENCES OF NUTRITIONAL DEFICIENCIES

Protein–Calorie Malnutrition and Immunity

The most complete information on the relationship of nutrition to immune function relates to macronutrient deficiency, specifically protein–calorie malnutrition. The role of malnutrition in increased susceptibility to infection has been recognized for centuries. Much of this information comes from observational studies in Third World countries, particularly in children, but, as Rudman and Feller (1989) stressed, these Third World studies have direct relevance to the health of residents of First World nursing homes, where the prevalence of protein–calorie malnutrition is similar to that seen among famine-striken populations. These two populations (nursing home residents and victims of famine) also have a high prevalence of anergy and other manifestations of impaired immunity (Newmann, Lawlor, Stiehm, et al., 1975). Although the causal relationship between malnutrition and depressed immunity in famine victims is both obvious and also well documented by prospective studies on the effect of refeeding (Chandra, 1972), there has been some reluctance to recognize malnutrition as a correctable cause of anergy among nursing home patients. Instead, both the malnutrition and the anergy are often cited as markers for an organism undergoing generalized decline. However, it is important to note that several studies have demonstrated marked improvements in immunity in malnourished older patients associated with programs to correct the nutritional deficiency (Lipschitz & Mitchell, 1982; Chandra, Joshi, Au, et al., 1982). An example of these is a study by Lipschitz and Mitchell (1982) in which nine elderly, anergic, malnourished (mean albumin = 2.8 g/dL) men were placed on oral or enteral alimentation at 35 kcal/kg/day, approximately 2500 kcal/day for a 70-kg man. After 3 weeks all subjects reacted to a battery of delayed hypersensitivity skin test antigens and showed marked improvements in a large panel of both nutritional and immunologic indices. A similar result was reported by Chandra et al. (1982). These studies complement earlier work in malnourished hospitalized patients showing improvements in immunity after parenteral nutrition.

MICRONUTRITENT DEFICIENCIES AND IMMUNITY

There is a considerable literature on the effects of single nutrient deficiency on immunity in experimental animals (reviewed in Chandra, 1988; Chernoff, 1991; Beisel, 1983). There is less information in humans, because controlled studies of single nutrient deficiencies in human volunteers have been quite rare. Thus, much of the human work involves multiple nutrient deficiencies, but sometimes with correction by single nutrient supplementation.

It is not surprising that various vitamins and minerals have been noted to play an important role in the maintenance of normal immune function. Vitamins by definition are essential micronutrients; many physiologic systems fail in the presence of a given micronutrient deficiency. The immune system, by virtue of being easily biopsied for in vitro study (a single tube of blood yields millions of lymphocytes, granulocytes, and macropages) perhaps receives more attention in nutritional studies than do equally important but less accessible organ systems that may be as sensitive to nutritional deficiency.

A summary of the effects of specific micronutrient deficiency on immune function is given in Table 18.1. The micronutrients listed are those that most clearly manifest immunologic dysfunction as one of the early or most obvious consequences of deficiency.

CHANGES IN NUTRITIONAL STATUS IN THE ELDERLY

The nutritional status of elderly individuals is at risk for several reasons. Energy expenditure tends to decrease in the elderly, as does total caloric intake. If the nutritional content of the diet is unchanged, then a decrease in total calories is accompanied by a proportionate decrease in intake of specific nutrients. Physiologic, medical, and social changes that frequently accompany aging can put an individual at risk for deficiency. This is perhaps most clearly seen in long-term care institutions, where a combination of chronic disease, depression, decreased sense of taste and smell, isolation, disability, anorexia-causing medications, unappetizing food, and poor dentition synergize to produce evidence of malnutrition in at least half of long-term nursing home residents (Goodwin, 1989). The prevalence of protein-calorie malnutrition among nursing home residents ranges from 10% to 40%. About half of nursing home residents lose weight throughout their stay (Rudman & Feller, 1989). Biochemical surveys have identified 20% to 50% of nursing home residents at risk for vitamin deficiencies (Drinka & Goodwin, 1991), most commonly involving pyridoxine and riboflavin, but also described with other water-soluble vitamins.

The nutritional status of noninstitutionalized elderly depends on the economic, social, and medical characteristics of the particular population studied. There are approximately 3 million home-bound elderly in the United States. Though we have very little information on this population, it would appear that they closely resemble nursing home residents in nutritional status. Conversely, the nutritional status of healthy, independently living elderly men and women is similar to what is found in younger populations (Garry, Goodwin, & Hunt, 1982; Garry, Goodwin, Hunt, & Gilbert, 1982; Garry, Goodwin, Hunt, Hooper, & Leonard, 1982). Thus, one's estimate of the "nutritional status of the elderly" is greatly dependent on the population chosen for study.

TABLE 18.1 Effect of Deficiency of Selected Micronutrients on Immune Function

Nutrient	Species	Immunologic Effect	Reference
Vit A	man	↑ infections	West (1989)
Vit A	mouse	↓ antibody prod.	Smith (1987)
	mouse	↓ T helper activity	Carman (1989)
	mouse	↑ interferon prod.	Carman (1991)
		↓ phagocytosis	Fischer (1982)
Vit E	mouse	↓ antibody prod.	Tangerdy (1980)
Pyridoxine	man	↓ antibody prod.	Hodges (1962)
	man	lymphocytopenia	Cheslock (1960)
	mouse	↓ antibody prod.	Axelrod (1971)
	mouse	↓ many T cell functions	Axelrod (1971); Ha (1984); Robson (1975)
Folate	man	↓ DTH	Gross (1975)
	rat	↓ many T cell functions	Newberne (1977)
	rat	↓ neutrophil phagocytosis	Youinou (1982)

Nutrient	Species	Effect	Reference
Cyanocobalamin	rat	↑ infections	Thomaskutty (1985)
	rat	↓ Ab prod.	Newberne (1977)
	rat	↓ T cell proliferation	Newberne (1977)
	rat	↓ neutrophil killing	Seger (1980)
Biotin	man	↓ T suppressor activity	Fischer (1982)
	rat	↓ thymus size	Rabin (1985)
	rat	↓ cellular immunity	Rabin (1985)
	rat	↓ antibody response	Rabin (1985)
Zinc	man	↓ NK activity	Tapazaglou (1985); Allen (1983)
	man	↓ DTH	Cunningham-Rundles (1981)
	man	↓ many T cell function	Cunningham-Rundles (1981, 1988)
	mouse	thymus atrophy	Fraker (1977)
	mouse	↑ infections	Tanaka (1978); Good (1980)
	mouse	↓ T helper function	Fraker (1978)
	mouse	↓ macrophage and PMN phagocytosis and killing	Cook-Mills (1991)

NUTRITION AND IMMUNITY IN THE ELDERLY

In the remainder of this chapter, we discuss three areas relevant to nutrition, immunity, and the aging process: (a) the possible contribution of nutritional deficiencies to the well-described decline in immune function with advanced age; (b) the role of "nutrients as drugs" and whether certain nutrients at levels of intake far exceeding the recommended daily allowance (RDA) reverse some of the decline in immune function seen in elderly organisms; and (c) the effect of caloric restriction in preventing age-associated declines in immunity and other physiologic functions.

Does Nutritional Deficiency Contribute to Immune Dysfunction in the Elderly?

As with essentially all the physiologic changes that have been found to be associated with old age, it has been difficult to prove that depressed cellular immune status is entirely secondary to the aging process itself and not to the many diseases that frequently accompany aging (Hess & Knapp, 1978). The increased variance in results of immunologic and other physiologic testing in the elderly suggests that age-related decreases in function are multiply determined and not simply a result of aging per se (Gutowski, Innes, Webster, et al., 1986).

One possible contributor to decreased immunity with age is inadequate nutritional status (Chandra, 1985; National Institute on Aging Research Planning Panel, 1982). In 1982 the Research Planning Panel of the National Institute on Aging called for an examination of a possible link between subclinical malnutrition and dysfunction of the immune system and other physiologic systems in the elderly. This concern was not without justification, in that previous studies have found a relationship between malnutrition and changes in other physiological systems with age. For example, clinically unrecognized malnutrition is associated with decreased cognitive function in some elderly adults (Brocklehurst, Griffiths, & Taylor, 1986; Goodwin, Goodwin, & Garry, 1983; Schorah, Newill, & Scott, 1979). In addition, reports demonstrating beneficial effects of vitamins supplementation on indices of cellular immunity have added to the interest in this area, even though the supplements were in the "megadose" range (see later). It should be clear that much or all of the immunosuppression seen in the elderly is indeed secondary to the aging process itself. Studies of experimental animals in controlled environments and of healthy human populations have all supported that conclusion. Nevertheless, many physiologic changes in elderly humans are multiply determined (Kinnel, 1974). The question then exists: Is part of the immunologic dysfunction seen in aged humans secondary to subtle nutritional deficiencies? This is a difficult question to answer, given the high degree of variance seen in both nutritional status and immune function in elderly populations. However, if inadequate nutrition does contribute to the immunodysfunction of aging, one would expect to find: (a) an association between immunologic and nutritional function within an elderly population, and (b) improvement in immune function associated with correction of nutritional deficiencies within an elderly population.

We addressed the first expectation in a population of 230 healthy elderly individuals who had received both comprehensive nutritional evaluations and testing of immune function (Goodwin & Garry, 1988). These subjects were older than age 65, fully ambulatory and living independently, on no prescription or routine nonprescription medication, and had no history or presence of serious illnesses after a comprehensive medical evaluation. Immunologic function was assessed with delayed-type hypersensitivity skin testing to four antigens, in vitro lymphocyte cultures with mitogens, lymphocyte count, and the presence of serum auto-antibodies and circulating immune complexes. Nutritional status was assessed by 3-day diet records and also biochemical analyses of blood for vitamins A, B12, C, D, E, riboflavin, folic acid, and the minerals iron, copper, and zinc. We had previously shown that this population contained substantial numbers of individuals with depressed immune function (Goodwin, Searles & Tung, 1982) and others with dietary or biochemical evidence of nutritional deficiency (Garry, Goodwin, and Hunt, 1982, 1984; Gary, Goodwin, Hunt, & Gilbert, 1982; Gary, Goodwin, Hunt, Hooper, & Leonard, 1982). Using a variety of analyses we found no association between malnutrition and depressed immunologic function in this population (Goodwin & Garry, 1988). The large size of the population provided sufficient power to find a relatively weak association between nutritional and immune status, had one existed.

The study described earlier would suggest that there is little or no association between nutrition and immunity among healthy elderly individuals. Chavance and associates (1985) found an association between vitamin A levels and results of some immunologic assays in a group of 100 healthy subjects older than age 60. However, no statistical adjustment was made for the many different analyses performed (comparing the levels of 6 different nutrients to the results of 14 different immunologic assays). Chance alone could produce several "statistically significant" results from the 84 potential analyses.

Many elderly are not healthy; it would appear that among chronically ill elderly inadequate nutrition does contribute to immune dysfunction, though, unfortunately, once again the database is rather meager. As we have noted previously, aggressive treatment of protein-calorie malnutrition in institutionalized elderly is associated with improvement in immunologic status (Chandra et al., 1982; Lipschitz & Mitchell, 1982).

Nutrients as Drugs

Many of the studies showing enhanced immune responses after nutritional supplementation have used supplemental intakes at levels far in excess of the RDA. For example, Talbott, Miller, and Kerkvliet (1987) found significant increases in lymphocyte responses to a variety of mitogens after 1 and 2 months of supplementation with 50-mg pyridoxine daily in 11 elderly individuals compared with controls taking placebo. This level of pyridoxine was 25 times the RDA. Similar results have been seen with short-term, high intakes of zinc (Duchateau, Delepesse, Vrijens, et al. 1981); vitamin C (Anderson, Dosthuizen, Maritz, et al., 1980; (Kennes, Dumont, Brohee, et al. 1983); vitamin E (Meydani, Meydani, Verden, et al. 1986; Meydani, Barkland, Liu, et al., 1990); beta carotene (Watson, Prabhala, Plezia, et al., 1991); and a combination of vitamins A, C, and E (Penn, Perkins, Kelleher, et al., 1991). The results, although impressive, allow for several possible interpretations: (a) the pyridoxine supplement was correcting a pyridoxine deficiency, and similar results would have been seen if the RDA for pyridoxine had been given; (b) the pyridoxine supplement was correcting a deficiency, but for reasons as yet unknown a high level of pyridoxine intake was required to correct that deficiency; and (c) the pyridoxine supplement was having an effect other than correcting a deficiency (i.e., it was a pharmacologic, not a nutritional intervention), perhaps resulting in a short-term stimulation of immunity similar to an adjuvant effect.

It is impossible with the information currently available to rule in or rule out any of those possibilities totally. This inability to determine which possibility is correct is an excellent demonstration of how little we actually know about this important area. There are clear public health implications to possibility one or two. The same points could be made about the interpretation of other demonstrations of immunologic enhancement with high-dose micronutrients (Duchateau et al., 1981; Meydani et al., 1986; Meydani et al., 1990; Penn et al., 1991; Watson et al., 1991).

Although the evidence is far from complete, there are some indications that the third possibility may explain the beneficial effects of high-dose pyridoxine and other nutrients on the immune response. For one thing, in the study by Talbott et al. (1987) there was no correlation between baseline plasma pyridoxal 5'-phosphate levels and improvements in mitogen responses with pyridoxine supplements; subjects with normal baseline plasma values had as much improvement as those with borderline or low values. Another line of evidence suggesting that the effects seen with high-dose single nutrient supplements might represent a short-term pharmacologic or adjuvant effect comes from our study of 270 healthy elderly New Mexicans. Approximately half of these subjects were ingesting some sort of vitamin or mineral supplement., many in the megadose range (Garry, Goodwin, Hunt, Hooper, & Leonard, 1982). For example, 10% of the subjects were ingesting more than 25 times the RDA for thiamine; more than 10 times the RDA for riboflavin, pyridoxine, niacin, and vitamin C; and more than 40 times the RDA for vitamin E. Thus, if high doses of any of these micronutrients resulted in a long-term increase in immune function, one might expect to see it in this population. In fact, we found no relationship between in vitro and in vivo assays of immune function and intake of large doses of any micronutrients (Goodwin and Garry, 1983). Once again, the large number of subjects generated sufficient power that, had difference in immune function of the magnitude previously reported (Anderson et al., 1980; Duchateau et al., 1981; Kennes et al., 1983; Talbot et al., 1987) with short-term, high-dose micronutrient supplements existed in this population, it almost certainly would have been detected. Finally, it is important to note that not all trials of high-dose micronutrient supplementation have shown beneficial effects on immune function (Brucker, Hollingsworth, Saltman, et al., 1988; Murphy, West, Greenough et al., 1992).

Caloric Restriction, Immunity and Longevity

Every review of nutrition in the elderly has to deal with the thorny issue of the benefits of caloric restriction. McKay and his colleagues (1935) showed that caloric restriction in early life resulted in substantial increases in life expectancy in several species of rodents. This work has been extended and refined over the years to include other mammals including vertebrates (reviewed in Hansen, Fernandez, & Good, 1982). Smaller but still significant effects are still seen if the caloric restriction is not started until adulthood. In addition to the fact that the animals live longer, they do not experience the expected physiologic changes with age. In particular, the immunologic changes with age reviewed earlier in this article are almost completely absent in these animals (Good, Fernandes, Yunis, et al., 1976).

The reason, of course, that this is a thorny issue is that it flies in the face of our clinical experience. Clinicians caring for children, adults, or the elderly know that severe caloric restriction is a major risk for increased mortality, not increased survival. And it is important to understand that the animal models require severe caloric restriction, such that its products are runts— long-lived runts but definitely runts. This can only be done in a controlled laboratory environment that eliminates potential pathogens that might wipe out the animals during their prolonged period of semistarvation. Thus, most investigators of nutrition in the elderly would agree with two statements relative to life extension by caloric restriction. (a) Caloric restrictions are by far the most powerful and best-described means of increasing life-span in experimental animals. As such, it is a powerful tool for studying the aging process. (b) The data from investigations of caloric restriction have absolutely no relevance to clinical geriatric nutrition. Prolonged caloric restriction in humans, for whatever reason, is associated with increases in morbidity and mortality.

SUMMARY AND CONCLUSIONS

In this final section we focus on the clinical significance of the information reviewed earlier. Immune function declines in the elderly, though there is great variability among individuals in the rate of decline. Otherwise healthy elderly individuals with depressed cellular immunity are at greater risk for morbidity and mortality in subsequent years than are those with more normal immune responses (Wayne, Rhyne, Garry, et al., 1990). Thus, any interventions that improve immunity in the elderly might be expected to affect health and longevity beneficially.

Nutritional interventions might beneficially affect immune function in the elderly in two ways. First, some elderly populations have a high prevalence of protein-calorie or micronutrient deficiencies. Correction of those deficiencies in many cases will improve immune function; indeed, such interventions should improve almost any physiologic function. Second, certain micronutrients in large doses may beneficially affect immune function through some pharmacologic effect rather than through correction of immune function.

It is fairly well established that attempts to correct protein calorie malnutrition result in improvements in immunity in the elderly. The experiments, though small and poorly controlled, produced impressive results that would be difficult to explain away by potential flaws in study methodology. In fact, one lesson to garner from those studies is that the nutritional intervention did not have to be heroic. Merely ensuring adequate micronutrient intake and increasing total caloric intake with supplements produced large improvements in immune function.

The question of what role micronutrient supplementation should have in enhancing immunity has not been answered. Most authorities are sufficiently concerned about micronutrient deficiencies in some elderly populations (e.g., institutionalized, homebound, chronically ill, socially isolated, impoverished, et c.) to recommend routine multiple vitamin supplements for these individuals. Two intriguing questions remain to be answered: (a) Do chronically ill elderly require intakes of certain micronutrients at levels exceeding the RDA to maintain adequate tissue levels (Baker, Frank, & Jaslow, 1980)? (b) Will high levels of intake of certain micronutrients (e.g., pyridoxine, vitamin C, vitamin E) produce lasting improvements in immune function in elderly subjects. If so, is this change beneficial?

These questions are not impossible to answer. However, they do involve extensive clinical trials in populations that are very difficult to study. We have no doubt, however, that the answers will eventually be forthcoming.

REFERENCES

Allen, J. J., Parri, R. T., McClain, C. J. & Kay, N. E. (1983). Alterations in human natural killer activity and monocyte cytotoxicity induced by zinc deficiency. *Journal of Laboratory and Clinical Medicine, 102,* 577.

Anderson, R., Dosthuizen, R., Maritz, R., Theron, A., & Van Rensburg, A. J. (1980). The effect of increasing weekly doses of ascorbate on certain cellular and humoral immune functions in normal volunteers. *American Journal of Clinical Nutrition, 33,* 71–79.

Axelrod, A. E. (1971). Immune processes in vitamin deficiency states. *American Journal of Clinical Nutrition, 24,* 265–71.

Baker, H., Frank, O., & Jaslow, S. P. (1980). Oral versus intramuscular vitamin supplementation for hypovitaminosis in the elderly. *Journal of the American Geriatrics Society, 28,* 42–45.

Beisel, W. R. (1983). Single nutrients and immunity *American Journal of Clinical Nutrition, 35,* 417–468.

Brocklehurst, J. C., Griffiths, C. C., & Taylor, F. (1986). The clinical features of chronic vitamin deficiency: A therapeutic trial in geriatric hospital patients. *Gerontological Clinics, 10,* 309–317.

Brucker, M. D., Hollingsworth, W., Saltman, P. D., Strause, L. C., Kleuber, M. R., & Lugo, N. J. (1988). Failure of dietary zinc supplementation to improve the antibody response to influenza vaccine. *Nutrition Research, 8,* 99–104.

Carman, J. A., Smith, S. M., & Hayes, C. E. (1989). Characterization of a helper T lymphocyte defect in vitamin A-deficient mice. *Journal of Immunology, 142,* 388.

Carman, J., & Hayes, C. E. (1991). Abnormal regulation of IFN-g secretion in vitamin A deficiency. *Journal of Immunology, 147,* 1247–1252.

Chandra, R. K. (1972). Immunocompetence in undernutrition. *Journal of Pediatrics, 81,* 1194–1200.

Chandra, R. K. (Ed.). (1988). *Nutrition and immunology* (pp. 1– 328). New York: Allan Liss.

Chandra, R. K. (1985). Nutrition, immunity and illness in the elderly. In R. K. Chandra (Ed.), *Nutrition, immunity and illness in the elderly* (pp. 3–5). New York: Pergamon.

Chandra, R. K., Joshi, P., Au, B. Woodford, G., Chandra S. (1982). Nutrition and immunocompetence in the elderly: Effect of short term supplementation on cell mediated immunity and lymphocyte subsets. *Nutrition Research, 2,* 223–232.

Chavance, M., Brubacher, G., Herberth, B., et al. (1985). *Immunological and nutritional status among the elderly* (pp. 137–142). New York: Pergamon Press.

Chernoff, R. (Ed.). (1991). Nutrition in immune function. *Clinics in Applied Nutrition, 1*, 1–94.

Cheslock, K. E., & McCully M. T. (1960). Response of human beings to a low vitamin B-6 diet. *Journal of Nutrition, 70,* 507–513.

Cook-Mills, S. M., Morford, G. L., & Fraker, P. J. (1991). Role of zinc in phagocytic function. *Clinics in Applied Nutrition, 1,* 25–34.

Cunningham-Rundles, S., & Cunningham-Rundles, W. F. (1988). Zinc modulation of immune response. In R. K. Chandra (Ed.), *Nutrition and immunology* (pp. 197–214). New York: Alan R. Liss.

Cunningham-Rundles, C., Cunningham-Rundles, S., Iwata, T., Inafy, G., Garofalo, J. A., Menendez-Botet, C., Lewis, V., Twomey, J. J., & Good, R. A. (1981). Zinc deficiency, depressed thymic hormones and T-lymphocyte dysfunction in patients with hypogammaglobulinemia. *Clinical Immunology and Immunopathology, 31*, 387.

Drinka, P. J., & Goodwin, J. S. (1991). Prevalence and consequences of vitamin deficiency in the nursing home: A critical review. *Journal of the American Geriatrics Society, 39*, 1008–1017.

Duchateau, J., Delespesse, G., Vrijens, R., Collet, H. (1981). Beneficial effects of oral zinc supplementation on the immune response of old people *American Journal of Medicine, 70*, 1001– 1004.

Fischer, A., Munnich, A., Saudubray, J. M., Mamas, S., Corde, F. X., Charpentier, C., Dray, F., Frezal, J., & Griscelli, C. (1982). Biotin-responsive immunoregulatory dysfunction in multiple carboxylase deficiency. *Journal of Clinical Immunology, 2*, 35–38.

Fraker, P. J., Haas, S. M., & Leucke, R. W. (1977). The effect of zinc deficiency on the young adult A/J mouse. *Journal of Nutrition, 107*, 1889.

Fraker, P. J., de Pasquale-Jarleu, P., Zwickl, C. M., & Leuke, R. W. (1978). Regeneration of T-cell helper functions in zinc deficient adult mice. *Proceedings of the National Academy of Sciences USA, 75*, 5660.

Garry, P. J., Goodwin, J. S., & Hunt, W. C. (1982). Nutritional status in a healthy elderly population: Riboflavin. *American Journal of Clinical Nutrition, 36*, 902–909.

Garry, P. J., Goodwin, J. S., & Hunt, W. C. (1984). Folate and vitamin B12 status in a healthy elderly population. *Journal of the American Geriatrics Society, 32*, 719–726.

Garry, P. J., Goodwin, J. S., Hunt, W. C., & Gilbert, B. A. (1982). Nutritional status in a healthy elderly population: Vitamin C. *American Journal of Clinical Nutrition, 36*, 332–339.

Garry, P. J., Goodwin, J. S., Hunt, W. C., Hooper, E. M., & Leonard, A. G. (1982). Nutritional status in a healthy elderly population: Dietary and supplemental intakes. *American Journal of Clinical Nutrition, 36*, 319–331.

Good, R. A., Fernandes, G., Cunningham-Rundles, C., Cunningham-Rundles, S., Garofalo, J. A., Rao, K. M. K., Incety, G. S., & Iwata, T. (1980). The relation of zinc deficiency to immunologic function in animals and man. In M. Seligman & W. H. Hitzig (Eds.), *Primary immunodeficiencies*. (Vol. 16, p. 223). *INSERM*. Amsterdam: Elsevier/North Holland.

Good, R. A., Fernandes, G., Yunis, E. J., Cooper, W. C., Jose, D. C., Kramer, T.R., &

Hansen, M. A. (1976). Nutritional deficiency, immunologic function and disease. *American Journal of Pathology, 84*, 599–614.

Goodwin, J. S. (1989). Social, psychological and physical factors affecting the nutritional status of elderly subjects: Separating cause from effect. *American Journal of Clinical Nutrition, 50*, 1201–1209.

Goodwin, J. S., & Garry, P. J. (1983). Relationship between megadose vitamin supplementation and immunological function in a healthy elderly population. *Clinical and Experimental Immunology, 51*, 647–653.

Goodwin, J. S., & Garry, P. J. (1988). Lack of effect of subclinical malnutrition on immune function in healthy elderly adults. *Journal of Gerontology, 43*, 46–50.

Goodwin, J. S., Goodwin, J. M., & Garry, P. L. (1983). Association between nutritional status and cognitive functioning in a healthy elderly population. *Journal of the American Medical Society, 249*, 2917–2921.

Goodwin, J. S., Searles, R. P., & Tung, K. S. K. (1982). Immunological responses of a healthy elderly population. *Clinical and Experimental Immunology, 48*, 403–410.

Gross, R. L., Reid, J. V. O., Newberne, P. M., Burgess, B., Marstrom, R., & Hift, W. (1975). Depressed cell mediated immunity in megaloblastic anemia due to folic acid deficiency. *American Journal of Clinical Nutrition, 28*, 225–232.

Gutowski, J. K., Innes, J. B., Webster, M. W., et al. (1986). Impaired nuclear responsiveness to cytoplasmic signals in lymphocytes from elderly humans with depressed proliferative responses. *Journal of Clinical Investigation, 78*, 40–43.

Ha, C., Miller, L. T., & Kerkvliet, N. E. (1984). The effect of vitamin B-6 deficiency on cytotoxic immune responses of T cells, antibodies, and natural killer cells, and phagocytosis by macrophages. *Cellular Immunology, 85*, 318–329.

Hansen, M. A., Fernandes, C., & Good, R. A. (1982). Nutrition and immunity. In W. J. Darby, H. P. Broquist, & R. E. Olson (Eds.), *Annual review of nutrition* (Vol. 2, pp. 151–177). Palo Alto, CA: *Annual Reviews*.

Hess, E. V., Knapp, D. (1978). The immune system and aging: A case of the cart before the horse. *Journal of Chronic Diseases, 31*, 647–649.

Hodges, R. E., Bean, W. B., Ohlson, M. A., & Bleiler, R. E. (1962). Factors affecting human antibody response: IV. Pyridoxine deficiency. *American Journal of Clinical Nutrition, 11*, 180–186.

Keenes, B., Dumont, I., Brohee, D., Hubert, C., & Neve, P. (1983). Effect of vitamin C supplements on cell-mediated immunity in old people. *Gerontology, 29*, 305–311.

Kinnel, D. C. (Ed.). (1974). *Adulthood and aging*. New York: Wiley.

Lipschitz, D. A., & Mitchell, C. D. (1982). The correctability of the nutritional, immune and hematopoietic manifestations of protein calorie malnutrition in the elderly. *Journal of the American College of Nutrition, 1*, 17–25.

McCay, C. M., Crowell, M. F., & Maynard, L. A. (1935). The effect of retarded growth upon length of life span and upon ultimate body size. *Journal of Nutrition* 10:63–79.

Meydani, S. N., Barklund, M. P., Liu, S., et al. (1990). Vitamin E supplementation enhances cell–mediated immunity in healthy elderly subjects. *American Journal of Clinical Nutrition, 52*, 557–563.

Meydani, S. N., Meydani, M., Verden, C. P., Shapiro, A. A., Blumberg, J. B., & Hayes, K. C. (1986). Vitamin E supplementation suppresses prostaglandin E_2

synthesis and enhances the immune response of aged mice. *Mechanisms of Aging & Development*, *34*, 191–201.

Murphy, S., West, K. P., Greenough, W. B., Cherot, E., Katz, J., Clement, L. (1992). Impact of vitamin A supplementation on the incidence of infection in elderly nursing home residents: A randomized controlled trial. *Age & Aging*, *21*, 435–439.

National Institute on Aging Research Planning Panel. (1982). *A national plan for research on aging*. (NIH Publication No. 82-2453). Bethesda, MD: National Institute on Aging.

Newberne, P. M. (1977). Effect of folic acid, B_{12}, choline and methionine or immunocompetence and cell mediated immunity. In R. M. Suskind (Ed.), *Malnutrition and the immune response* (pp. 375–386). New York: Raven Press.

Newmann, C. G., Lawlor, G. J., Stiehm, E. R., Swenseid, M. E., Newton, C., Herbert, J., Ammann, A., & Jacob, M. (1975). Immunologic responses in malnourished children. *American Journal of Clinical Nutrition*, *28*, 89–104.

Penn, N. D., Purkins, L., Kelleher, J., Heatley, R. V., Mascie-Taylor, B. H., & Belfield, P. W. (1991). The effect of dietary supplementation with vitamins A, C and E on cell-mediated immune function in elderly long-stay patients: A randomized controlled trial. *Age & Aging*, *20*, 169–174.

Rabin, B. S. (1983). Inhibition of experimentally induced autoimmunity in rats by biotin deficiency. *Journal of Nutrition*, *13*, 2316–2322.

Robson, S., Schwarz, M. R. (1975). Vitamin B-6 deficiency and the lymphoid system I effects on cellular immunity and in vitro incorporation of ^{3}H-uridine by small lymphocytes. *Cellular Immunology*, *16*, 135–144.

Rudman, D., & Feller, A. (1989). Protein-calorie undernutrition in the nursing home. *Journal of the American Geriatrics Society*, *37*, 173–183.

Schorah, C. J., Newill, A., & Scott, D. L. (1979). Clinical effects of vitamin C in elderly inpatients with low blood vitamin C levels. *Lancet*, *1*, 403–406.

Seger, R., Frater-Schroeder, M., Hitzig, W. H., Wildfeuer, A., & Linnel, J. C. (1980). Granulocyte dysfunction in transcobalamin II deficiency responding to leucovorin or hydroxycobalamin-plasma transfusion. *Journal of Inherited Metabolic Diseases*, *3*, 3–9.

Smith, S. M., & Hayes, C. E. (1987). Impaired immunity in vitamin A-deficient mice. *Proceedings of the National Academy of Sciences USA*, *84*, 5878.

Talbott, M. C., Miller, L. T., & Kerkvliet, N. I. (1987). Pyridoxine supplementation: Effect on lymphocyte responses in elderly persons. *American Journal of Clinical Nutrition*, *46*, 659–664.

Tanaka, T., Fernandes, G., Tsao, C., Pih, K., & Good, R. A. (1978). Effects of zinc deficiency on lymphoid tissues and immune function of A/Jax mice. *Federation Proceedings*, *37*, 931.

Tapazoglou, E., Prasad, A. S., Hill, G., Brewer, G. F., & Kaplan, J. (1985). Decreased natural killer cell activity in patients with zinc deficiency with sickle cell disease. *Journal of Laboratory and Clinical Medicine*, *105*, 19.

Tangerdy, R. P. (1980). Effect of vitamin E on immune responses. *Basic and Clinical Nutrition*, *1*, 429–445.

Thomaskutty, K. G., & Lee, C. M. (1985). Interaction of nutrition and infection: Effect of vitamin B$_{12}$ deficiency on resistance to *Trypanosoma lewisi*. *Journal of the National Medical Association, 77*, 289–299.

Watson, R. R., Prabhala, R. H., Plezia, P. M., & Alberts, D. S. (1991). Effect of beta-carotene on lymphocyte sub-populations in elderly humans: Evidence for a dose-response relationship. *American Journal of Clinical Nutrition, 53*, 90–94.

Wayne, S., Rhyne, R., Garry, P. J., & Goodwin, J. S. (1990). Cell mediated immunity as a predictor of morbidity and mortality in the aged. *Journal of Gerontology, 45*, 45–49.

West, K. P., Howard, G. R., & Sommer, A. (1989). Vitamin A and infection: Public health implications. *Annual Review of Nutrition, 9*, 63.

Youinou, P. Y., Garre, M. A., Menez, J. F., Bales, J. M., Morim, J. F., Pennee, Y., Mossec, P. J., Morin, P. P., & LeMenn, G. (1982). Folic acid deficiency and neutrophil dysfunction. *American Journal of Medicine, 73*, 652–657.

Options for Control of Influenza in Long-Term Care Facilities

19

Stefan Gravenstein, Barbara A. Miller, and Paul J. Drinka

Influenza A is virulent in people of all ages, especially in those with immunocompromising disease or at either age extreme. Approximately 80% to 90% of deaths attributed to pneumonia and influenza occur in persons 65 years old or older. Influenza and pneumonia rank fifth as a leading cause of death in elderly people. When an influenza outbreak occurs in long-term care facilities (LTCFs), up to 70% of the residents may become ill, and the case fatality rate may be as high as 30%. Influenza epidemics in the United States alone result in billions of dollars in added costs to society and tens of thousands of deaths annually.

The primary means of influenza prevention has been through the use of vaccination. Within a LTCF, another relatively inexpensive strategy of yet unproved efficacy is isolation of symptomatic residents. The use of aman-

48

tadine, both a therapeutic and immunoprophylactic agent, has also been promoted and is currently recommended for prevention and control of influenza A in this setting. Despite these measures, outbreaks of influenza occur in LTCFs annually. This chapter describes the current recommendations for the control of influenza as promoted by the Advisory Committee on Immunization Practices (ACIP) (Centers for Disease Control, 1992) and our application of these recommendations in the long-term care setting.

RECOMMENDATIONS FOR THE PREVENTION AND CONTROL OF INFLUENZA BY THE ACIP

Prevention is the first and most important step to reduce the impact of influenza in a long-term care setting, and is primarily instituted through comprehensive influenza vaccination programs. The ACIP targets high-risk persons and their close contacts for influenza vaccination. At high-risk are all individuals aged 65 years or older, patients who are residing in LTCFs, or those with a chronic medical, metabolic, cardiac, or respiratory disorder requiring hospitalization in the previous year or regular medical follow-up (diabetes, renal dysfunction, hemoglobinopathy, or primary or secondary immunosuppression). Close contacts are those individuals who have contact or live with high-risk individuals (family members, physicians, nurses, clinical staff, and LTCF employees and volunteers). Vaccination is ideally done between mid-October and mid-November. Earlier vaccination in an institution is discouraged because the postvaccination antibody titer declines within a few months after vaccination, leaving individuals who receive premature vaccination unprotected during the latter half of the influenza season. Early vaccination is only recommended when influenza activity is expected to begin before December. Persons admitted to LTCFs after the facility-wide vaccination program has been completed but during the influenza season (December to March in most states) should be vaccinated on admission.

To implement these recommendations in the LTCF, the ACIP proposes that individual vaccination orders for each resident be avoided and that their physicians concur that all residents without a specific history suggesting vaccine hypersensitivity be vaccinated annually with the influenza vaccine. Resident consent for annual influenza vaccination should be obtained on admission to the facility and remain valid for the duration of the resident's stay there. As part of the institutional vaccination program, education of personnel and easy access to vaccine is encouraged. Ready vaccine access may enhance compliance and could be achieved by using a mobile cart to take vaccine to nursing units during different shifts including nights and weekends.

The ACIP acknowledges that influenza outbreaks occur even in LTCFs where vaccination programs are successful in immunizing a large proportion of the resident and staff populations. Antigenic drift or shift of the influenza virus may occur, allowing the virus to escape vaccine-induced antibody defenses. Their recommendations for influenza prevention and control, therefore, also include the use of chemoprophylaxis against influenza A. Amantadine and rimantadine are the two antiviral agents currently licensed in the United States for the prevention or treatment of influenza A infections and are ineffective against influenza B or C. Amantadine is approximately 70% effective in preventing influenza A illnesses (prophylactic use). When given to young healthy persons within 48 hours of influenza A infection, amantadine can reduce the duration of fever and other symptoms (treatment use). Amantadine is principally cleared through the renal system and has the potential for significant CNS toxicity should it accumulate. The majority of LTCFs serve a chronically ill, elderly population with a high prevalence of renal dysfunction. Thus, the dose of amantadine must be adjusted based on estimated renal function (see later).

Within these limitations, amantadine is recommended for influenza A outbreak control. The initiation of amantadine both for treatment and prophylaxis is to "begin as early as possible to reduce the spread" of influenza A, and amantadine "should be administered to all residents of the . . . institution regardless of whether they received influenza vaccine the previous fall . . . for the duration of influenza activity in the community" (Centers for Disease Control, 1992). Amantadine prophylaxis should be offered to unvaccinated staff caring for high-risk residents. However, there are some reasons to limit amantadine use, which are discussed later.

Vaccination

Vaccine-induced antibodies protect against morbidity and mortality from influenza strains similar to those in the vaccine. The degree of protection is directly correlated to the antibody titer. The amount of antibody produced following influenza vaccination tends to be considerably less in elderly people, especially those who are frail or have underlying medical conditions such as malignancy or cardiopulmonary disease (Ershler, Moore, & Socinski, 1984; Gravenstein, Duthie, Miller, et al., 1989; Laver & Valentine, 1969). Despite receiving an influenza vaccine, up to 50% of elderly individuals may not achieve the fourfold increase in antibody titer or have titers greater than or equal to 1:40 by hemagglutination inhibition assay, and are therefore considered susceptible to influenza infection by conventional standards (Hobson, Curry, Beare, et al., 1972; Potter & Oxford, 1979). In elderly people, the antibody response to split virus vaccine peaks 6 to 8 weeks after vaccination, lasts a few months, and then rapidly falls to prevaccination levels (Arden, Patriarca, & Kendal, 1986; Gravenstein et al., 1989; Levine, Beattie, McLean, et al., 1987). Lower postvaccination antibody titers or failure to retain protective antibody could explain influenza infection in individuals who had received a vaccine closely representing the circulating influenza strains.

A change in the prevalent influenza virus such as that produced by antigenic drift or shift can also render a vaccinated person relatively or completely unprotected from the prevalent strain. Because of intense surveillance efforts and generally accurate predictions by epidemiologists, this type of failure is uncommon. Even when there is significant antigenic drift or the vaccine response is limited, the vaccine appears capable of reducing mortality, hospitalization, and invasive disease. The vaccine is up to 47% effective in reducing the number of hospitalizations, 58% effective in preventing the occurrence of radiologically diagnosed pneumonia, and 76% effective in preventing mortality as a direct consequence of influenza-like illness (Arden et al., 1986; Kendal, Patriarca, & Arden, 1985). The protective effect of vaccination can be even greater in a LTCF. When most of the institution's staff and residents have been vaccinated against influenza, the transmissibility of the virus in the facility is further limited (herd immunity). A target vaccination rate of 80% is achievable and should suffice to induce herd immunity in a LTCF.

There are many deterrents to achieving an 80% influenza vaccination rate. Vaccination programs may fail because of the unfounded concern that the influenza vaccine causes an influenza illness. Because the current vaccine contains only noninfectious virus particles, preservatives, and trace amounts of egg protein, it *cannot* cause an influenza infection. Occasional cases of respiratory disease following vaccination represent coincidental illnesses unrelated to the vaccine (Centers for Disease Control, 1992). Vaccine recipients may need reassurances that less than one third of them will complain of mild injection site tenderness and that fever, malaise, or myalgia occurs in fewer than 10%. The rate of the systemic reactions in elderly people is similar to that in saline placebo recipients (Margolis, Nichol, Poland, et al., 1990). The risk for an allergic-type response to the vaccine components like residual egg proteins or vaccine preservatives is rare. Only the 1976 influenza vaccine was associated with the Guillian-Barré syndrome (six cases), and this relationship is not expected to recur. The influenza vaccine is contraindicated in persons with *anaphylactic* hypersensitivity to eggs. Persons with an acute febrile illness (temperature greater than 100 °F orally) may be vaccinated when the fever abates. Pregnancy (in care providers or family members) is not a contraindication for vaccination (Centers for Disease Control, 1992), although it may be prudent to wait until the second trimester.

For vaccination programs to be successful, the health care providers must be convinced that the vaccine is safe and useful, and the vaccine must be readily available. Despite general resistance of staff to influenza vaccination, some unique approaches have proved successful. For example, an "influenza cart" moved between nursing stations during different shifts daily over several weeks has been associated with a much higher employee vaccination rate than the previous technique where free vaccination was available only at a central location. Education of personnel combined with effortless access to vaccine seem to be important in promoting staff vaccination.

Chemoprophylaxis

Many retrospective reports claim success at controlling influenza A outbreaks with rapid administration of amantadine to residents on outbreak detection. Even though the efficacy of amantadine in the treatment of influenza A is established for specific situations, its value and safety in the nursing home setting has yet to be proved. The policy of administering amantadine to all nursing home residents is based on studies testing amantadine in mostly young healthy community-based adults who self-reported influenza-like illness. When given prophylactically to children with cystic fibrosis, there was no difference in incidence or severity of illness compared with that in placebo recipients (Wright, Khaw, Oxman, et al., 1976). The failure to demonstrate amantadine efficacy in these high-risk subjects may be partially explained by its immunosuppressive properties (Clark, Woodson, & Nagasawa, 1992; Jackson, 1986). Results in other studies of high-risk individuals are equally disappointing. Mate and coworker (1970) found a reduction in the number of acute lower respiratory tract complications when amantadine was administered to a large group of military recruits, but there have been no controlled clinical trials that demonstrate reduced complications of influenza in high-risk individuals by amantadine therapy.

Efficacy in the Elderly

Amantadine has only been demonstrated to be effective when administered near the onset of illness. Elderly people may present atypically with influenza, making early onset diagnosis difficult. Influenza-like illness as defined by the Centers for Disease Control is either a cough, runny nose, or sore throat accompanied by an oral temperature of at least 100 °F. The Centers for Disease Control definition used for surveillance may be too insensitive and nonspecific for an elderly population. In one prospective study, the definition was only 51% sensitive and 63% specific in accurately diagnosing influenza in an elderly institutionalized population (Gravenstein, Miller, Ershler, et al., 1990). Cases may not be diagnosed in a timely fashion, and outbreak detection may therefore be late. Individuals susceptible to influenza may have already been infected or ill for some time before amantadine is initiated. Amantadine administration late in illness may contribute to the development of amantadine resistant influenza strains; subjects who receive amantadine more than 48 hours after illness onset may have a large enough viral load permitting opportunity for resistant virus to emerge (see later).

Toxicity

Amantadine has been clearly associated with adverse drug events related to the drug's action on the CNS. These include hyperexcitability, tremors, slurred speech, insomnia, lightheadedness, irritability, difficulty concentrating, dry mouth, as well as gastrointestinal upset, nocturia, and urinary retention, which occur in 5% to 33% of healthy adults taking this drug (Dolin & Bentley, 1986; Goodman & Gilman, 1982; Kilbourne, 1987; Monto, Gunn, Bandy, et al., 1979). In summarizing clinical trials involving more than 11,000 subjects receiving amantadine, investigators of the National Institutes of Health (1980) have reported that 7% had transient CNS-related adverse drug events. Among 88 college students, dizziness, nervousness, and insomnia occurred in 33% of those receiving amantadine and in 10% of those receiving placebo (Bryson, Monahan, Pollack, et al., 1980). CNS-related adverse drug events are particularly worrisome in the elderly. Institutionalized residents tend to be frail, have numerous underlying medical conditions, receive multiple prescription medications, and are consequently at a high risk for adverse drug events. The frailer residents of LTCFs may experience unacceptably high rates of amantadine-associated adverse reactions (Stange, Little, & Blatnik, 1991). In Wisconsin nursing homes, similar to those of other states, 30% of residents have some form of mental illness that may predispose them to CNS toxicity. Furthermore, nursing home residents receive on average more than five prescription medications daily, and it is believed that the number of prescription medications is directly related to the risk for adverse drug events (Bryson et al., 1980; May, Stewart, & Cluff, 1977).

Of the more serious amantadine-associated adverse drug events, falls have been reported in 3% of elderly subjects (Arden, Patriarca, Fasano, et al., 1988). In our experience with nearly 900 institutionalized subjects, there is no significant difference between fallers and nonfallers regarding underlying medical disorders, osteoarthritis, or medication usage. However, our data suggest that adverse drug events may be significantly more prevalent in the setting of prophylaxis than previously recognized. We noted that falls increased fourfold to eightfold during prophylaxis, an important observation when one considers that 5% of falls result in hip fracture. Residents were more likely to be agitated and physically restrained during the amantadine course, and seizures occurred more frequently. Additionally, adverse drug events may mimic other disease states, making it difficult to distinguish a drug effect from exacerbation or progression of existing diseases. This could lead to unnecessary interventions (Vestal, 1990). For example, in a population where confusion is already prevalent, increased confusion may result in prescription of additional psychoactive medications, further increasing the likelihood of adverse drug events. Perhaps amantadine should not be given to residents with underlying mental disorders or balance disturbances. Shorter duration of prophylaxis may also reduce the risk for adverse effects.

Adverse drug events are often due to drug accumulation. Renal function declines with age (Rowe, 1976). Amantadine is principally cleared by the kidneys (Bleidner, Harmon, Hewes, et al., 1965). As the extent of drug toxicity is directly related to dose and blood levels (Jackson, 1986), risk for amantadine-related toxicity increases with age. The likelihood for adverse reaction and the clinical consequences resulting from amantadine are worrisome when prophylaxis is indiscriminately prescribed in the LTCF.

Cost

Amantadine is expensive. The direct administration costs for 21 days at $1.75 per dose to 200 individuals is $7,350. This underestimates overall costs because it does not include the nursing care and those incurred by adverse drug events. The use of amantadine prophylaxis throughout the influenza season costs at least 650% more than alternatives (Patriarca, Arden, Koplan, et al., 1987). In each of the last 10 years, influenza A has been isolated in Wisconsin over at least a 2-month span. If the Centers for Disease Control recommendation of prophylaxis is for all subjects in LTCFs where influenza A is detected, for the duration of its persistence in the community, then in Wisconsin 52,000 institutionalized residents (Sirrocco, 1988) might receive amantadine for more than 21 days, at a cost of $1.91 million annually. Wisconsin residents fill fewer than 4% of the country's LTCF beds.

Resistance

Another concern raised by antiviral use for influenza A outbreak control is the possible emergence and transmission of resistant virus strains. Resistant influenza A viruses have been demonstrated to emerge readily in vitro in the the presence of amantadine. Studies in humans have documented emergence of resistant viruses in children and young adults who were receiving rimantadine treatment (Belshe, Smith, Hall, et al., 1988; Hayden, Belshe, Clover, et al., 1986). Transmission of resistant viruses has been observed in animal studies (Bean, Threlkeld, & Webster, 1989), and among humans in household settings (Hayden, et al., 1989), and in nursing homes. Only two naturally occurring amantadine resistant strains of influenza virus are documented (personal communication, Nancy Cox, Centers for Disease Control, January 1993), but this may be in part due to the failure to look for them (Belshe, Burke, Newman, et al., 1989). The clinical importance of resistant strains has not been determined, but we believe that all cases of influenza arising during the use of amantadine must be resistant. In a study we performed in a LTCF, 29% (35 of 119) of influenza-like illnesses (fever and at least one respiratory symptom) occurred during amantadine prophylaxis, and *all* culture-confirmed influenza cases presenting during amantadine prophylaxis were resistant (Mast, Harmon, Gravenstein, et al., 1992). This observation has again been made by other investigators during the 1989 to 1990 influenza season where amantadine prophylaxis and treatment was initiated (Degelau, Somani, Cooper, et al., 1992).

CURRENT IMPLEMENTATION OF RECOMMENDATIONS

Inexpensive, additional, or alternative steps must be easily implemented to control the transmission of influenza in the institutional setting. Effective institutional influenza outbreak prevention and control is currently under study by our research group. We are prospectively studying whether (a) isolation of ill residents or geographic areas of a LTCF and (b) the duration of amantadine prophylaxis can affect the spread of influenza within the facility during an influenza outbreak. The first year results of this 5-year study are promising and, if confirmed, will support the following implementation of the current CDC recommendations.

Influenza Vaccination

The primary preventive measure of annual influenza vaccination should be carried out as recommended by the ACIP. In our study setting, all residents receive an admission order for annual influenza vaccination unless contraindicated. Physicians admitting their patients to the facility have concurred with this policy. A one-time consent for annual influenza vaccination is obtained at admission from the resident or legal medical guardian. Influenza vaccine is also available to all facility employees and recommended for those with direct resident contact. An annual vaccination program occurs during the week before Thanksgiving. One nurse coordinates the program and administers most of the vaccination. If a person is admitted and does not remember having received the influenza vaccine, they are vaccinated. With this program our vaccination rate among residents is at least 85%.

The vaccine is also offered free to staff and brought to all nursing units during all shifts concurrent with the resident influenza vaccination program and remains available for employees at the employee health office thereafter. The vaccination rate among staff is growing annually but is still low at just over 35%. Vaccine is administered to newly admitted residents and employees through March of the following year. Annual fall inservice education programs that include a discussion of influenza vaccination and control immediately followed by a vaccination workshop also appear to improve staff compliance. Other facilities send thank you notes to vaccinated staff for doing their part in helping prevent an influenza outbreak.

Influenza Surveillance

Once vaccination has been performed, the only additional step available to prevent influenza from entering the LTCF is reducing exposure of individuals within the facility from individuals who are shedding live virus. To prevent exposure of residents from infected individuals, the LTCF first must determine when respiratory illness is likely to be influenza. Tracking respiratory illnesses within the LTCF allows influenza cases to be readily identified.

The likelihood of a respiratory illness to be caused by influenza can be assessed using several criteria (see Table 19.1). Two of the criteria depend on the incidence of respiratory illness and influenza in the LTCF and elsewhere and therefore depend on active influenza surveillance.

We in the United States are fortunate to have a strong national influenza surveillance network coordinated by the Centers for Disease Control in Atlanta. The goals of this surveillance system are to identify influenza cases and track their clinical severity, determine how the circulating influenza viruses have drifted or shifted from those represented in the vaccine, report on the use of antiviral medication, and report on the impact of influenza illnesses on hospitalizations and or death. To meet these goals the Centers for Disease Control receives reports from (a) each of the 50 states' Departments of Health on influenza-like illness activity in that region; (b) the 150 sentinel physicians scattered across the United States on office visits and hospitalizations for influenza-like illness; (c) more than 100 cities on pneumonia or influenza-related mortality; and (d) approximately 60 viral laboratories on viral culture results. The Centers for Disease Control makes this influenza surveillance information available through the Centers for Disease Control Voice Information System for Disease Control and Prevention (telephone: 404-332-4555), and can provide specific information or

TABLE 19.1 Respiratory Illness: Is It Influenza?

More likely	Less likely	Unlikely
Winter	Late fall, early spring	Late spring, summer or early fall
Febrile (>100° F) or hypothermic	Low grade fever (temperature above baseline but <100° F)	Temperature at baseline
Bronchitis or pneumonia; other respiratory symptoms	No respiratory symptom	Not ill
Influenza reported within the community or state	No influenza in the community or state	No influenza in the country or no other respiratory virus at facility
Only influenza virus within the community or state	Some other respiratory virus(es) is known to be circulating within the community or state	Only other respiratory virus is known to be circulating within the community or state
Not vaccinated this season and facility vaccination rate low	Vaccinated this season and facility vaccination rate high (>80%)	
Major holiday in the last few weeks	No major holiday in the last few weeks	
Other close contacts have/had respiratory illness in last weeks	No close contacts with respiratory illness	No other respiratory illness at facility (residents or staff)

contact telephone numbers. This source can quantitate influenza activity in your area.

Within the LTCF, surveillance can be instituted in a variety of ways. In our setting, we have made surveillance part of a larger infection control program that tracks respiratory illnesses, hospitalizations, and deaths on a daily basis. The attention to respiratory symptoms is heightened during the influenza season. Beginning in December, attention is directed at identifying individuals with new respiratory symptoms. Our experience has repeatedly demonstrated the difficulty in clinically diagnosing influenza. Fewer than 50% of serologically or culture-confirmed cases ever develop fever greater than 100 °F. Also, influenza is clinically indistinguishable from other viral illnesses that are prevalent during the influenza season. For example, during an influenza outbreak (32 culture-confirmed cases), an outbreak caused by respiratory syncytial virus (9 culture-confirmed cases) was discovered. The cases were clinically indistinguishable. However, neither outbreak would have been detected in a timely fashion if we did not have surveillance in place. Simple isolation of the index case may make the difference between having a killer versus a manageable influenza outbreak (Degelau et al., 1992), but the cases cannot be isolated unless active surveillance is in place.

Active surveillance should begin with the influenza season (early or mid-December in most of the United States). We post signs on building entrances and elevator doors telling individuals with new respiratory symptoms to report to a designated person before entering the building. The designee person determines if the visitor should leave or provides the visitor with a respiratory mask to be worn at all times while in the facility. Ward surveillance is accomplished by asking residents about new respiratory or clinical complaints at the time their medication is dispensed. This facilitates detection of residents who have or can transmit the virus. Individuals who are unable to express clinical complaints but have behavioral changes are considered to have new symptoms that potentially may represent influenza. Those individuals identified with new symptoms are noted on a 24-hour report that is sent daily to the nursing supervisor or a designated infection control person. If the resident also has an oral temperature at least 100 °F, the finding is reported without delay and viral nasopharyngeal and throat cultures are performed.

With internal institutional and national Centers for Disease Control influenza surveillance every LTCF has timely access to community and national influenza surveillance data. When influenza is detected in the community, opportunity for its introduction into the nursing home can be minimized by screening visitors and employees, educating employees, and encouraging absenteeism for employees who have influenza-like illness. Our index of suspicion for influenza is low until influenza is present in the state and the incidence of respiratory illness within the facility is rising. When influenza is detected within the LTCF, we reoffer vaccination to remaining unvaccinated residents and staff, institute several infection control measures, and consider limited treatment and prophylaxis with amantadine.

Infection Control

Whether influenza is principally transmitted by aerosol or formite is still debated. Most experts believe the aerosol route is most important, and thus we have focused on separating ill residents by distance or barriers. Once influenza has been detected within the LTCF, all newly symptomatic individuals (illness onset less than 5 days previously) are encouraged to wear masks when out of their rooms and limit their out-of-room activities. If they are febrile, they are instructed to eat their meals in their room or in the hall outside their room instead of a general dining room area. Group activities between residents who reside in geographically distinct areas of the facility are curtailed.

These restrictions have been associated with a high compliance rate when implemented with the consent or "vote" of the competent residents who are informed of influenza within the LTCF. Staff have been frequently reluctant to wear masks but appear more willing when residents self-impose these restrictions. We currently *require* symptomatic individuals to wear masks, and encourage others, especially those who have direct resident contact, to wear them.

Antiviral Use

We initiate selective creatinine-adjusted amantadine prophylaxis and therapy when 10% or more of newly symptomatic residents of a nursing unit or cohort of individuals who dine together have illness onsets within a 7-day period, and there is culture-proven influenza A in the LTCF. Amantadine prophylaxis is offered to all asymptomatic residents and staff on that unit for 7 days after the last new influenza-like illness is identified on that unit or the last culture-proven case of influenza is identified within the LTCF, whichever is longer. Treatment is offered to symptomatic individuals only if they have been symptomatic for less than 48 hours, and then only for 5 days. All residents have age, serum creatinine level, and weight available on their medical charts. Using the Cockroft-Gault equation (Cockroft & Gault, 1976) we estimate creatinine clearance and adjust the amantadine dose according to Table 19.2.

Rimantadine has been recently approved for the prevention and treatment of influenza A and has the advantage of reduced toxicity. However, it

TABLE 19.2   Amantadine Treatment for Influenza A in the Elderly*

Creatinine Clearance (ml/min)	>40	20-40	10-20	Dialysis
Amantadine	100 mg daily	100 mg every other day	100 mg alternating with 200 mg weekly	100 mg with each dialysis treatment

*These guidelines are based on a body surface area of 1.72 m^2.
Adapted from Mostow, 1987).

provides no advantage in the development of resistant influenza strains. Neither drug is effective against influenza B.

We are attempting to determine the efficacy of antiviral use and isolation in controlling influenza outbreaks and have observed that influenza outbreaks may be contained within a geographic region of LTCF. During the 1991 to 1992 influenza season, influenza A was culture proven on only 7 of 13 floors in the four buildings of the 706-bed facility. Only patients on these 7 floors received amantadine prophylaxis. Patients on 4 of these floors received amantadine prophylaxis for 14 days, and others on 3 floors received amantadine prophylaxis for 21 days. Amantadine prophylaxis given for a shorter duration than for the time that influenza is circulating within the community may be warranted because the facility may be isolated from circulating influenza in the community at large, reducing the potential for reintroduction of influenza once it has been cleared from the home. During the 1992 to 1993 season we had an influenza B outbreak. The inexpensive strategies noted earlier (distance between residents, reduced activities, use of barriers such as masks) were employed, and the outbreak was again geographically restricted. The contribution of each of these measures to containing influenza has yet to be determined. These outbreaks indicate that influenza is not so contagious that its presence in a LTCF automatically predicts its spread throughout the entire facility. Rather, there are a variety of measures that may limit its spread.

Influenza remains an important disease for LTCFs. Primary prevention (vaccination) and preparation for outbreak detection and control (surveillance and policy) need to occur if the impact of influenza is to be minimized. Although many of the approaches we are promoting remain unproved, they are inexpensive and logical. Current prospective studies should help establish their efficacy, and perhaps refine the CDC recommendations for influenza surveillance and outbreak control.

REFERENCES

Arden, N. H., Patriarca, P. A. S., Fasano, M. B., Lui, K. J., Harmon, M. W., Kendal, A. P., & Rimland, D. (1988). The roles of inactivated influenza vaccine and amantadine hydrochloride in controlling an outbreak of influenza A (H3N2) in a nursing home. *Archives of Internal Medicine, 148*, 865–868.

Arden, N. H., Patriarca, P. A., & Kendal, A. P. (1986). Experiences in the use and efficacy of inactivated influenza vaccine in nursing homes. In A. P. Kendal & P. A. Patriarca (Eds.), *Options for the control of influenza*. New York: Alan R. Liss.

Bean, W. J., Threlkeld, S. C., & Webster, R. G. (1989). Biologic potential of amantadine-resistant influenza A virus in an avian model. *Journal of Infectious Diseases, 159*, 1050–1056.

Belshe, R. B., Burk, B., Newman, F., Cerruti, R. L., & Sim, I. S. (1989). Resistance of influenza A virus to amantadine and rimantadine: Results of one decade of surveillance. *Journal of Infectious Diseases, 159,* 430–435.

Belshe, R. B., Smith, M. H., Hall, C. B., Betts, R., & Hay, A. J. (1988). Genetic basis of resistance to rimantadine emerging during treatment of influenza virus infection. *Journal of Virology, 62,* 1508–1512.

Bleidner, W. E., Harmon, J. B., Hewes, W. E., Lynes, T. E., & Hermann, E. C. (1965). Absorption, distribution and excretion of amantadine hydrochloride. *Journal of Pharmacology and Experimental Therapy, 150,* 484–490.

Bryson, Y. J., Monahan, C., Pollack, M., & Shields, W. D. (1980). A prospective double blind study of side effects associated with the administration of amantadine for influenza A virus prophylaxis. *Journal of Infectious Diseases, 141,* 543–547.

Centers for Disease Control. Prevention and control of influenza. (1992). Recommendations of the Immunization Practices Advisory Committee (ACIP). *Morbidity and Mortality Weekly Report, 41,* RR-9.

Clark, C., Woodson, M. M., & Nagasawa, H. T. (1990). Inhibition of lymphocyte proliferation by amantadine and its isomer, 2-aminoadamantane; impact on LYT-2[+] T cells while sparing L3T4[+] T cells. *Immunopharmacology, 21,* 41–50.

Cockroft, D. W., & Gault, M. H. (1976). Prediction of creatinine clearance from serum creatinine. *Nephron, 16,* 31–41.

Degelau, J., Somani, S. K., Cooper, S. L., Guay, D. R. P., & Crossley, K. B. (1992). Amantadine-resistant influenza A in a nursing facility. *Archives of Internal Medicine, 152,* 390–392.

Dolin, R., & Bentley, D. W. (1986). Amantadine and rimantadine: Prophylaxis and therapy of influenza A in adults. In A. P. Kendal & P. A. Patriarca (Eds.), *Options for the control of influenza.* New York: Alan R. Liss.

Ershler, W. B., Moore, A. L., & Socinski, M. A. (1984). Influenza and aging: Age-related changes and the effects of thymosin on the antibody response to influenza vaccine. *Journal of Clinical Immunology, 4,* 445–454.

Goodman, L. S., & Gilman, A. (Eds.) (1982). *The pharmacological basis of therapeutics.* New York: MacMillan.

Gravenstein, S., Duthie, E. H., Miller, B. A., Roecker, E., Drinka, P., Prathipati, K., & Ershler, W. B. (1989). Augmentation of anti-influenza antibody response in elderly men by thymosin alpha one: A double-blind placebo controlled clinical study. *Journal of the American Geriatrics Society, 37,* 1–8.

Gravenstein, S., Miller, B. A., Ershler, W. B., Brown, C. S., Mast, E., Circo, R., Duthie, E. H., & Drinka, P. (1990). Low sensitivity of CDC case definition for H3N2 influenza in elderly nursing home subjects. *Clinical Research, 38,* 547A.

Hayden, F. G., Belshe, R. B., Clover, R. D., Hay, A. J., Oakes, M. G., & Soo, W. (1989). Emergence and apparent transmission of rimantadine-resistant influenza A virus in families. *New England Journal of Medicine, 321,* 1696–1702.

Hobson, D., Curry, R. L., Beare, A. S., & Ward-Gardner, A. (1972). The role of hemagglutination-inhibiting antibody in protection against challenge infection with influenza A2 and B viruses. *Journal of Hygiene, 70,* 767–777.

Jackson, G. G. (1986). The development and clinical evaluation of amantadine for prophylaxis and treatment of influenza A. In A. P. Kendal & P. A. Patriarca (Eds.), *Options for the control of influenza.* New York: Alan R. Liss.

Kendal, A. P., Patriarca, P. A., & Arden, N. H. (1985). Policies and outcomes for control of influenza among the elderly in the USA. *Vaccine, 2,* 274–276.

Kilbourne, E. D. (1987). Control of influenza. In E. D. Kilbourne (Ed.), *Influenza.* New York: Plenum.

Laver, W. G., & Valentine, R. C. (1969). Morphology of the isolated hemagglutinin and neuraminidase subunits of influenza virus. *Virology, 38,* 105–119.

Levine, M., Beattie, B. L., McLean, D. M., & Corman, D. (1987). Characterization of the immune response to trivalent influenza vaccine in elderly men. *Journal of the American Geriatrics Society, 35,* 609–615.

Margolis, K. L., Nichol, K. L., Poland, G. A., & Pulhar, R. E. (1990). Frequency of adverse reactions to influenza vaccine in the elderly: A randomized, placebo-controlled trial. *Journal of the American Medical Association, 264,* 1139–1141.

Mast, E. E., Harmon, M., Gravenstein, S., Wu, S. P., Arden, N. H., Circo, R., Tyska, G., Kendal, A. P., & Davis, J. P. (1992). Emergence and possible transmission of amantadine-resistant viruses during nursing home outbreaks of influenza A (H3N2). *American Journal of Epidemiology, 134,* 988–997.

Mate, J., Simon, M., Juvancz, E., Takatsy, G. Y., Hollos, I., & Farkas, E. (1970). Prophylactic use of amantadine during a Hong Kong influenza epidemic. *Acta Microbiologica Academica Scientifica Hungarica, 17,* 285–296.

May, F. E., Stewart, R. B., & Cluff, L. E. (1977). Drug interactions and multiple drug administration. *Clinics in Pharmacological Therapy, 22,* 322–328.

Monto, A. S., Gunn, R. A., Bandyk, M. G., & King, C. L. (1979). Prevention of Russian influenza by amantadine. *Journal of the American Medical Association, 241,* 1003–1007.

Mostow, S. R. (1987). Prevention, management and control of influenza: Role of amantadine. *American Journal of Medicine, 82,* (Suppl. 6a), 35–41.

National Institutes of Health. (1980). Amantadine: Does it have a role in prevention and treatment of influenza? A NIH Consensus Development Conference. *Annals of Internal Medicine, 92,* 256–258.

Patriarca, P. A., Arden, N. H., Koplan, J. P., & Goodman, R. A. (1987). Prevention and control of type A influenza infections in nursing homes: Benefits and costs of four approaches using vaccination and amantadine. *Annals of Internal Medicine, 107,* 732–740.

Potter, C. W., & Oxford, J. S. (1979). Determinants of immunity to influenza infection in man. *British Medical Bulletin, 35,* 69–75.

Rowe, J. W. (1976). The effect of age on creatinine clearance in man: A cross-sectional and longitudinal study. *Journal of Gerontology, 31,* 155.

Sirrocco, A. (1988). Nursing and related care homes as reported from the 1986 inventory of long term care places. *Vital and Health Statistics of the National Center for Health Statistics, 147,* 1–3.

Stange, K. C., Little, D. W., & Blatnik, B. (1991). Adverse reactions to amantadine prophylaxis of influenza in a retirement home. *Journal of the American Geriatrics Society, 39,* 700–705.

Vestal, R. E. (1990). Clinical pharmacology. In W. R. Hazzards, R. Andres, E. L. Bierman, & J. P. Blass (Eds.), *Principles of geriatric medicine and gerontology.* New York: McGraw-Hill.

Wright, P. F., Khaw, K. T., Oxman, M. N., & Shwachman, H. (1976). Evaluation of the safety of amantadine HCL and the role of respiratory viral infections in children. *Journal of Infectious Diseases, 134,* 144–149.

Strategies for Improving Vaccine Delivery to Targeted Groups

20

Cassandra M. Wade, Jurgis Karuza,
Evan Calkins, and John Feather

Although influenza vaccination has been marketed in the United States since the 1940s, the vaccine has never experienced widespread acceptance or demand by either the public or health professionals. Each year during the 1970s only about 10% of the general population and 20% of the medically high-risk population received influenza vaccination, even though specific recommendations have been provided on repeated occasions by the Advisory Committee on Immunization Practices (ACIP) of the Centers for Disease Control since 1963 (Fedson, 1987). Annual vaccination against influenza, using vaccine developed against the specific strain or strains known to be prevalent in a given year is recommended for the following target groups at high risk of serious illness:

1. Persons age 65 years and older
2. Residents of nursing homes and other chronic care facilities housing persons of any age with chronic medical conditions

3. Adults and children with chronic disorders of the pulmonary or cardiovascular systems (including asthma)
4. Adults and children who have required medical follow-up or hospitalization during the preceding year because of chronic metabolic diseases, renal dysfunction, hemoglobinopathies, or immunosuppression
5. Children and teenagers (6 months to 18 years) who are receiving long term aspirin therapy (Morbidity and Mortality Weekly Report, 1990).

Despite clear evidence of the protective effectiveness of influenza vaccine and the intensive efforts by the Centers for Disease Control, the American College of Physicians, and other organizations to enhance use of vaccines, overall vaccination rates against influenza have remained low. Tracing the immunization rates and overall use of supplies of flu vaccine employed over the 16-year period between 1968 to 1969 and 1984 to 1985, except for the period of the "swine flu epidemic" in 1976 to 1977, the total number of persons immunized in this country has steadily decreased. Although there has been a slight increase in the immunization rates for elderly persons, from 18% to 22% or 23%, the immunization rates for high-risk patients, ages 20 to 64, have declined, thus leading to the decrease in use of flu vaccine materials (Fedson, 1987). Other reports agree, estimating vaccination rates for the elderly and for high-risk adults at approximately 20% (Kavet, 1976; Ennes & Tully, 1976).

FACTORS AFFECTING RATE OF INFLUENZA VACCINATION IN OLDER ADULTS

Patient-Based Factors

Older patients' beliefs about the influenza vaccine effectiveness and its side effects are significantly related to prior vaccination history and are strongly influenced by physician recommendations and physician behavior. Several investigators have used the Health Belief Model as a framework to assist in understanding response to vaccination from the patients' point of view. According to this model (Larson, Olson, & Shortell, 1979; Sivert, Elsea, Bohan, & Sikes, 1988; Buchner, Carter, & Inui, 1985), the likelihood of a patient's acceptance of flu vaccination depends on their intention to get vaccinated. Intention is based on a comparison of the perceived threat from possible infection with influenza (i.e., the perceived susceptibility to infection and its perceived severity) against "costs," such as discomfort and side effects, compared with "benefits," such as the effectiveness of the vaccine. Four factors consistently stand out as related to patient acceptance of the influenza vaccination.

- Perceptions of or history of adverse reactions associated with the influenza vaccination
- Importance of physician recommendation for the vaccination
- Previous immunization history
- Schedule of clinic visits.

In a study of high-risk patients of a Family Medicine Center, conducted by Larson and his colleagues (1979), the persons who obtained vaccination believed that the infection is a severe disease, that they had a reasonable likelihood of being infected, and that vaccination would reduce the chance of infection or lessen its severity. Patients not complying were less impressed with the protective benefits of vaccination. Similarly, in studies by Frank, McMurray, & Henderson (1985) and Buchner et al. (1985), the perception that adverse reactions occurred with previous vaccinations was related to not receiving the influenza vaccination. Sivert et al. (1988) of the Division of Physical Health of the DeKalb County Board of Health, Georgia, report a somewhat similar survey of residents of two counties in Georgia who were age 65 and older. Among factors that might be associated with receiving the influenza vaccine, the most important was a recommendation for a vaccination by a health care provider. Of the 596 respondents, 75% reported that their health care provider had recommended influenza vaccination and 75% of these individuals reported being vaccinated within the previous year. The importance of physician recommendation for vaccine was replicated in studies by Frank et al. (1985), Cummings, Jette, Brock, and Haefner (1979), and Buchner et al. (1985). In keeping with the health belief model they found that physician recommendation for being vaccinated was related to ultimately receiving the vaccine. In the Buchner et al. (1985) study, which followed patients longitudinally, 50% of the patients underwent attitude changes regarding influenza vaccination, suggesting that physicians' efforts in patient education can be effective in increasing patient compliance with influenza vaccination.

Nationally, vaccination rates range from 20% to 40% among high-risk groups, but there is a debate over the number of older adults who could be expected to change their behavior and accept the influenza vaccine. Estimates of intractable noncompliance range from 50% according to Frank et al. (1985) to 9% of patients refusing vaccination after a physician recommended vaccination according to McKinney and Barnes (1989). Even taking the pessimistic figure of Frank et al. (1985), the potential exists of doubling of vaccination rates among older adults. The reliance of many, possibly most, patients on the recommendation of their physician as their primary health care provider, combined with the exceedingly poor overall compliance rates noted earlier, identifies the physician as a focal point of the problem.

Physician-Based Factors

Several studies indicated that physicians have reasonable knowledge of the influenza immunization recommendations and about the effects of the influenza vaccination. In many studies physician knowledge and attitudes do not predict actual immunization rates (McKinney & Barnes, 1989). This is paralleled by the findings that simple educational interventions aimed at enhancing physicians' knowledge are ineffective in increasing the rate of immunization. A frequent strategy reported in the literature is to couple the educational intervention with another treatment, such as a chart reminder or checklist. There is evidence that such approaches do increase physician compliance. The review of the literature also indicates that the predominant style of physician education tends not to be involving or requiring extensive commitment on the part of the physician. This suggests that a fruitful area of investigation to examine would be the effectiveness of more active and participatory styles of physician education.

Fedson (1987) reported on a survey of physicians' attitudes toward influenza and influenza vaccine conducted by the Centers for Disease Control. More than 80% of the respondents recognized influenza as a very serious threat to the health of the elderly, especially those with high-risk conditions; 98% agreed that all high-risk persons should be immunized; 90% agreed that this should be done annually. By contrast, the actual performance of primary care physicians in immunizing their own patients older than age 65 ranged from 6.7% to 12.3%.

Stetia, Serventi, and Lorenz (1985), conducted a survey of the medical staff of a county hospital in New Jersey. The results indicate a high degree of awareness on the part of the physicians of the benefits of influenza vaccine in reducing the otherwise high rate of risk associated with influenza. About 80% of the physicians agreed that vaccination would decrease morbidity, 71% felt it would decrease mortality, and 80% felt that it was cost effective. Despite this, only one third of the residents of the hospital's extended care facility received vaccination. Following discussion with the staff, at which there was general agreement concerning the need for better compliance, and the submission of letters sent to individual physicians citing the names of their patients who had not yet been vaccinated, the level of compliance only increased by an additional 4%.

McKinney and Barnes (1989) surveyed physicians in a primary care clinic at the Milwaukee County Medical Center. Eighty percent of the physicians knew the time of year when flu vaccine should be administered; 75%

knew that vaccination would be contraindicated if the patient was either febrile or sensitive to eggs; and 69% felt that vaccination was effective in preventing infection in between 70% and 90% of cases. There was, however, a slight overestimation of the incidence of side effects—25% of the physicians felt that anaphylaxis would occur in more than 1% of cases and 15% felt the Guillain-Barré syndrome might occur in more than 1% of cases. About 41% of the 854 patients age 65 and older were offered the vaccine. Physician compliance ranged from 0% to 90%. *However, accuracy of knowledge about influenza vaccine and its effectiveness was not related to actual immunization rates.* Thus, the study showed that physicians' perception of the efficacy of vaccine is high, and confirmed their strength and conviction to offer vaccination. However, their knowledge and conviction were not used in their practice as is evidenced by continually low vaccination rates. This suggests that mere dissemination of knowledge may not be a sufficient way of increasing physician influenza vaccination rates.

INTERVENTION STUDIES

The following three approaches, often in combination, have been frequently reported in the literature to enhance physician compliance with influenza vaccination guidelines:

- Educational programs
- Various forms of checklists or reminders, attached to patient charts or appearing on a computer at the time of the patient's visit
- Feedback concerning physician performance either as a group or individually.

Some evidence suggests that combinations of interventions (e.g., education with reminders) are more likely to have an impact on physician compliance with prevention guidelines than education by itself, although the evidence is mixed.

Korn, Schlossberg, and Rich (1988) described one of the few instances in which an educational program alone yielded enhanced compliance with influenza vaccination on the part of physicians. In this instance, there was an increase from 9% in 1983 to 28% the following year. Mandel, Franks, and Dickinson (1985), however, found that an educational program per se failed to achieve any enhancement in performance by medical house staff. The intervention involved "specific educational feedback about preventive medicine deficiencies found in their charts as well as routine comments on the content of their progress notes." Both before and after this intervention, residents immunized 40% of their patients. Because no difference was noted before or after the intervention it was suggested that physicians are relatively resistant to changing their behavior in response to this type of educational intervention.

Belcher (1990), working at the Seattle Veterans Administration Medical Center, attempted three interventions in four groups. The first was an initial training session, followed by introduction of a "reminder" sheet attached to the chart, listing recommended preventive modalities and the frequency with which they should be employed. The second intervention involved mailing to patients, annually, an informational packet regarding preventive activities, with a request that patients would discuss this information with their physicians. The third intervention was the creation of a separate clinic devoted to screening, health counseling, and preventive measures. A fourth group served as a control.

Neither of the specific techniques designed to enhance physician compliance with immunization guidelines yielded any further increases compared with the control group of physicians. A combined program, including both the reminder sheet and patient informational material, also led to no improvement in compliance with preventative measures. The establishment of a Health Promotion Clinic, however, was markedly successful, and led to a threefold enhancement of preventive activities.

A study by Cohen, Littenberg, Wetzel, et al. (1982) examined physician compliance with preventive medicine guidelines as a function of implementing a checklist reminder system and scheduling physician information seminars. However, poor attendance at the seminars led the authors to conclude that the checklist was more effective in changing the practice patterns of physicians than the educational intervention. This was replicated by Tierney, Hui, and McDonald (1986), who found a sevenfold enhancement of compliance with pneumococcal vaccine guidelines was achieved by institution of a computerized reminder system for physicians.

The effectiveness of providing physician feedback as an adjunct to educational sessions was employed by Winickoff, Coltin, Morgan, et al. (1984). The results showed that physician performance could be improved through peer comparison feedback. The topic chosen to evaluate quality assurance was the hemmocult test. Three interventions that were sequentially employed in an attempt to improve performance comprised:

1. A 1-hour educational meeting at which the standard was discussed and agreed on.
2. Another meeting at which the rate of group compliance with the standard before and after the educational meeting was presented.
3. Computer-based peer comparison feedback.

Following the educational meeting the compliance level increased but not significantly by 1.2% for the contiguous 6-month posteducation period. Another departmental meeting was held devoted to colorectal cancer. The results of the posteducation period were presented as well as results from a retrospective study demonstrating that a 90% level is optimal. Physicians were surprised with their poor performance and agreed to try harder. However, performance for the next 2 months was 68.5%, statistically unchanged.

The next intervention, that of peer comparison feedback, was implemented. Physicians were given a computer printout with an arrow pointing to a number that represented the physician. Results of this intervention did show significant improvement, both in the feedback and control groups, with a significantly greater increase in compliance in the feedback group. Follow-up showed that the improvement in compliance "held over" for the following year, although to a reduced extent.

Barton and Schoenbaum (1990) attempted to increase the rate of influenza vaccination performance in a health maintenance organization (HMO) setting by using both computer-generated reminders and peer comparison feedback. Three different interventions were implemented sequentially between the years 1983 to 1987.

1. In the first year the intervention involved postcard reminders to HMO members, educational materials, and a reminder message to clinicians at the front of the summary of the computerized record, which was prepared for each scheduled primary care visit for a high-risk patient under age 65.
2. In the second year this was supplemented by chart reminders for persons older than age 65 and feedback of performance to service chiefs.
3. In the third year these interventions were further supplemented by feedback of performance to individual physicians and by the periodic distribution of lists of patients who had not yet been immunized by the physicians.

Vaccination rates increased substantially after the physician feedback intervention in the third year of the study (1986 to 1987). Immunization rates at the center without the automated record remained stable throughout the three flu seasons. Patients on the reminder list were more likely to be vaccinated if they had a visit to their primary care physician. The difference in rates is probably attributable to the effect of the postcard reminder on encouraging flu season visits. The difference in influenza vaccination rates of 73% for patients for whom a reminder was generated versus 42% for those not getting the reminder reflect the effect of the computer-generated chart reminder on the physician. This report demonstrated that it is possible to achieve an improvement in annual influenza vaccination performance in a practice setting using a combination of reminder and feed-back techniques.

A specific variant of the reminder technique, patient reminders, was studied by Larson, Bergman, Heinrich et al. (1982). They examined whether postcard reminders mailed to patients improved influenza vaccination rates. Patients were randomly assigned to one of four groups: a control group receiving no postcard, a group receiving a neutral postcard (reminder of a vaccine clinic), a group receiving a postcard telling of importance of influenza vaccine, and a personal postcard (note from patients' doctor advising them to get a flu vaccine). Patients receiving the postcard telling of the importance of influenza vaccine had a higher vaccination rate (51.4%) than control patients (20.2%) or patients receiving a neutral postcard. Patients receiving a personal postcard also had a higher vaccination rate (41.0%) than control patients. This study supports the hypothesis that the combination of a cue postcard and a message emphasizing the elements of the health belief model are more effective than a postcard containing a neutral message or no message.

WESTERN NEW YORK GERIATRIC EDUCATION CENTER MODEL

A new strategy for improving influenza vaccination compliance has been developed by the Western New York Geriatric Education Center (WNY GEC) in contract with the Bureau of Health Professions. This particular strategy is aimed at changing physician practice patterns so as to achieve a lasting effect on patient care. In general, the aforementioned interventions are "one-shot" efforts that will temporarily alter vaccine rates so long as someone is available to put the system in place. Also, given the varied cultures and structures of physician practice sites, it is not plausible to generalize one specific method of increasing vaccinations to each setting. The proposed method of the WNY GEC is to allow physicians in their own settings to determine what they feel will work best for them to fit into the structure or culture of the practice setting.

Rationale

The logic of the intervention integrates the findings from the literature of knowledge transfer, continuing medical education, attitude change, and the group dynamics. The knowledge transfer literature makes a useful distinction between four functions of knowledge dissemination (e.g., Backer, 1991; Hutchins, 1989): spread, choice, exchange, and implementation. *Spread* is one way of broadcasting knowledge to increase awareness. *Choice* is the dissemination of knowledge in formats that provides users with options in the obtaining of information. *Exchange* is the interactive exchange or feedback between users and disseminators. *Implementation* is putting knowledge to use. Critiques from a variety of disciplines make the similar point that it is imperative for knowledge transfer systems and research to focus more on ways to enhance implementation of knowledge, that is, the translation and penetration of knowledge into practice (Backer, 1991; Greer, 1988; Klein & Gwaltney, 1991). Review of the compliance with influenza vaccination guidelines literature suggests that merely broadcasting information and ensuring its availability does not guarantee use in practice.

A similar theme is sounded in the continuing medical education (CME) literature. Reviews of the CME literature have long called into question the effectiveness of standard CME formats, such as lectures, journal articles, or conferences, in changing practice (Bertram & Brooks-Bertram, 1977; Greer, 1988). More specifically, recent critiques have focused on the usefulness of consensus conferences. As several studies indicate, major problems remain with distribution of the guidelines to practicing physicians and, more important, having these guidelines incorporated into practice (Lomas, Anderson, Domnick-Pierre, et al., 1989; Mullan & Jacoby, 1985).

On a more general level, the attitude change literature makes a parallel point. Starting with the classic work of LaPierre around 1932 through the current theory of reasoned action (Fishbein & Ajzen, 1975), the empirical data clearly show that a change in knowledge or attitude does not necessarily lead to a change in behavior. The implication is that change in knowledge and attitude about a practice guideline is necessary but not sufficient to lead to a change in medical practice pattern. A dissemination effort that has as its goal the actual implementation of the medical technology into practice must also have a mechanism that enables the translation of knowledge into a change in behavior. Current conceptualizations of attitude and behavior (Fishbein & Ajzen, 1975) highlight the importance of considering the social context and social expectations as factors influencing the behavior pattern of individuals. For example, in the theory of reasoned action, a person's perception of *social norms* to perform an act and the attitude the person holds about the *act*, independently and directly influence the intention to perform the act which, in turn, predicts behavior. Considerable empirical evidence supports this logic (Fishbein & Ajzen, 1975).

A similar theme is found in the group dynamics literature. Starting with Kurt Lewin (1951), group dynamics has focused on the use of group process as a technique to bring about changes in individual behavior. Recent applications of this can be found in the development and increased use of participatory management styles and quality improvement approaches in industrial organizations to improve worker productivity (Lawler & Drexler, 1978). As a management style, these methods adopt a decentralized approach in which the workers most involved with the operating system or process form "quality teams" with the responsibility and authority to troubleshoot problems, develop solutions and evaluate their effectiveness. The changes made by the team are products of group discussion and consensus building among the individuals. Currently, several demonstrations are in place that specifically attempt to apply these quality improvement techniques, including the use of quality teams, in medical clinics (Berwick, 1989).

Although a multitude of variants can be found, these approaches converge on a core set of principles (Dietrich, et al., 1990; Lewin, 1951).

1. Social norms and expectations influence an individual's behavior.
2. The use of a group process can be effective in changing normative expectations and the subsequent behavior of an individual because it is easier to change behavioral patterns of groups than those of individuals.
3. Behavioral change is facilitated in groups that are composed of individuals who are directly concerned with the issue.
4. Behavioral change is facilitated in groups that are democratically led by a natural group leader who is respected and accepted by the group members.
5. Behavioral change is facilitated by having sufficient accurate information about the problem the group is discussing.
6. Behavioral change is facilitated by having group discussion that follows a systematic process, sufficiently defines problems and tasks, analyzes the problem, explores alternative solutions to it, and generates a recommended course of action.
7. Behavioral change is facilitated by having a group consensus decision-making process.
8. Behavioral change is facilitated by having a public commitment to accept the group decision.

Although not specifically testing group process approaches in CME, a body of literature has emerged that suggests that involving physicians in discussions about medical information or feedback about practice patterns, either in groups (Dietrich, Barrett, Levy, et al., 1990) or a one-on-one basis (Avorn & Soumerai, 1983), leads to changes in primary care practice patterns. These approaches share a common dynamic of having physicians become more actively and socially involved in the dissemination process. If effective, the involved physicians "buy into" the intervention and create an emotional commitment to improved outcome (Eisenberg, 1985; Fox,

1990). Studies typifying this approach often combine techniques designed to increase the amount of information about the medical technology with a physician "buy-in" process. In Cohen et al. (1982), use of a participatory or "buy-in" approach to education was supplemented by a reminder or checklist. It was one of the few studies in which an educational intervention led to improved compliance. Winickoff et al. (1984) demonstrated that a "buy-in" approach that was supplemented by individualized feedback was effective in increasing overall physician compliance with preventive medicine. This can also be seen in the Barton and Schoenbaum (1990) study in a HMO context.

Core Model and Hypothesis

In keeping with the knowledge dissemination literature, we conceptualize the dissemination and implementation of medical technology as a four-stage process beginning with physician awareness of the medical technology, formulating a decision, adopting the decision, and, finally, implementing the decision.

Adoption of an innovation *is more than an exercise in information processing*. As several critics of the CME literature point out (Lomas & Haynes, 1988), a rational information processing or cognitively based model of adoption of an innovation is not sufficient in leading physicians to adopt an innovation. Reviewers such as Lomas and Haynes (1988); Fox (1990); Greer (1977); Backer (1988), Backer, Liberman & Kuehnel (1986); and Rogers (1968) all point to the importance of considering professional, social, and personal forces for change in physicians. An effective innovation dissemination strategy should capitalize on these other forces.

The hypothesis is that the dissemination and adoption of medical technology by physicians is enhanced when the dissemination effort occurs in a social context that actively involves the physician in the dissemination process—the so-called buy-in approach. Based on the earlier review, a *core* set of minimal features can be defined for the intervention.

Clear and Complete Information About the Medical Technology

In the case of a formed (i.e., well defined) medical technology (Greer, 1988), this information should include the existence of official guidelines, adherence to guidelines, the effectiveness of the technology, and problems associated with implementing the technology. In the case of "dynamic" medical technology in which the technology is being developed, the information process is similar to the quality improvement team approach. Because the medical technology to be disseminated is the set of guidelines for influenza vaccination of older adults over age 65, the technology is a "formed" one.

Study Population

A total of 214 physicians from the Western New York area was surveyed in this study. More than 3,000 charts of patients 65 and older were reviewed to collect data relating to influenza vaccination status between the years 1990 to 1991 and 1991 to 1992. Participants were sampled from a heterogeneous mix of practice sites including: family medicine clinics, internal medicine clinics, managed care physician groups, a fee-for-service group, a rural physician network, and a Veteran's Affairs Hospital.

Subject Selection Process

To be included in this study, physicians must have met the following criteria: a resident or licensed physician of a primary care discipline with formal affiliation with the selected practice sites, had at least five older adults (age 65 and older) in the active practice panel, and saw patients during the 1990 to 1991 and 1991 to 1992 influenza season. Patients whose charts were selected must have been: 65 or older as of October 1, 1991; an active patient (defined as being seen by the physician at least once during February 1, 1990, and January 31, 1991); formally assigned to the physician as the attending physician; and residing in an ambulatory or community dwelling.

A total of 101 physicians and 2,404 patients met this criteria. The mean age of patients in the study was 75 with 35% being male and 64% being female.

Chart Review Procedure

Approximately 40 charts per physician were reviewed to achieve an appropriate level of statistical power. In cases in which the practices had less than 40 charts, all charts were reviewed. If the practice had more than 40 charts, the charts to be reviewed were randomly selected to obtain a minimum of 40 charts. Twelve medical and graduate students were trained to conduct the chart reviews. Pearson product moment correlations showed greater than 95% reliability of the chart reviewers.

Information regarding influenza immunization practices was collected twice. Data were first collected during the summer months of 1991. Patient records were reviewed to determine vaccination rates for the 1990 to 1991 influenza season (October 1, 1990 to January 31, 1991) to establish base line compliance rates (preintervention). Follow-up data collection occurred during the spring months of 1992 to determine if vaccination rates had increased for the 1991 to 1992 influenza season (postintervention).

Method

Small-Group Process

The small-group process has as its specific aim the achievement of enhanced adherence to accepted standards for the provision of influenza vaccine to elderly patients, especially those with chronic diseases that are known to put these patients at greater risk for serious illness or death from influenza and its complications. Although physicians seem to know the importance of influenza vaccine, vaccination rates are strikingly low. With the following method of intervention, it is hoped that physician interest will be generated enough to improve vaccination rates.

The small-group process intervention has three phases.

Phase 1

A brief 5-minute introduction to the physicians by the facilitator stressing the following points: organization of the meeting, the philosophy of the approach as a decentralized, grass-roots effort by physicians as a way of disseminating medical technology and implementing it into practice, and the importance of the physicians to play active roles as agents of change in shaping their practice.

Phase 2

A "technical" lecture is presented on the medical technology (i.e., influenza vaccination guidelines). The technical lecture takes 10 minutes to cover the following points:

- National guidelines for vaccination including vaccinating those older than age 65 as a special priority group
- Effectiveness of the vaccine in reducing mortality and morbidity
- Low compliance rate historically, nationally, and locally
- Background on how the vaccine is prepared
- Contraindications (i.e., sensitivity to eggs)
- Misconceptions about negative side effects (e.g., vaccine does not cause influenza)
- Review of the literature on why patients do not receive vaccine with special consideration given to the importance of physician recommendation to patients.

Standardized audio-visual materials are used in all groups. In addition, print material, a copy of *Morbidity and Mortality Weekly Report* (1990) outlining the influenza vaccination guidelines, and a published review (Fedson, 1987) are distributed to the physicians.

The technical lecture is given by one of three expert physicians. To ensure generalizability, all the physicians are given the same audio-visual aids and have the same 1-hour training before the presentation. All presenting physicians are given a summary paper of the pertinent information they need to present. They are also provided with some key articles with which they need to be familiar (Fedson, 1987; Morbidity and Mortality Weekly Report, 1990).

This curriculum remains constant for all of the sites regardless of which physician is presenting the lecture. After the material has been presented, the speaker poses a few questions to the physicians regarding their usage of influenza vaccine. This sets the scenario for the group discussion.

Phase 3

The group processes for approximately 40 minutes. After the "technical" lecture, the speaker leaves so that they are not introducing any type of bias to the outcome. The facilitator then leads the group in discussion.

Before starting the discussion, a "recording secretary" is selected to record the comments of the group. The record of the comments and decisions is collected at the end of the session. This record serves as a "check" on the group process to make sure the critical features are followed.

The role of the facilitator is not to make a decision for the group but to keep the group focused on the topic of interest (i.e., increasing compliance with influenza vaccination guidelines). The facilitator leads the group through the following set sequence:

1. Restatement of the problem of compliance with the influenza vaccination guidelines in the physicians practice setting.
2. Problem-finding stage—identifying potential barriers to implementation of guidelines.
3. Solution generation stage—where possible techniques to increasing vaccination rate are proposed.
4. Solution evaluation stage—where techniques are evaluated as to their practicality.
5. A consensus to adopt the proposed means of implementing the medical technology is reached.
6. A verbal public commitment is obtained from each physician that they will increase the influenza vaccination rates in their patients

older than age 65 and will support the means to increase influenza vaccination.

Once a consensus is reached as to what method the physicians would like to implement to increase influenza vaccination rates, it is the responsibility of the WNY GEC contract to provide technical support (within reason) to the practice sites. No payment is given to physicians to participate in the small-group process.

Preliminary Results

Physician Attitudes and Knowledge

Physicians were required to complete a questionnaire whose objective items measure knowledge about influenza vaccine, side effects, and effectiveness. Additionally, the questionnaire had general attitudinal questions regarding the importance of primary prevention behaviors including influenza vaccination. The questionnaires were to be completed before the small-group process, 1 month after the small-group process, and again 3 months later.

Pretests of physician knowledge and attitudes showed that 12% of participating physicians were not aware of the Centers for Disease Control influenza vaccination recommendations. Also, physicians tended to overestimate their vaccination rates. Physicians were reporting, on average, that they vaccinated 48% of their patients age 65 and older last year. However, chart reviews showed that the average vaccination rate of patients age 65 and older last year was 39%. Additionally, 60% of the physicians participating in this study did not receive the influenza vaccine last year even though they are targeted as one of the groups that should receive vaccine. Of the physicians who did receive vaccine, results showed that their patients were more likely to receive vaccine than those patients whose physicians did not receive vaccine.

Evaluation of Small-Group Process

The 1990 to 1991 average vaccination rate for the control group was 38% and 43% for the experimental group. The small-group process increased the influenza vaccination rates to 49% in the experimental group ($F = 4.96$, $p < .03$). There was no change in the control group. A total of 1100 patients were seen by physicians who did not participate in the small-group process. Of these patients, only 448 received influenza vaccine. A total of 1,304 patients were seen by physicians who did participate in the small-group process. Of these patients, 707 received vaccine ($\chi^2 = 43.5$, $p < .0001$).

Much of the data analysis has yet to be completed at the time of this writing. In addition, there are two contracting sites that are part of this project. The two sites are the Birmingham, Alabama Geriatric Education Center (GEC) and the San Antonio, South Texas GEC. The objective of these GECs is to target the age 65 and older African- and Mexican-American populations for increasing influenza vaccine compliance using the small-group process.

REFERENCES

Avorn, J., & Soumerai, S. B. (1983). Improving drug-therapy decisions through educational outreach. *New England Journal of Medicine, 308,* 1457–1462.
Backer, T. (1988). Research utilization and managing innovation in rehabilitation organizations. *Journal of Rehabilitation, 54,* 18–22.
Backer, T. (1991). *Drug abuse technology transfer.* Rockville, MD: National Institute on Drug Abuse, Office of Policy and External Affairs, Professional Education Branch.
Backer, T., Liberman, R. P., & Kuehnel, T. G. (1986). Dissemination and adoption of innovative psychosocial interventions. *Journal of Consulting and Clinical Psychology, 54,* 111–118.
Barton, M., & Schoenbaum, S. (1990). Improving influenza vaccination performance in an HMO setting: The use of computerized reminders and peer comparison feedback. *American Journal of Public Health, 80,* 534–536.
Belcher, D. (1990). Implementing preventive services. *Archives of Internal Medicine, 150,* 2533–2541.
Bertram, D. A., & Brooks-Bertram, P. A. (1977). The evaluation of continuing medical education: A literature review. *Health Education Monographs, 5,* 330–362.
Berwick, D. M. (1989). Health services research and quality of care: Assignments for 1990's. *Medical Care, 27,* 763–771.
Buchner, D. M., Carter, W. B., & Inui, T. S. (1985). The relationship of attitude changes to compliance with influenza immunization. *Medical Care, 23,* 771.
Cohen, D., Littenberg, B., Wetzel, C., & Neuhauser, D. (1982). Improving physician compliance with preventive medicine guidelines. *Medical Care, 20,* 1040–1045.
Cummings, K. M., Jette, A., Brock, B., Haefner, D. P. (1979). Psychosocial determinants of immunization behavior in a swine influenza campaign. *Medical Care, 17,* 639–649.
Dietrich, A. J., Barrett, J., Levy, O., Carney-Gersten, P. (1990). Impact of an educational program on physician cancer control knowledge and activities. *American Journal of Preventive Medicine, 6,* 346–352.
Eisenberg, J. (1985). Physician utilization. *Medical Care, 23,* 461–483.
Ennes, F. A., & Tully, M. (1976). Acceptance of vaccination by the elderly. In P. Selby (Ed.), *Influenza: Virus, vaccines, and strategy* (pp. 311–318). New York: Academic Press.
Fedson, D. S. (1987). Influenza prevention and control: Past practices and future prospects. *American Journal of Medicine, 82,* 42.

Fishbein, M., & Ajzen, I. (1975). *Belief, attitude, intention, and behavior: An introduction to theory and research.* Reading, MA: Addison-Wesley.

Fox, R. D. (1990). New horizons for research in continuing medical education. *Academic Medicine, 65,* 550–555.

Frank, J., McMurray, L., & Henderson, M. (1985). Influenza vaccination in the elderly: The economics of sending reminder letters. *Canadian Medical Association Journal, 132,* 516–521.

Greer, A. L. (1977, Fall). Advances in the study of diffusion of innovation in health care organizations. *The Milbank Memorial Fund Quarterly: Health and Society, 505–532.*

Greer, A. L. (1988). The state of the art versus the state of the science: The diffusion of new medical technologies into practice. *International Journal of Technology Assessment in Health Care, 4,* 5–26.

Hutchins, C. (1989). A brief review of federal dissemination activities, 1958–1983. *Knowledge: Creating, Diffusion, Utilization, 11,* 10–27.

Jacoby, I. (1985). The consensus development program of the National Institutes of Health. *International Journal of Technology Assessment in Health Care, 1,* 420–432.

Kavet, J. (1976). Trends in the utilization of influenza vaccine: An examination of the implementation of public policy in the US. In P. Selby (Ed.), *Influenza: Virus, vaccines and strategy* (pp. 297–308). New York: Academic Press.

Klein, S., & Gwaltney, M. (1991). Charting the education dissemination system. *Knowledge: Creating, Diffusion, Utilization, 12,* 241–265.

Korn, J. E., Schlossberg, L. A., & Rich, E. C. (1988). Improved preventive care following an intervention during an ambulatory care rotation: Carry over to a second setting. *Journal of General Internal Medicine, 3,* 156.

Larson, E. B., Bergman, I., Heinrich, F., & Schneeweir, R. (1982). Do postcard reminders improve influenza vaccination compliance? A prospective trial of different postcard "cues." *Medical Care, 20, 6,* 639–648.

Larson, E. B., Olson, W. C., & Shortell, S. (1979). The relationship of health beliefs and a postcard reminder to influenza vaccination. *Journal of Family Practice, 8,* 1207.

Lawler, E. E., & Drexler, J. A. (1978). Dynamics of establishing cooperative quality-of-worklife projects. *Monthly Labor Review,* 23–28.

Lewin, K. (1951). *Field theory in social science.* New York: Harper.

Lomas, J., Anderson, G. M., Domnick-Pierre, K., Vayda, E., Enkin, M. W., & Hannah, W. J. (1989). Do practice guidelines guide practice? *New England Journal of Medicine, 321,* 1306–1311.

Lomas, J., & Haynes, R. B. (1988). A taxonomy and critical review of tested strategies for the application of clinical practice recommendations: From "official" to "individual" clinical policy. *American Journal of Preventive Medicine, 4* (Suppl.), 77–94.

Mandel, I. I., Franks, P., & Dickinson, J. (1985). Improving physician compliance with preventive medicine guidelines. *Journal of Family Practice, 21,* 223.

McKinney, W. P., & Barnes, G. P. (1989). Influenza immunization on the elderly: Knowledge and attitudes do not explain physician behavior. *American Journal of Public Health, 79,* 1422.

Morbidity and Mortality Weekly Report. (1990). Prevention and control of influenza: Recommendations of the Immunization Practices Advisory Committee. *Morbidity and Mortality Weekly Report, 39*, 1–15.

Mullan, H., & Jacoby, I. (1985). The consensus development program of the National Institutes of Health. *International Journal of Technology Assessment in Health Care, 1*, 420–432.

Rogers, E. M. (1968). *Diffusion of innovations.* New York: The Free Press.

Sivert, A. J., Elsea, W. R., Bohan, G. N., & Sikes, R. K. (1988). Adult immunization: Knowledge, attitudes, and practice. Leads from the *Morbidity and Mortality Weekly Report. Journal of the American Medical Association, 260*, 3253.

Stetia, U., Serventi, I., & Lorenz, P. (1985). Clinical report: Factors influencing the use of influenza vaccine in the institutional elderly. *Journal of the American Geriatrics Society, 33*, 856.

Tierney, W. M., Hui, S. L., & McDonald, C. J. (1986). Delayed feedback of physician performance versus immediate reminders to perform preventive care. *Medical Care, 24*, 659–666.

Winickoff, R. N., Coltin, K. L., Morgan, M. M., Buxman, R. C., & Barnett, G. O. (1984). Improving physician performance through peer comparison feedback. *Medical Care, 22*, 527–534.

Withholding Antibiotics as a Form of Care: An Ethical Perspective

21

Douglas K. Miller

Aggressive diagnosis and treatment of all infections can cause a great deal of pain and discomfort for patients, and often for their loved ones and care-givers who have to watch their suffering. Consider, for example, a female nursing home resident with underlying dementia and pneumonia. If she is to receive full curative care, even is she is not moved to the hospital, she will be obligated to receive venipunctures, to be moved about for radiographs, to undergo suctioning and percussion and postural drainage, and painful administration of antibiotics if they are given intramuscularly or intravenously. These procedures are difficult enough for cognitively intact individuals; they can be horrifying for the cognitively impaired. Add to this all the potential side effects of antimicrobials including pruritic rashes, diarrhea, toxicities to kidneys, liver, bone marrow, hearing, and so on. The situation could be worse if she is moved to hospital. There, she is in strange surroundings with unfamiliar people wearing austere clothing, both of which can be very frightening, especially to patients with cognitive disturbances such as dementia or delirium. She is very likely to be put into restraints to keep her from pulling out her intravenous line or urinary catheter. She may well be strapped down and wired for cardiac monitoring and perhaps given cardiac poisons for the irregular rhythms that develop while she is sick. She may be put on a ventilator and further strapped down. Then if she develops resistant organisms, she will go through the whole scenario all over again but at a higher level of intensity. This is the negative side of aggressive care. Conversely, we know that treatment of infections can often prolong a patient's life. Thus we have a basic ethical conflict between preventing suffering and prolonging life, and the question becomes when is the suffering associated with treatment worth the benefit to be gained? This issue also arises frequently. Marin and colleagues (1989) surveyed 448 nonpsychiatric physicians in Wales and found that 77% of them had managed a terminally ill patient within the past year. In the event that such a patient would become febrile, only 16% would treat with antibiotics, and a mere 9% of the respondents would take blood cultures.

ETHICAL GUIDELINES

Given that the consideration of whether to withhold antibiotics at the end of life is both difficult and a common occurrence, are there guidelines for addressing the issue in an ethically sound way? To address this question, it is useful to start with basic ethical principles. Physicians have a moral and ethical obligation to do what is best for the patient, *as viewed by the patient*, from a social context. The goal of medical care is to help each patient pursue life's goals as he or she defines them (as long as they are not illegal, of course). The issue then becomes "what is meaningful life" without presuming to judge for the individual patient. In other words, it means assessing benefits and burdens from the patient's point of view.

To meet the operational demands of this ethical paradigm requires a combination of medical knowledge, understanding of the patient's viewpoint, some common sense, and a willingness to negotiate the best alternative for a specific patient in a specific situation. When the benefits of a therapy definitely outweigh the imposed burdens, the therapy is said to be "proportionally beneficial." When the burdens definitely outweigh the benefits, the therapy is said to have "disproportional benefit" (President's Commission for the Study of Ethical Problems, 1983).

All of us will die sooner or later. Unless we die from cardiac causes, most of us will experience infection as our final cause of death. The actual demise of most patients with any form of end-stage chronic disease—whether the chronic disease is cancer, pulmonary disease, dementia, chronic malnutrition, or di⸺tes—is most likely to be caused by an infection. Obviously there comes a time when aggressive treatment of all infections no longer offers the patient benefits that outweigh the burdens of therapy. The question is how to recognize that point.

Withholding Treatment

Currently there are two situations for which withholding antibiotics is considered ethically sound. The first obtains when antibiotics have no benefit to offer the patient, that is, they provide neither comfort nor life prolongation. The second situation occurs when the patient's quality of life has deteriorated to such a degree that the *patient* would not consider prolongation of that life to be beneficial.

If the available treatments of infection offer no reasonable hope of life prolongation, physicians have no obligation to offer them. In the parlance of medical ethics, truly futile treatment may be withheld based on a unilateral decision by the health care team, but that decision and the reasons for it should be communicated clearly to the patient and his or her loved ones (Youngner, 1990). Conversely, withholding antibiotics because of *poor quality of life* must revolve around the patient's values and life goals. Thus the decision to withhold antibiotics based on poor quality of life should be made either by the patient or by others acting for the patient using the patient's value system, an activity that is known as substituted judgment.

A third situation arises in which the diagnosis and treatment of an individual may be important for the community in which the individual lives. An obvious example is the evaluation and treatment of contagious diseases such as influenza and tuberculosis in close living situations such as a nursing home. This recently occurred in two nursing homes that experienced epidemics of influenza with several fatal cases (Andrus, Ostroff, Kobayashi, et al., 1992). It was important for other residents and staff of the nursing homes to undergo amantadine prophylaxis to protect not only themselves but also other residents in the facilities. In addition greater use of influenza immunization was encouraged during the next influenza season in both homes.

As the field of medical ethics matures, recognition that individuals have some responsibility to their communities is becoming more common (Ashley & O'Rourke, 1989; Loewy, 1992). We all grow, mature and gain sustenance from the communities in which we live, and we all have some obligation to help maintain the strength and integrity of those communities. The problem is that in the setting of treatment of contagious diseases part of the benefit of an individual's treatment goes to the community, but the individual assumes essentially all the treatment's burdens and risk. The question than becomes who will make the decision for or against treatment considering the benefits (and sometimes risk) of treatment for the community in addition to the benefits and burdens for the patient? Here our ethical paradigms fail to give us firm direction at this time (Miller, in press). However, the issue will not go away just because we have incomplete paradigms. Although the ethical community works on the development of proper paradigms, it is reasonable for individuals to assume some (reasonable level) of risk to gain some additional benefit for the community and the community be willing to assume some (reasonable level) of risk for an individual to avoid a severe burden or gain a large benefit. As examples a nursing home resident might take isoniazid prophylaxis for a low risk to tuberculosis reactivation to spare other residents on the outside chance that she or he does reactivate, and the medical community assumes some risk of HIV infection to care for AIDS patients.

MAKING THE PARADIGMS WORK: DATA ON FUTILITY

Despite the unresolved issues involving responsibility to community, in most practical situations the ethical paradigm for use of antibiotics at the end of life is clear, using the concept of benefits and burdens from the patient's viewpoint. What does one need to operate the paradigm effectively? For the criterion of no life prolongation, one needs data documenting those situations in which therapy is truly futile. The best evidence on the futility of antibiotics toward the end of life relates to severe dementia. In an important study by Fabiszewski, Volicer, and Volicer (1990), 104 nursing home residents who had either moderate or severe dementia were followed for an average of 10.4 months. Management meetings were held with the family of the nursing home resident to determine levels of care including whether to take a curative or palliative approach to infections. In the palliative approach, antibiotics could be given only in the occasional instance in which antibiotics improved the resident's comfort. Seventy-two percent of residents developed fever during the observation period, and those who developed fever had severer dementia than those who experienced no febrile episodes. Not surprisingly most of the residents who developed fever also had difficulties with mobility, swallowing, and double incontinence. Thus, conclusion 1 is that most dementia patients late in the course of their illness develop fever for a variety of reasons related to decreased host defense. Of those residents who developed fever, about one half were in the curative, antibiotics-use group and the other half were in the palliative, antibiotics-withheld group. Even when the fevers were fully evaluated, in 30% of episodes no source of infection could be found, and nearly 80% of those fevers in the palliative group resolved spontaneously. Thus, conclusion 2 is that most fevers in this setting are either not bacterial in origin or self-limited bacterial infections. Finally and most telling are the survival

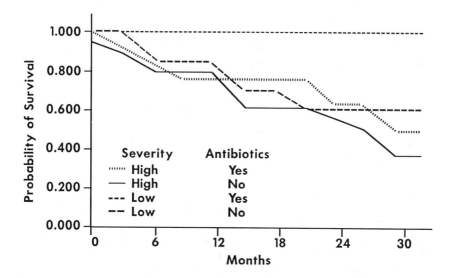

FIGURE 21.1   Survival analysis of patients with Alzheimer's disease by severity of disease and antibiotic use. Adapted from Fabiszewski et al. (1990), with
permission. Severity of dementia is measured by the Social Contact subscale of
the MAAC Behavioral Adjustment Scale (Ellsworth, 1971).

curves (Figure 21.1). Patients with severe dementia had nearly identical
curves whether they received antibiotics or not. The survival curves of
those with more moderate severity dementia demonstrate a different
point. Although residents treated with antibiotics lived somewhat longer
than those without antibiotic treatment, the families of one half of them
nevertheless chose no antibiotics for their family member.

More data are needed to identify other situations where antibiotics offer
no useful life prolongation. Additional clinical settings where this situation may pertain include persistent vegetative state, late metastatic disease, and end-stage cardiomyopathy, but the absence of data makes any
conclusions purely speculative.

EFFECTIVE COMMUNICATION

Next we examine the criterion for withholding treatment of infections because of poor quality of life. Recall that the guiding principle is benefits and
burdens *from the patient's viewpoint*. Many patients will be able to commu-

nicate and reason well enough to make this decision on their own, but many others will not. In the latter situation what is the evidence that either families or physicians make decisions on patients' behalf as the patients would themselves? Most data that exist relate to cardiopulmonary resuscitation (CPR), mechanical ventilation, and dialysis, rather than use of antibiotics, and they are not particularly encouraging. Uhlmann, Pearlman, and Cain (1988) used standardized scenarios to ask patients whether they would like to undergo CPR or ventilator support given specific situations described in each of the scenarios. They used the same scenarios to obtain decisions from the patient's spouses and personal physicians about whether the patient would want to undergo these procedures. The authors demonstrated that spouses and personal physicians incorrectly estimated the patients' resuscitation decision 25% to 50% of the time. Using a similar design Tomlinson, Howe, Notman, et al. (1990) showed that small changes in wording of instruction to the surrogate decision makers made important differences in their concordance with the patients' decisions. When the designated surrogates were asked "what should be done?," they demonstrated less concordance than when they were queried "what would the patient want done?" However, even in the improved situation, disagreement levels approximated 40%. These are not trivial differences in these life-and-death decisions.

It is possible that greater use of advance directives will help improve concordance between patients and their alternate decision makers. A complete exploration of advance directives is not possible here, but suffice it to say that the term usually refers to a document that patients can complete while able to make their own decisions to give guidance for times, either temporary or permanent, when they are unable to make decisions themselves. The documents can either give specific guidelines or designate an individual (known as the proxy or surrogate) to make those decisions on the patient's behalf. Alternatively the patient can give advance direction verbally. In any of these cases it is *essential* that the physician or designated surrogate go through "what-if" scenarios with the patient to clarify his or her intent. For example patients will commonly say, "No, no. Don't put me on any breathing machine. I don't want to live like a vegetable." It is necessary and often extremely revealing to follow up by asking questions such as, "What if you had a pneumonia from which you might recover completely, but you might need the breathing machine a week or so to help you recover and then you could return nearly to your previous state of health. Would you want the breathing machine then?" These what-if scenarios can be based either on standardized situations (Emanuel & Emanuel, 1989) or individualized to the patient's most likely problems.

Sometimes the patient or family requests that antibiotics be withheld, but the physician feels that the decision may be inappropriate. Issues to explore include whether the patient is severely depressed and making poor decisions on that basis, whether the patient has fears based on incorrect or correctable assumptions (e.g., that he or she will be inadequately treated for his or her cancer pain), or whether the proxy has any conflict of interest.

So far we have discussed the situation where the benefits are minimal from one of two perspectives: life prolongation or quality of life, and the only options that have been considered have been a curative approach involving aggressive diagnosis and therapy, or a palliative approach that uses antibiotics only to enhance comfort. A third approach is possible and often advisable. Situations frequently arise in which the benefit of treatment is real but small and easily overwhelmed by a burdensome therapy such as a very aggressive approach to diagnosis and treatment. In this situation there is room for an intermediate approach between fully aggressive and strictly palliative. That approach emphasizes limited investigation; empiric, easily administered medications; and comfort over diagnostic and treatment precision. This can be used as an empiric "test of functional reserve"; that is, if the patient is able to help fight off the infection or the infection is not too severe or overwhelming, then some reasonable quality of life may yet be possible. Although this approach has not been tested rigorously, it does have the advantage of avoiding very painful and burdensome therapy and may offer some benefits. In practice it has been a comforting middle ground for families and other loved ones.

CASE EXAMPLES OF DECISION MAKING

Regardless of who is involved in the decision and the specific life support being discussed, accurate and sensitive communication is essential. We have recently collected data about effective and ineffective methods of making decisions regarding withholding or withdrawing life support. The setting is the medical intensive care unit at Saint Louis University Hospital, and the issue is usually whether to withdraw mechanical ventilator support. Although both female and male physicians are involved, masculine pronouns will be used consistently here to protect their confidentiality. In similar fashion the distinction between attendings and fellows in training (both of whom are involved) will be obscured.

The first case demonstrates that the patient or family often needs prognostic information in simple, understandable terms and reassurance regarding comfort and support. Physicians, wrapped up in the attempt to help the patient improve, often give too much medical detail that can obscure the main points of interest for the family. The patient is a 78-year-old woman with severe underlying lung disease on a mechanical ventilator with respiratory failure when the diagnosis of lung cancer is made. The physician   initiates the following discussion with the family.

> Doctor: *How do you do? I just want to update you on what was going on and discuss new information after today's cytology report. . . . Okay. You heard about the report that came back, the one test showing that there is lung cancer there on the right lung.*
>
> Husband: *Yeah, lung cancer.*
>
> Doctor: *Which, as I told you when we went down there last week, that we were suspicious of it. Interestingly, the samples that we got during that procedure came back suspicious. It was the samples that we got back in the secretions after the procedure that turned positive. And that happens sometimes because you open up some areas during the bronchoscopy. . . .*

After more information and discussion, a decision not to do cardiopulmonary resuscitation if the heart stops is confirmed, and the conversation moves to use of the mechanical ventilator. The following interaction ensues.

> Daughter: *If you took the tube out like that, what would happen?*
>
> Doctor: *If we took her tube out right now, yeah—*
>
> [All talking at once]
>
> Doctor: *Well, if we took the tube right now, . . . I think her blood oxygen, even if we gave her some oxygen, might not be high enough, and the carbon dioxide would build up and she would slip into respiratory failure. And I think that would probably happen within a matter of hours just based on . . . I could be wrong. As I said, there's at least a 5% or 10% chance that she could make it. If we shut it off and give her good suction and try to do all this other, lots of other things and put her on a lot of oxygen by mask after we took the tube out.*

Although this physiologic information is of some help, the family appears more interested in knowing whether the patient would suffer or not. Postdiscussion notes from one daughter indicated that the most helpful information was regarding "her cancer and the fact that nothing could *reasonably* [italics added] be done to cure the cancer" and "the results when removing ventilator."

A second case demonstrates the conflict families can feel withdrawing life support from loved ones and their need for reassurance that the patient's comfort will be protected during the process of withdrawing life support. It involves a 75-year-old woman with a newly diagnosed large stomach cancer, who experienced cardiac arrest and presently is on a mechanical ventilator with postanoxic encephalopathy. The physician is speaking with the patient's daughter and grand-daughter.

Daughter: *We understand it better. It's hard to understand, you know, medical terms for us, but we understand what you're saying, and we don't feel that that she would want that* [continuation on the ventilator]. . . . *We just decided we don't want to prolong the agony. It* [their removing her from the ventilator] *has nothing to do with love, it's just that we* [becoming emotional] . . . *we know that, uh, the end, what the end results are.*

A nurse who knew the patient and family and attended the conference indicated in a postdiscussion note, "the family's main concern was the method used to remove lines. . . . It was important to explain the weaning process. It was helpful to use layman's terms to explain the 'death with dignity' and 'no pain'—using all comfort measures available.

A third case demonstrates that when a physician pushes for decisions made a priori, results are often counterproductive. It is known from other arenas of inquiry (Fisher & Ury, 1981) that other methods for negotiating decisions have greater likelihood for generating enduring, satisfying conclusions.

The patient is an 86-year-old woman, who has been limited to bed and chair before her current illness and is now in the intensive care unit with severe pneumonia, malnutrition, congestive heart failure, and renal insufficiency. The physician convenes a conference with the patient's husband and niece and uses the first 5 minutes of the discussion to detail the number and severity of the patient's problems. The husband responds, and the following interaction occurs.

Husband: *You trying to tell me that she's going to die or something?*

Doctor: *I'm trying to say that her likelihood of coming off the ventilator is low. Extremely low, in fact. The likelihood that she will be on the ventilator for a prolonged period of time and continue to develop one complication after the other like infections, sepsis, . . .*

The physician spends several more minutes listing the potential complications, leading to the following summary and exchange:

Doctor: *So the point I'm making is, I'm asking you with all this informa-*
tion, you know, what would you like us to do should her heart
stop beating. Would you like us to give her chest compressions
and revive it?

Husband: *Yes, sure, sure would.*

Doctor: *Even though you feel that,—even though you know it's not go-*
ing to change anything for her. It is only going to prolong things.

Husband: *It can't hurt. . . .*

The physician focuses again on the malnutrition and raises the specter that
the patient may have cancer, resulting in the following exchange.

Husband: *I don't believe it. I don't believe she has cancer. TB either. Her*
heart may be bad. I could see that part. I would say, I'd like you to
do anything you can to try and keep her going.

Doctor: *Even though you realize that it's not going to change things. Her*
body's not strong enough.

Husband: *How could it hurt? Sure couldn't hurt.*

Doctor: *It just prolongs things.*

Husband: *Well, there's always a chance that if you rest awhile you may*
come back.

Doctor: *Only temporarily.*

Husband: *I wouldn't care if it was only for a day or for a week, a month.*

In the field of mediation and negotiation, these exchanges represent
what is known as "bargaining from positions," which is notorious for leading to hardening of positions and preventing movement toward identification of reasonable solutions (Fisher & Ury, 1981). A better method for
creative problem solving involves focusing on interests rather than positions and inventing options for satisfying those interests (Fisher & Ury,
1981).

In this case the physician attempts again to convince the family of the futility of the situation. The husband tells about his wife's unusual sleeping
positions and that a little sleep has often returned her to health in the past.
The physician then states the following:

Doctor: *I just feel it's my duty to let you know where things stand*
today. . . . They look pretty dismal, and without meaning to be

*discouraging, I do feel that you need to make some informed deci-
sions, and what decisions you make are totally yours. . . .*

The physician apparently expects that by providing the family with a
shaded view of the patient's poor prognosis, they will come to the conclusion he wants them to draw, and he becomes very frustrated when they resist. Several more exchanges occur, during which physician's and family's
positions are restated. During one of the exchanges, the husband makes the
following comment:

Husband: *Well, at least we could try. That's my answer. I couldn't give no
            other.*

Doctor: *Well, you—it's your decision and if you would like for us to try,
            you know, we can do that. We can't deny her that.*

Here the husband states his interest to give his best effort for his wife, and
the physician fails to explore his concerns, returning instead to discussing
positions.

Now that his original argument has failed, the physician tries another
approach, nearly 15 minutes into the discussion:

Doctor: *What do you think she would have wished. Have you ever had an
            opportunity to discuss this with her in the past?*

The family indicates that she never discussed these issues, and this approach goes nowhere. They are about ready to disband, when the physician asks the niece if she has any questions, and she responds:

Niece: *I would like to ask how long they leave them on the ventilator.*

Doctor: *As long as she—*[needs it.]

Niece: *I mean she'll just stay on it—indefinitely?*

Doctor: *Yeah. Yes.*

Husband: *Shouldn't she be propped up, have that* [the endotracheal tube]
            *taken out for a while? Seems to me like if she was . . . sit up
            straight more, she could breath better.*

Niece: *And take the ventilator out?*

Husband: *Yeah.*

Doctor: *I can't do that. Like I said, if I take the ventilator off, she'll stop breathing within less than five minutes. You just said you wanted to keep her going, right?*

Husband: *Not on the ventilator.*

Doctor: *You do not want her on the ventilator?*

Niece: *You just want them to take it out and sit her up?*

Husband: *Yeah, let's try something, anything.*

Doctor: *What if she stops breathing within 5 minutes?*

Husband: *You don't know that any more than I do, do you?*

Doctor: *I'm reasonably certain she won't be able to breath on her own. Assuming she does. Let's take a scenario. If she does, what would you like us to do?*

Husband: *Oh, I would come down and be witness—I'd come down and witness. I really would. If you want to do it that way. I would come here and watch it.*

Doctor: *We usually don't do that in the presence of relatives.*

Husband: *Well, in fact that's probably the only way I would consent to it.*

Doctor: *I don't think we'd be able to do it in your presence.*

Husband: *Mmm.*

Doctor: *So, which means you're telling us we've got to keep her on the ventilator.*

Now that the physician has been pushing for a specific conclusion rather than exploring concerns and solutions, he is in a poor position to follow up on the family's clear misperception about the severity of the patient's pulmonary condition. Further the physician's inflexibility prevents him from considering an innovative approach to the problem, such as allowing the husband to observe the results of extubation.

Another case demonstrates a more successful approach. It involves a 46-year-old woman who had severe systemic lupus erythematosus, chronic renal failure on continuous ambulatory peritoneal dialysis (CAPD), thrombocytopenia, and leukopenia who was admitted to another hospital with a stroke and seizures. She was transferred to the present hospital, where she suffered an intracerebral hemorrhage. The physician and the patient's husband meet to discuss her current situation and decide what to do.

Doctor: *Alright, well let me sort of go through it again as I understand it, okay? When your wife went home last month, it looked as if things were a lot better, okay? And she was doing okay for a while, and we got her back on the CAPD, etc. And then she took ill some weeks ago or days ago and was hospitalized at [another local hospital], correct? And she had seizures after that, if I remember correctly.*

The physician then details the patient's transfer to the present hospital and her improvement over the first several days, leading up to the following.

Doctor: *And then something happened this morning. She was found in her bed sort of in a coma-like, so to speak. Unresponsive.*

The physician than indicated that they put her on a mechanical ventilator and obtained a computed tomographic scan of the brain, which showed a huge intracerebral hemorrhage. She was seen by the neurologist, and the conclusion was that there was "very little if any hope that she will ever be able to do anything again. Can't breathe for herself again. Can't eat. [etc.]" Continuing:

Doctor: *. . . so, I guess the question is, would it be appropriate to continue these artificial life support measures when you know that there is no hope for recovery, or would it be more appropriate to simply turn them off and let nature take its course.*

Husband: *Yeah, I think, um, I know she would. She would want us to turn them off. Because she expressed to me she's just not interested in even a low, low quality of life.*

Doctor: *I see. . . . so then, you would request that we turn off all the mechanical equipment and, uh—*

Husband: *Yeah. I request you cut it off. . . . I've got one question, though.*

Doctor: *Mm-hmm.*

Husband: *When you cut off all the equipment, how long do you think? Do you think she'll die right away?*

Doctor: . . . *Once the ventilator's stopped, then what happens is there is no more breathing. Okay, breathing stops. Within a matter of a minute or two, there is no more fresh oxygen, and the heart will stop beating in a normal matter. It will start doing something we call fluttering or fibrillation and within another 3 minutes to 5 minutes, the heart will stop completely.*

Husband: . . . *Well, the way I look at it, she's not in any pain, is she?*

Doctor: *Oh, no. There's so much destruction in the brain that she's totally unaware of what is going on.*

Husband: *Okay. That's my only concern. I just don't want her in any pain.*

Here the husband's concerns surfaced and were satisfactorily responded to by the physician, facilitated by the husband's ability to express his concerns clearly and directly as well as by the physician's responses.

To summarize, in end-of-life decision making patients and families need prognostic information and reassurance regarding the provision of full comfort care in simple, clear language. Often (but not always) they are willing to hear what are reasonable expectations rather than focusing on the rare or unusual. Frequently it is important to explain the actual processes used during withholding or withdrawing therapy that help keep the patient comfortable. Families in particular often feel internal conflict. They do not want to give up hope on someone they love, and yet they do not want to extend the patient's misery to no useful purpose. They also struggle with their own needs (e.g., "I can't live without her") and sense of loss. In this setting a focus on concerns, an alert ear to recognize internal conflicts, and a search for creative methods for meeting identified needs works much better than any hard and fast rules about when to continue and when to stop therapy. Finally an ability to empathize (Spiro, 1992) is an invaluable asset.

CONCLUSION

When to withhold or withdraw antibiotics is a difficult, complex issue that arises often toward the end of life, and this issue occurs particularly frequently in older patients. These are difficult decisions to make, and they should be; when to allow someone to die peacefully and when to fight hard and long requires careful thought and discussion among the people who really care about the patient—the patient, the family and other loved ones, and the physicians and other health care providers.

It is difficult to improve on the description of this issue in the *New Eng-*

land Journal of Medicine article on the physician's responsibility toward hopelessly ill patients (Wanzer, Adelstein, Cranford, et al., 1984): "Few topics in medicine are more complicated, more controversial, and more emotionally charged than treatment of the hopelessly ill. Technology competes with compassion, legal precedent lags, and controversy is inevitable" (p. 959). One does well not to fear conflict in this situation. Conflict indicates that people care, in this case that they care about the patient. Rather one should fear the situation where no one really cares about the patient, and the decision to withhold or withdraw antibiotics becomes too easy.

Wanzer et al. (1984) made another important observation about this situation, specifically: "The physician has a special obligation to listen to the doubts and fears expressed by patients who are hopelessly or terminally ill" (p. 957). The ethical paradigm for use of antibiotics at the end of life is clear, although the social justice component needs additional work. What is most needed now are (a) better data about situations where antibiotics offer no life prolongation and (b) methods for improving communication between health care providers and patients and their families.

REFERENCES

Andrus, J. K., Ostroff, S. M., Kobayashi, J. M., Horan, J. M., & Fleming, D. W. (1992). Patient-care directives and infection control: The potential conflict of interest during epidemics in long-term care facilities. *American Journal of Preventive Medicine, 8*, 203–206.

Ashley, B. M., & O'Rourke, K. D. (1989). *Healthcare ethics: A theological analysis* (3rd ed.). St. Louis, MO: Catholic Health Association of the United States.

Ellsworth, R. B. (1971). *The MACC Behavioral Adjustment Scale* (rev. 1971 manual). Los Angeles, CA: Western Psychological Services.

Emanuel, L. L., & Emanuel, E. J. (1989). The Medical Directive: A new comprehensive advance care document. *Journal of the American Medical Association, 261*, 3288–3293.

Fabiszewski, K. J., Volicer, B., & Volicer, L. (1990). Effect of antibiotic treatment on outcome of fevers in institutionalized Alzheimer patients. *Journal of the American Medical Association, 263*, 3168–3172.

Fisher, R., & Ury, W. (1981). *Getting to yes: Negotiating agreement without giving in.* Boston: Houghton Mifflin.

Loewy, E. H. (1992). Advance directives and surrogate laws: Ethical instruments or moral cop-out [Commentary]? *Archives of Internal Medicine, 152*, 1973–1976.

Marin, P. P., Bayer, A. J., Tomlinson, A., & Pathy, M. S. J. (1989). Attitudes of hospital doctors in Wales to use of intravenous fluids and antibiotics in the terminally ill. *Postgraduate Medical Journal, 65*, 650–652.

Miller, D. K. (in press). Ethical principles [Chapter K22]. In J. E. Morley (Ed.), *Geriatric care.* St. Louis, MO: G. W. Manning.

President's Commission for the Study of Ethical Problems in Medicine and

Biomedical and Behavioral Research (1983). *Deciding to forego life-sustaining treatment: A report on the ethical, medical, and legal issues in treatment decisions.* Washington, DC: U.S. Government Printing Office.

Spiro, H. (1992). What is empathy and can it be taught? *Annals of Internal Medicine, 116,* 843–846.

Tomlinson, T., Howe, K., Notman, M., & Rossmiller, D. (1990). An empirical study of proxy consent for elderly persons. *Gerontologist, 30,* 54–64.

Uhlmann, R. F., Pearlman, R. A., & Cain, K. C. (1988). Physicians' and spouses' predictions of elderly patients' resuscitation preferences. *Journal of Gerontology, 43,* M115–M121.

Wanzer, S. H., Adelstein, J., Cranford, R. E., Federman, D. D., Hook, E. D., Moertel, C. G., Safar, P., Stone, A., Taussig, H. B., & van Eys, J. (1984). The physician's responsibility toward hopelessly ill patients. *New England Journal of Medicine, 310,* 955–959.

Youngner, S. J. (1990). Futility in context [Editorial]. *Journal of the American Medical Association, 264,* 1295–1296.

Index

A

Accidents, death from, 153
Acquired immunity, 4
Acquired immunodeficiency syn-
    drome (AIDS), 27, 68, 154–155
  age-diferences in progression of
    illness, 68
  gender differences in, 154–155
  stressful life events and, 115
Acute prostatitis, 183
  treatment of, 186–187
Age and stress, animal studies on,
    143–147
Age-related thymic involution,
    97–109
  plasticity of thymus-neuroendo-
    crine interactions in aging,
    103–105
  role of nutritional elements, 103
  thymus rejuvenation in old age
    by hormonal or nutritional
    treatment, 105–107
Aging
  age-related changes in NK activ-
    ity, 67, 76, 141
  changes in factor release and re-
    ceptor expression in, 78t
  and elevated sympathetic activ-
    ity, 141–147

gender, immunity and, 155–159
host defense in, 57–62
immune dysfunction and, 66–81
infections that increase with, 2t
inflammatory factors and, 72–76
Metchnikoff's theory of, 4–5
relationship of infectious
    mortality and, 3t, 68
stress and, 137f
AIDS. *See* Acquired immunode-
    ficiency syndrome
al-Razi, Aku Bekr Mohammad ibn
    Zakariya, 4
Alzheimer's disease, 158
  survival analysis of patients
    with, 287f
Amantadine, 196, 248–249, 250,
    252
  cost of, 254
  in influenza treatment in elderly,
    260t
  prophylaxis, 259–261, 285
  resistance to, 254–255
  timing of administration,
    252–253
  toxicity of, 253–254
Aminoglycosides, 195
Anergy, 234
Antibiotic pharmacokinetics, 7

Antibiotic therapy, diarrhea and, 225

Antibiotics. *See Clostridium difficile* infections in elderly, *and* Withholding antibiotics

Antibody response to influenza vaccine, 49, 250

Antigenic variation or "drift" of influenza viruses, 43, 250–251

Arginine, 103

Asymptomatic bacteriuria, 181–182

Atypical pneumonia, 193

Autoimmune disease, 154
  in women, 157

Autoimmunity, 5

Autonomic nervous system, 116

Azithromycin, 195

Aztreonam, 195–196

B

Bacteriuria, 181–182

"Ball-point pen" technique, 19

"Bargaining from positions," 292

Beta carotene, 240

Beta-endorphin
  effects of, on immune system, 136t
  and immune function, 134–137
  NK cell activity and, 134
  physiologic effects of, 136–137
  stress and, 137–138

Bismuth subsalicylate, 225–226

Brain regions, in neural modulation of immune reactivity, 116–117

C

Caloric restriction, 241–242

Cancer, 153
  exercise and, 136–137

Cardiovascular diseases, 153

Caregivers, women as, 155

Caregiving, mental health impairments and, 158

Catecholamines
  macrophages and, 119–120
  in NK cell activity, 119–120
  physical stressors and, 141, 146

Catheter-related urinary tract infection, 187–189
  prevention of, 188
  treatment of, 188–189

Cellular, or cell-mediated, immunity, 28–31, 42, 56–57
  classic role for, 56–57
  theory of, 4

Central nervous system, immune system and, 116

Cerebrovascular diseases, 153

Chronic obstructive pulmonary diseases, 153

Circumlunar rhythms, 168

Clairithromycin, 195

Clindamycin, 196, 217

Clostridium difficile infection in elderly, 216–227
  abdominal radiograph of patient with recurrent diarrhea, 222f
  age-related prevalence rate of, 219–220
  diagnosis of, 217–219
  historical perspective on, 216–217
  in nursing home patients, 221–224
  problem with tissue culture assay for, 218–219
  relapses of, in elderly, 221
  spectrum of diseases among elderly, 219–224
  treatment of, 224–227

Cockroft-Gault equation, 259
Colon. *See Clostridium difficile* infection in elderly
Community, responsibility to, 285–286
Concanavilin A (Con A), 72, 83
Congenital hypopituitarism, 101
Consensus conferences, 273
Continuing medical education (CME) literature, 273
Cystic fibrosis, 252
Cystitis
    pyelonephritis versus, 182–183
    treatment of, 184
Cytotoxic T lymphoctes (CTL), 42, 43, 57
    age and, 45–49
    in aged versus young mice, 62
    responses to vaccination, 47–49

D
Depression, gender and, 157–159
Diabetes, experimentally induced, 101
Diarrhea
    antibiotic therapy and, 225
    following antibiotics, 217
    in pseudomembranous colitis, 220
    recurrent, 221
    treatment for, 220
"Disproportional benefit," 284
Distal ileum, 217
DNA synthesis, decline in, 70
Down's syndrome, 103

E
Elderly, infections in the, 68
Electronic thermometers, 223–224
Endocrinopathies, 101
Endogenous opioids, 133–138

Beta-endorphin and immune function, 134–137
    physiological changes and decline in opioid system, 135t
Epinephrine (EP)
    CRH in, 143–146
    in immune reactivity, 120
Erythromycin, 195, 196
Estrogens, gender differences and, 156–157
Ethambutol (EMB), 22, 23
Ethical guidelines, 284–286
    withholding treatment and, 285–286
Extrapulmonary tuberculosis, 24–25

F
Falls, amantadine as cause of, 253

G
Gamma interferon (IFN-γ), 29, 33, 45, 72
Gender
    aging, immunity and, 153–159
    depression and, 157–159
    health and, 153–155
    hormones and, 155–157
    immunity and, 155–157, 157–159
    NK activity and, 76
Gerontology, 152
Granulocytes, 79
Group dynamics/group process, 273–274
Growth hormone (GH)
    gender differences and, 156
    hypersecretion of, 102
Growth hormone treatment, 100
    thymulin and, 101
Guillain-Barré syndrome, 251, 269

H
Health, gender and, 153–155

Health Belief Model, 266, 267
Hemagglutinin (HA) glycopro-
teins, 43
Heterotypic immunity, 57, 58–61
Hippocratic school theory of dis-
eases, 4
HIV infection, age-related pattern
of, 68
"Homing" molecules, 35f
Homotypic immunity, 57, 58
Hormones, gender and, 155–157
Hospital acquired bacterial pneu-
monia, 194
Humoral immunity, 42
"Hyperadaptosis," 169
Hyperthyroidism, 101
Hypothalamus-pituitary axis,
97–98
Hypothyroidism, 101

I

Immune deficiency of aging, 66–80
cross-sectional studies of, 67
genetic influences on immune
function, 69
IL-6 production by mouse
spleen cells, 74
inflammatory factors and aging,
72–76
longitudinal versus cross-sectional studies of, 67
morbidity and mortality of infectious diseases in elderly, 68
nonimmune host defense functions, 76–79
problem of studying, 66–67
T-cell function in aging host,
69–72
Immune dysfunction in elderly,
malnutrition and, 238–239
Immune function
Beta-endorphin and, 134–137
characteristics of, 79t

genetic influences on, 69
Immune-neuroendocrine pathways, 99f
Immune system
arginine and, 103
Beta-endorphin's effect on, 136t
central nervous system and, 116
loss and loneliness and, 115
stressful life events and, 115–116
zinc and, 103
Immunity
aging and, 5
caloric restriction and longevity,
241–242
effect of micronutrient deficiency on, 236–237t
gender and, 155–157, 157–159
historical perspective on, 3–4
micronutrient deficiencies and,
234–235
nutritional deficiencies and,
233–234
prospects, 7–9
Immunity to influenza in elderly,
41–52
age and CTL activity, 45–47
cellular, or cell-mediated, immunity against influenza, 42
effectiveness of vaccines against
influenza in elderly, 49–52
effect of aging and vaccination
on influenza-specific cytotoxicity, 48t
humoral immunity against influenza, 42
nasal wash antibody response to
vaccine, 51t
serum antibody response to vaccine, 50t, 250–251
susceptibility of elderly to influenza, 41–45
Immunization, reduced responses
to in the elderly, 49, 68, 250

Immunogerontology, 82
Immunosenescence
  characteristics of, 153
  definition of, 152–153
Infections
  frequency of, with age, 2t
  prospects, 7–9
  relationship of infectious
    mortality and aging, 3t
Infectious diseases
  historical perspective on, 1–3
  morbidity and mortality of, el-
    derly, 68
Infective endocarditis, 6
Influenza, 153, 154, 196
  acquisition of, 193–194
  amantadine treatment for, 260t
    cost of, 254
    toxicity of, 253–254
  as cause of death, 41, 248
  chemoprophylaxis for, 252
  current recommendations for
    control of epidemics in insti-
    tutional settings, 255–261
  host defense against, 42–43,
    56–57
  incidence of, 41
  respiratory illness and, 257t
  timing of administration of,
    252–253
  vaccination for, 41, 196–197, 249,
    250–252, 255–256
  vaccination rates against, 266
Influenza in aged mice, 56–62
  heterotypic immunity, 58–61
  homotypic immunity, 58
  host defense in aging, 57–62
  vaccines and aging, 62
  viral shedding from nose and
    lungs, 61t
Influenza in long-term care facili-
    ties (LTCFs), 248–261
  antiviral use, 259–261

infection control, 259
  prevention and control recom-
    mendations for, 249–255
  surveillance of, 256–259
  transmission of, 259
INH (Rifamate), 22, 23, 24, 25
  side effects/toxicity of, 23–24
Innovation, adoption of, 275
Insulin, in thymic function,
    102–103
Intraabdominal sepsis, 6

K
Knowledge dissemination, four
    functions of, 272–273

L
Lactobacillus theory of aging, 5
Latex agglutination test, 219
Life expectancies, 1–2
  in men versus women, 153
Liver function tests (LFTs), 22–24
Longevity
  caloric restriction and immunity
    and, 241–242
  increase in, 2
Lymphoid organs
  age-related decline in NA in-
    nervation of, 121–123
  innervation of, 117–121

M
Macrophages, 119–120
Major histocompatibility complex
    (MHC) molecules, 42
Malnutrition, 233–234
  immune dysfunction in elderly
    and, 238–239
Marital status and satisfaction,
    158–159
Melatonin, 166–167
Memory T cells, 82–84
Menopause, 157

"Metabolic aging," 169
"Metabolic immunosuppression," 169
Metchnikoff, Elie, 4–5
Methicillin-resistant *Staphylococcus aureus* (MRSA), 199–212
  acute care institutions, 200
  aged patient, 200–201
  in chronic care facilities, 202–203t
  as endemic organism in long-term care, 204–205
  as epidemic organism in long-term care, 205–206
  in long-term care, prevalence of, 201–204
  management of outbreaks in long-term care, 208
  methods of control in chronic care facilities, 210–211
  role of antimicrobial decolonization in long-term care, 208–209
  and role of nursing homes, 201
  routine management of carrier in long-term care, 206–208
  significance of, 200–201
Metroidazole, 223, 226
Micronutrient deficiencies, immunity and, 234–235, 236–237t
Mind-body interactions, 133
MRSA. *See* Methicillin-resistant *Staphylococcus aureus*
"MRSA reservoirs," 201

N

Naive T cells, 82–84
Natural killer (NK) cell activity
  age-related changes in, 141
  age-related decrease in, 142
  Beta-endorphin and, 134, 137–138
  depression and, 158
  exercise and, 136–137
  mind-body interactions and, 133
  neuropeptide Y in reduction of, 142
  stress and, 137, 138
  stressful mental activity and, 136
  in young and old rats, 126
Natural killer (NK) cell function, 67, 119–120
  age-related pattern of activity, 76–79
  factors influencing, 76
Natural killer (NK) cells, definition and description of, 155–156
Neural-immune interactions, 115–117
Neuraminidase (NA) glycoproteins, 43
Neuroendocrine system, 116
  age-associated alterations in, 105
Neuroendocrinimmune interactions, 97–98
Neuroendocrinologic pathways, 98
Neuropeptide Y
  age-related increase in, 141–142
  CRH in, 144–147
  in NK cell activity, 142
Niacin, 241
NK cells. *See* Natural killer (NK) cell *entries*
Noradrenergic sympathetic innervation, 114–127
  of aged rat spleen, 123–125
  complex role for, 119
  evidence for neural-immune interactions, 115–117
  innervation of lymphoid organs, 117–121
  of lymphoid organs, age-related decline in, 121–123

NK cell activity and antibody
   response in young and old
   rats, 126
other lymphoid organs and aging, 125
plasticity of NA nerves in aged
   rodent spleen, 126
Norepinephrine
   age-related increase in, 141
   CRH and, 143–147
Nutrients, as drugs, 240–241
Nutrition
   C. difficile infection and, 221
   change of nutritional status in
      elderly, 235
   immunity in elderly and,
      238–242
Nutritional deficiencies, 233–234

O

Oral contraceptives, 157
Oral rehydration therapy, 225, 226

P

Parental immunization, 49
Pasteur, Louis, 4
Periarteriolarlymphatic sheath
   (PALS), 117–118
Peripheral blood lymphocytes, 71t
Pharmacodynamics, age in, 7
Phosphoproteins (PPNs), 87–89
"Pineal aging clock" hypothesis,
   169
"Pineal clock," 168
"Pineal complex," 167–168
Pineal gland, 166–172
   adaptability and, 167
   as adaptive process, 167–169
   general mechanism of, 170–172
"Pineal interventions," 169
Pineal peptides, 169
Pirazinamide (PZA), 22, 23

Pneumonia, 56, 153, 154
   as cause of death, 248
   mortality due to, 58
   in older patient, 5–7
Pneumonia in elderly, 191–197
   community-acquired pneumo-
      nia, 192–194
   hospital-acquired bacterial
      pneumonia, 194
   prevention of, 196–197
   treatment of, 194–196
"Ponce de Leon" hypothesis, 62
Postantibiotic pseudomembranous
   colitis, 217
Primaxin, 195
Prolactin-secreting tumors, 102
"Proportionally beneficial," 284
Protein-calorie malnutrition and
   immunity, 233–234
   in nursing home residents, 235
Protein kinase function, 87–89
Protein kinase system, 87
Pseudomembranous colitis, 218,
   220–221
Psychoneuroimmunology (PNI),
   152
Psychosomatic diseases, 115
Pyelonephritis
   antibiotics in management of,
      186t
   cystitis versus, 182–183
Pyridoxine, 24, 235, 240, 241

Q

Quality improvement techniques,
   274
"Quality teams," 274
Quinolones, 186, 196

R

Reasoned action theory, 273
Respiratory illness, 257t
Rheumatoid arthritis, 154, 157

Rhinotracheitis, 56
Riboflavin, 235
   high intake of, 241
Rifamate. *See* INH
Rifampin (RIF), 22, 23, 25
Rimantadine, 259

S

Schizophrenia, 155
Selye, Hans, 137
Smallpox, 4
"Spread," 272
Stress
   gender differences in, 154
   NK cell activity and, 137, 138
   types of, 137
Stressful life events, depression
      and, 157
Suppressor T cells, 155

T

T-cell proliferative response,
      69–72, 82–84
   gender differences in, 155
   GH and, 156
T cells
   age-dependent increase in
      P-glycoprotein in, 85f
   age-dependent loss in, 82
   calcium-resistant, 83–84
   function of, in aging host, 69–72
   gender differences in, 68
   growth hormone (GH), 155, 156
   Heterogeneity and responsive-
      ness in aging mice, 82–93
   IL-4 production by, 84–87
   naive-to-memory cell transition
      in, 82–84
   proliferative ability of, 70–72, 83
   response to Anti-CD3 and Anti-
      CD2, 73t

   thymus and, 69–70
   in tuberculosis, 36f, 37f
Theory of cellular immunity, 4
Theory of old age, 4–5
Thymic epithelial cells, 100
Thymic peptides, 100
Thymulin, 101–103
   age-dependent decline of, 104f,
      104–105
   alterations of, in disendocrino-
      pathies, 102f
   recovery of secretion, 105–107
Thymus
   description and definition of, 100
   insulin and, 102–103
   NA innervation, 126
   in neuroendocrine interactions,
      98
   pineal gland and, 170–171
   rejuvenation by hormonal or
      nutritional treatments,
      105–107
   in T-cell system, 69–70
   zinc bioavailabilty and, 100
Thymus-neuroendocrine interac-
      tions, 100–103
   plasticity of, in aging, 103–105
Thyroidectomy, 101
Thyrotropin-releasing hormone
      (TRH), 170–172
T-lymphocyte, 57–58
T-lymphocyte function, 121–122
Toxic megacolon, 222f
Trimethoprim-sulfamethoxazole,
      189
Tuberculin skin test in elderly,
      18–19
   positive reaction to, 19–20
Tuberculosis (TB)
   in aging patients, 6

acquired cellular response in
    young mice to infection with,
    28–31
case rate among elderly, 16–17,
    17t, 18t
drug toxicity, monitoring for,
    22–23
elderly at risk for, 20–21
in elderly patients, 15–25
extrapulmonary tuberculosis,
    24–25
increased resistance in elderly
    mice to, 35
increased susceptibility of old
    mice to, 31–35
later retesting of nonreactors in
    nursing homes, 21
positive tuberculin skin test,
    19–20
preventive therapy, 23–24
prospects for elderly persons
    with, 35–38
recrudescence of, 16
rise in incidence of, 27–28, 38
T-cell response and young mice,
    28–31
T cells in old mice, 31–35
treatment considerations in el-
    derly, 21–22
tuberculin skin test in elderly,
    18–19
Two-step method, of tuberculin
    skin test, 19

U

Urinary tract infection in elderly,
    179–189
acute prostatitis, 183
bacteriuria in older persons,
    181t
catheter-related, 187–189

cystitis versus pyelonephritis,
    182–183
factors predisposing to, 180t
incidence of bacteriuria, 181–182
microbiology of, 180–181
in older patients, 6, 7
pathogenesis of, 179–180
treatment of, 184, 185t
treatment of acute prostatitis,
    186–187
treatment of cystitis, 184
Urosepsis, 186t

V

Vaccination for influenza, 249,
    250–252, 255–256
contraindications for, 251
effectiveness of, 251
Vaccine delivery, 265–280
combination intervention pro-
    gram, 270, 271–272
core model and hypothesis, 275
education programs alone for
    physicians, 269–270
health maintenance organiza-
    tion (HMO) intervention pro-
    gram, 271–272
Health Promotion Clinic inter-
    vention program, 270
intervention studies, 269–272
patient-based factors in, 266–268
patient reminder intervention
    program, 272
peer comparison feedback inter-
    vention program, 270–271,
    274–275
physician-based factors in,
    268–269
physician feedback intervention,
    271
target groups for, 265–266

Western New York Geriatric
    Education Center Model,
    272–280
Vaccines, aging and, 62
Vancomycin, 223, 226
Von Behring, Emil, 4
Vitamins, 234
    deficiencies of, in nursing home
        residents, 235
    high intakes of, 240, 241
    in malnutrition and immunity
        of elderly, 238, 239–241

W
Western New York Geriatric
    Education Center Model,
    272–280
    chart review procedure, 276–277
    core model and hypothesis, 275
    evaluation of small-group pro-
        cess, 279–280
    information on medical technol-
        ogy, 275–276
    method, 277–279

physician attitudes and knowl-
    edge, 279
preliminary results, 279–280
rationale, 272–275
small-group process, 277–279
study population, 276
subject selection process, 276
Withholding antibiotics, 283–297
    bargaining, 292
    buy-in approach, 275
    case examples of decision mak-
        ing, 289–296
    data on futility, 286–287
    effective communication,
        287–289
    ethical guidelines, 284–286
    poor quality of life as criterion
        for, 287
Women, as caregivers, 155

Z
Zinc, 240
    deficiency of, 103

Springer Publishing Company

MEMORY FUNCTION AND AGING-RELATED DISORDERS

John E. Morley, MD, **Rodney M. Coe,** PhD,
Randy Strong, PhD, and
George T. Grossberg, MD,
Editors

Up-to-date, authoritative material on basic mechanisms of memory processes. The text is divided into sections covering fundamentals of memory function, human memory and approaches to Alzheimer's Disease, and the diagnosis and management of dementing disorders.

Part I. Fundamentals of Memory Function
Role of Tropic Factors in Neuronal Development and Aging / Molecular Biology of Information Storage in the Nervous System During Aging / Interaction of Hormones and Neurotransmitters in the Modulation of Memory Storage / Neuropeptides as Modulators of Memory / Age-Related Changes and Spreading Activation: Implications for Connectionist Models of Cognitive Aging.

Part II. Animal and Human Memory Approaches to Alzheimer's Disease
Age-related Changes in the Physiology and Cognitive Ability of Senescence Accelerated Mice / Defective Axonal Transport: A Mechanism in the Degeneration of Neurons in Alzheimer's Disease / Cerebrovascular Disease in Dementia / Corticotropin Releasing Factor, Adrenocorticotropic Hormone, and Cortisol in Alzheimer's Disease: Diagnostic and Therapeutic Implications / Autonomic Nervous System Dysfunction in Alzheimer's Disease: Implications for Pathophysiology and Treatment / Hormonal Alterations in Alzheimer's Disease / Nutritional Aspects of Memory Dysfunction.

Part III. Diagnosis and Managment of Demanding Disorders
Possible Biologic Basis for a Major Memory Disorder / Detection of Early (Very Mild) Alzheimer's Disease / Diagnosis of Depression in Demented Patients / Neuropharmacological Modeling of Memory Disorders / New Cholinesterase Inhibitors for Treatment of Alzheimer's Disease / Behavioral Intervention in the Dementias by a Multiple-Therapist Team / Psychotherapy for Patients with Demantia.

1992   352pp   0-8261-7710-7   hardcover

536 Broadway, New York, NY 10012-3955 • (212) 431-4370 • Fax (212) 941-7842

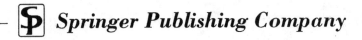

AGING AND MUSCULOSKELETAL DISORDERS

Concepts, Diagnosis, and Treatment

Horace M. Perry III, MD, **John E. Morley,** MD, BCh, and **Rodney M. Coe,** PhD, Editors

Describes the biomedical and environmental issues surrounding the loss of muscle and bone strength with age. Also covered are strategies for managing and decreasing risk of frailty, including exercise, nutritional, and hormonal interventions.

Contents:

Part I. Epidemiology of Frailty in Older People. Epidemiology of Frailty: Scope of the Problem • Age Related Changes in Bone • Longitudinal Study of Physical Performance and Frailty at Age 70 and Above

Part II. Age-Related Changes in Skeletal Muscle, and Bone. Changes in Muscle Strength with Age • Cellular Basis of Aging in Skeletal Muscle • Changes in Bone Mass and Their Contribution to Fractures • Changes in Mineral and Bone Metabolism with Age • Osteoporosis in Post-Menopausal Women

Part III. Prediction and Prevention of Falls. Factors Contributing to Falls and Fractures • Epidemiology and Prevention of Falls in the Nursing Home • Adrenergic Receptors: Implications for Falls • Age-Related Changes in Balance: Rehabilitation Strategies • Novel Interventions to Prevent Falls in the Elderly

Part IV. Exercise, Nutrition, and Hormonal Interventions with the Frail Elderly. Effect of Exercise on Muscle Mass in the Elderly • Effect of Exercise on Bone Mass in the Elderly • Benefits of Exercise for the Elderly • Nutritional Intervention in the Frail Elderly • Meal-Associated Hypotension • Growth Hormone in Elderly Men • The Effects of Testosterone and Growth Hormone Therapy in Frail Elderly Individuals

Part V. Rehabilitation of the Frail Elderly. An Update on The Diagnosis and Management of Musculoskeletal Disease in Older People • Nursing Rehabilitation of the Elderly Stroke Patient • Frailty and Physical Restraints • Posture Improvements in the Frail Elderly • Reimbursement for Rehabilitation of the Elderly

1993   392pp   0-8261-7930-4   hardcover

536 Broadway, New York, NY 10012-3955 • (212) 431-4370 • Fax (212) 941-7842